Milestones in Drug Therapy
MDT

Calcium Channel Blockers

T. Godfraind
with a contribution by E. Ertel

Springer Basel AG

Théophile Godfraind
Université Catholique de Louvain
Avenue Hippocrate 54 - UCL 5410
B-1200 Bruxelles
Belgium

Library of Congress Cataloging-in-Publication Data
Godfraind, T. (Théophile)
Calcium channel blockers / T. Godfraind ; with a contribution by Eric Ertel.
p. cm.-- (Milestones in drug therapy)
Includes bibliographical references and index.
ISBN 978-3-0348-9599-6 ISBN 978-3-0348-7859-3 (eBook)
DOI 10.1007/978-3-0348-7859-3
1. Calcium--Antagonist--Mechanism of action. I. Title. II. Series.

RM666.C243G63 2003
615'.739--dc22 2003063565

Bibliographic information published by Die Deutsche Bibliothek
Die Deutsche Bibliothek lists this publication in the Deutsche Nationalbibliografie; detailed bibliographic data is available in the Internet at <http://dnb.ddb.de>.

ISBN 978-3-0348-9599-6

Originally published by Birkhäuser Verlag in 2004
Softcover reprint of the hardcover 1st edition
Printed on acid-free paper produced from chlorine-free pulp. TCF ∞
Cover illustration: Model of voltage-operated Ca^{2+} channel flanked with typical calcium channel blockers.

ISBN 978-3-0348-9599-6

9 8 7 6 5 4 3 2 1 www.birkhasuer-science.com

Contents

Preface

The drugs named calcium channel blockers (CCBs) were initially termed calcium antagonists (see Chapter 1). They are also designated as calcium entry blockers (CEBs), calcium blockers, calcium channel antagonists, calcium channel inhibitors (and in French anticalciques). As this is reported in several chapters of this book, their main effect is a blockade of calcium entry into cells through voltage operated calcium channels (VOCCs). Chemically related drugs, such as Bay K 8644, exert the opposite effect by increasing the probability of calcium channel opening. One of the subcommittees of the Nomenclature Committee (NC-IUPAR) of the International Union of Pharmacology has been devoted to the classification of calcium channels and the site of action of drugs modifying channel function. The members of this Committee are noted for their significant contribution to the field (Tab. 1). A report has been published in 1992 in *Pharmacological Reviews* [3].

A list of criteria was approved for the identification of distinct drug binding sites on Ca^{2+} channels. It included: (a) the demonstration of a stereoselective binding site supported by drug interaction studies (competition with other drugs, non-competitive interactions with other sites, reversal of inhibitory effects by channel activators); (b) demonstration of the electrophysiological effects of the drug and selectivity of action compared to other sites; (c) determination of the affinity for the type and subtype of ion channel. These criteria have identified different classes of Ca antagonists (see Chapter 2). When recommending a drug nomenclature, the Committee mentioned that the terms "calcium antagonist" or "calcium entry blocker" have gained historic pharmacological and clinical acceptance when applied to agents inhibiting L-type channel function by acting at specific sites and that these terms will undoubtedly continue to be used to describe the classic pharmacological properties of this type of agent. However, it was clear at that time that new pharmacological profiles were expected from interactions with other types of calcium channel, or even from new binding sites on the L-type channel, quite different from the profile associated with, for example, nifedipine. For the Committee, the term "calcium channel modulator" was preferred for agents interacting with calcium channels. The term "calcium agonist" was considered inappropriate, and agents such as Bay K 8644 were referred to as calcium channel activators and inhibitory compounds were referred to as calcium channel blockers. More recently NC-IUPHAR has established a new subcommittee devoted to calcium channels classification (Tab. 2), which has published a Compendium in 2002 [1]. The IUPHAR recommended classifications have been followed in this book, which is divided in ten chapters. All chapters can be independently read.

Table 1. Composition of the temporary section of the Nomenclature Committee (NC-IUPAR) of the International Union of Pharmacology devoted to the classification of calcium channels and the site of action of drugs modifying channel function

R. Paoletti President: Institute of Pharmacol. Sciences, Via Balzaretti 9 20133 Milan, Italy	J. Moss Professor of Anesthesia and Critical Care The University of Chicago Medical Center Chicago, IL 60637, USA
M. Spedding Institut de Recherches Servier Suresnes, France	S. Murata Department II Pharmacological Research Laboratory Tanabe Seiyaku Co Ltd 2-2-50, Kawagishi, Toda-Shi Saitama, Japan
F. R. Buhler Department of Internal Medicine University Hospital CH-4031 Basel, Switzerland	J. Olesen Department of Neurology Gentofte Hospital University of Copenhagen 2900 Copenhagen, Denmark
M. O. Christen Lab. de Therapeutique *Medeme* L. T. M Latema Sarbach 42, Rue Rouget-de-Lisle 92151 Suresne Cedex, France	L. H. Opie University of Capetown Heart Research Unit and Hypertension Clinic Department of Medicine Medical School, Observatory 7925, South Africa
S. Ebashi Director-General and Professor National Institute for Physical Sciences Myodaiji, Okazaki 444, Japan	A. Schwartz Professor and Chairman Department of Pharmacology and Cell Biophysiology University of Cincinnati College of Medicine Cincinnati, OH 45267-0575, USA
C. Fieschi Cattedara di Clinica Neurologica Viale dell'Universita 90 University of Rome	B. Siesjo University of Lund Laboratory for Experiment Brain Research, Lund Hospital S-22185 Lund, Sweden
A. Fleckenstein (†) and G. Fleckenstein-Grun Albert Ludwigs Universität Physiologisches Institut Herman Herder Strasse 7 D-78oo Freiburg, Germany	R. W. Tsien Department of Molecular Cell Physiology Stanford University B 105 Beckman Centre Stanford, CA, USA
T. Godfraind Laboratoire de Pharmacodynamie Generale et de Pharmacologie Universite Catholique de Louvain Avenue Mounier 73-U. C. L 7350 B-1200 Bruxelles, Belgium	P. M. Vanhoutte Baylor College of Medicine Centre for Experimental Therapeutics One Baylor Plaza Houston, TX 77030, USA
B. E. G. Johansson AB Hassle Research Labs 8-431 83 Molndal Sweden	J. M. Van Nueten International Research Council Janssen Research Foundation Turnhoutseweg 30 B-2340 Beerse, Belgium

(Continued on next page)

Table 1. (Continued)

S. Kazda Bayer A. G.-Institute fuer Pharmacologie Postfach 10 1709 D-5600, Wuppertal, Germany	P. A. Van Zwieten Departments of Pharmacotherapy, Pharmacology and Cardiology Academic Medical Centre and Academic Hospital University of Amsterdam 1105 AZ Amsterdam, The Netherlands
R. J. Miller Department of Pharmacology University of Chicago 947 E. 58th Street Chicago, IL 60637, USA	

Chapter 1 deals with an historical perspective: from early steps on calcium research to the identification of calcium antagonist prototypes and of the signaling functions of Ca^{2+}. Chapter 2 is a review dealing with the various identified calcium channels: receptor-activated, ligand-gated, and voltage-operated. Special attention is devoted to voltage-operated calcium channels that are targets of calcium antagonists. Chapter 3 deals with the action of calcium antagonists on Ca^{2+} movements in isolated vessels. Our initial hypothesis [2] was that the reduction of blood pressure by calcium antagonists is the result of a decrease of peripheral resistance due to vasodilatation within the arterial beds. Therefore, a large body of experimental work has been concerned with studies of the mechanism of action of CCBs in arteries. Earliest studies have addressed the mechanism of action of calcium antagonists in the vasculature by considering their interaction with Ca^{2+} activator of the contractile machinery. Such approaches have required the characterization of calcium movements in the absence and in the presence of calcium antagonists. Chapter 4 deals with the tissue selectivity of calcium antagonists, which has some interest for pharmacotherapy. Analytical pharmacology studies of various CCBs that have supported the concepts of tissue and action selectivity are reported in this chapter. Chapter 5 deals with acute haemodynamic effects of calcium channel block-

Table 2. NC-IUPHAR Subcommittee on calcium channels

William A. Catterall (Chairman), Department of Pharmacology, University of Washington School of Medicine, Box 357280, Seattle WA 98195-7280, USA; E-mail: wcatt@u.washington.edu
Joerg Striessnig, Abteilung Pharmakologie und Toxikologie, Institut für Pharmazie, Universität Innsbruck, A-6020 Innsbruck, Austria
Terrance P. Snutch, Biotechnology Laboratory, University of British Columbia, Vancouver, British Columbia V6T 1Z3, Canada
Edward Perez-Reyes, Department of Pharmacology, University of Virginia, Charlottesville VA 22908, USA

ers. The examples taken in this chapter are illustrative of the actions of CCBs in general, even if all drugs have not been examined. Owing to the complexity of haemodynamic reflexes and the tissue selectivity of CCBs at the level of the various vascular beds, it might be anticipated that those drugs may exhibit variations in action according to the vascular bed or the species so far considered. Because of the importance of CCBs for the therapy of coronary diseases, hypertension and stroke, their actions have been studied in coronary, renal and cerebral circulations. Chapter 6 deals with calcium channels and the regulation of vascular tone in hypertension. Regulation of the contractile activity of vascular smooth muscle cells in the systemic circulation is dependent on a complex interplay of vasodilator and vasoconstrictor stimuli from circulating hormones, neurotransmitters, endothelium-derived factors, and blood pressure. All these signals are integrated by vascular muscle cells to determine the activity of the contractile apparatus of the muscle cells and hence resistance of a blood vessel. Calcium antagonists produce a hypotensive effect more pronounced in hypertensive than in normotensive humans and animals. How the disease modifies the target is the purpose of this chapter. Chapter 7 deals with long-term effects of calcium antagonists. Indeed, patients are treated for life with those drugs, which prevent both in hypertensive humans and animals the alterations of various organs including heart and kidneys. Analysis of the long-term effects has been done in experimental animals showing how calcium channel blockers prevent tissue remodeling and the activation of endothelin and renin-angiotensin systems in salt-sensitive species. Such studies raise the question of whether the reduction of blood pressure is the sole mechanism responsible for the therapeutic long-term effects. Therefore, in Chapter 8 we examine the blood pressure-independent effects of calcium channel blockers as potential mechanisms of tissue protection, which have not reached full acceptance because of poor evidence from clinical studies. Evidence for such mechanisms is provided by various studies: analytical pharmacology showing that prevention of cardiac remodeling is not directly related to reduction of blood pressure, effects on hypertrophic stimuli in cardiac cells in culture, blockade of the renin-angiotensin system, inhibition of the translocation of protein-kinase, interaction with the L-arginine-NO pathway and the anti-oxidant properties of some molecules that could account for a therapeutic action in atherosclerosis. Chapter 9 deals with early clinical trials and with randomized control trials (RCTs) in cardiovascular medicine, considering cardiac ischaemia, cardiac arrhythmias, hypertension and atherosclerosis. Questions raised by meta-analyses are also examined in the light of results obtained from ALLHAT, the largest RCT so far organized in the treatment of hypertension. Chapter 10 is entitled 'Beyond the cardiovascular system'. Blockade of L-type calcium currents by dihydropyridines, phenylalkylamines and benzothiazepines forms the basis for treatment of cardiovascular diseases. A number of other agents that either unselectively or selectively target neuronal and other calcium channels have been described. Some of them have been introduced in therapy to treat gastro-intestinal or neuronal disorders and more recently, some blockers have become the subject of intense interest regarding their potentiality for the treatment of chronic and neuropathic pain. This appears promising for a variety of pain conditions. Those various aspects are examined. In the final section of this chapter it is assumed that although the future is by definition imperceptible, it is likely that powerful medicines will be identified within a novel generation of calcium channel blockers. New chemical and biological technologies are emerging in the field of calcium channels pharmacology that may help the discovery of novel compounds more active in diseases insufficiently controlled by the actual calcium channel blockers.

References

1 Catterall WA, Chandy KG and Gutman GA. *The IUPHAR Compendium of voltagegated ion channels*. Leeds: IUPHAR Media, 2002
2 Godfraind T. Nouveaux aspects de la pharmacologie du muscle lisse vasculaire. *Prod Probl Pharmac* 26: 117–125, 1971
3 Spedding M and Paoletti R. Classification of calcium channels and the sites of action of drugs modifying channel function. *Pharmacol Rev* 44: 363–376, 1992

Acknowledgements

The publication of this book provides an opportunity to acknowledge Colleagues who furthered over the past 40 years my research on Calcium Signaling Pharmacology. They include members of NC-IUPHAR subcommittees (see Preface, Tabs 1 and 2), co-editors of books dedicated to calcium and calcium antagonists [1–8] and some others*. I am pleased to quote several Senior and Junior Colleagues including Ph.D. students for their contribution, within the Laboratory of Pharmacology of the Catholic University of Louvain, to advance in the pharmacology of calcium channel blockers. They now hold positions in Universities or private sector in Europe, Africa, Australia, North and South America**.

Most of the experimental work of the author and his co-workers was supported by grants from the Fonds National de la Recherche Scientifique (FNRS), from the Fonds de la Recherche Scientifique Médicale (FRSM), from the Communauté française de Belgique and from the Belgian Government. Scientific initiatives were made possible through grants from the Belgian Centre Biomédical pour la Recherche et le Développement (A.S.B.L.), the Fondation Professeur Lucien Dautrebande, the Lorenzini Foundation and private companies including Bayer, GlaxoWellcome, Janssen Pharmaceutica and Pfizer.

I wish also to thank Sir John Vane, Sir James Black, Professors S. Ebashi, B. Furchgott, P. Janssen (†) and P. Munson (†) for their esteem and friendship. Last but not least, I am indebted to my wife Professor Anne Godfraind-De Becker for initiating with me the research on the role of calcium in Pharmacology and for her continuous attention to calcium channel blockers pharmacology after her moving to another field of research.

* (Atkinson J, Bianchi A, Bianchi C P, Bowman W, Ertel E, Gaviraghi G, Hofmann F, Karaki H, McGrath JC, Napoli C, Nayler W, Netter K, Reuter H, Ruegg U, Stoclet JC, Taira N, Triggle D, Weiss G.)

** (Alosachie I, Balligand JL, Bravo G, Broekaert A (=), Buryi V, Castaneda-Hernandez G, Costa R, De Pover A, Delfosse I, Demesy F, DeRoth L, Dessy C, Dieu D, Donckier J, Duong AT, Ebeigbe AB, Egleme C, Fagoo M, Feron O, Finet M, Ghisdal P, Ghysel-Burton J, Goffin A (†), Gomez JP, Hajo-Tello N, Hardy JP, Kaba A (=), Khoury G, Koch MC, Kolar F, Krenek P, Krippeit-Drews P, Kyselovic J, Leonardy G, Lutete DN, Mennig D, Miller R, Morel N, Noel F, Polster P, Pousti A, Rojas R, Salomone S, Schleiffer R, Schoeffter P, Silva CL, Simon P, Socrates Lima J, Sotnikova R, Sturbois X, Van Dorsser W, Verbeke N, Wibo M, Zheng L.)

References

1 Casteels R, Godfraind T, and Rüegg JC. *Excitation-Contraction Coupling in Smooth Muscle.* Amsterdam, New York, Oxford: Elsevier/North-Holland Biomedical Press, 1977

2 Christen MO, Godfraind T, and McCallum RW. *Calcium Antagonism in Gastrointestinal Motility*. Amsterdam, New York, Oxford, Paris: Elsevier, 1989
3 Godfraind T, Albertini A, and Paoletti R. *Calcium Modulators*. Amsterdam, New York, Oxford: Elsevier/North-Holland Biomedical Press, 1982
4 Godfraind T, Govoni S, Paoletti R, and Vanhoutte PM. *Calcium Antagonists. Pharmacology and Clinical Research.* Dordrecht/Boston/London: Kluwer Academic Publishers, 1993
5 Godfraind T, Herman AG, and Wellens D. *Calcium Entry Blockers in Cardiovascular and Cerebral Disfunctions*. The Hague, The Netherlands: Martinus Nijhoff Publishers, 1984
6 Godfraind T, Mancia G, Abbrachio MP, Aguilar-Bryan L, and Govoni S. *Pharmacological Control of Calcium and Potassium Homeostasis*. Dordrecht/Boston/London: Kluwer Academic Publishers, 1995
7 Godfraind T and Meyer P. *Cell Membrane in Function and Dysfunction of Vascular Tissue*. Amsterdam, New York, Oxford: Elsevier/North-Holland Biomedical Press, 1981
8 Godfraind T, Vanhoutte PM, Govoni S, and Paoletti R. *Calcium Entry Blockers and Tissue Protection*. New York: Raven Press, 1985

Calcium Channel Blockers
T. Godfraind

Historical perspective: from early steps on calcium research to the identification of calcium antagonist prototypes and of the signaling functions of Ca^{2+}

The role of calcium for the maintenance of cellular activity was observed by Ringer [55] as early as 1883. Some years later, Stiles reported that calcium activates smooth muscle contraction [61]. The key role of calcium in intracellular functions was not perceived until 70 years later by Heilbrunn in the United States (1947) [39] and by Kamada in Japan (1943) [43].

Nowadays, it is recognized that calcium is responsible for regulating a wide range of cellular processes, being generally considered as the ubiquitous second messenger. At the beginning of life, it mediates the process of fertilization. As cells differentiate to perform specific functions, Ca^{2+} is regulating processes as diverse as muscle contraction, exocytosis, energy metabolism, chemotaxis, neurotransmission and synaptic plasticity during learning and memory. It is also involved in pathological processes such as cardiac hypertrophy and vascular hypertrophy. Irreversible damage as occurs during cardiac or cerebral ischaemia results from prolonged elevations of $[Ca^{2+}]$. The intracellular level of Ca^{2+} in resting cells is normally held within a narrow range of 20–100 $nmol \cdot l^{-1}$, avoiding this cytotoxicity. The signaling functions of Ca^{2+} have to be performed against a tightly controlled Ca^{2+} homeostasis. It is believed that dysregulation of this homeostasis has pathological consequences in cardiovascular diseases such as hypertension, atherosclerosis, coronary insufficiency, cardiac failure. The mechanisms involved are multiple and complex; therefore, the therapeutic mechanism of action of drugs used in order to manage those diseases might involve various targets.

The main steps in calcium research as summarized by Ebashi [17] are reported in Table 1. This shows that investigations into the pharmacology of calcium have only begun in the last 40 years. On examination of the literature of the end of the 1950s and of the early 1960s, it appears that the role of calcium in pharmacological processes was initially quantified in smooth muscle studies [16, 22]. Edman and Schild [19–21], for example, showed that depolarization of rat uterus rendered the membrane of the smooth muscle cell permeable to extracellular calcium and that the force of the contraction developed by the preparation was proportional to the concentration of calcium in the extracellular fluid. In addition, they provided evidence that acetylcholine-evoked contractions of smooth muscles were dependent on both intracellular and extracellular calcium. Similar observations were made with serotonin, his-

Table 1. Chronology of calcium research (as from [17])

Without Ca in bathing medium, the frog heart does not contract	1983	Ringer
Ca activates smooth muscle contraction	1901	Stiles
The first proposal of the Ca concept	1940	Heilbrunn
Ca injection into myoplasm elicits local contraction	1943 1947	Kamada and Kinosita Heilbrunn and Wiercinski
Discovery of relaxing factor	1951	Bozler
EDTA mimics the relaxing factor	1954	Bozler
The relaxing factor is identical with microsomal ATPase	1955	Kumagai et al.
Activation of myofibrillar ATPase requires about 1 μM Ca^{2+}	1959–61	Ebashi Weber
The mechanism of the relaxing factor	1960–62	Ebashi and Lipman
Native tropomyosin is essential for Ca regulation	1963	Ebashi
Cardiac actomyosin requires Ca^{2+} like skeletal muscle one	1964	Otsuka et al.
The sensitivity to Ca^{2+} in smooth muscle is the same than in heart and skeletal muscle	1965	Filo, Bohr and Ruegg
Discovery of troponin	1965	Ebashi and Kodama
Ca activates Phosphorylase b kinase	1967	Ozawa et al.
Ca-induced Ca release	1968	Endo
The concept of Ca^{2+} antagonist emerges	1969	Fleckenstein Godfraind
Discovery of calmodulin	1969 1970	Kariuchi and Yamazaki Cheung
Myosin-linked regulation	1970	Kendrick-Jones
Phosphorylation of myosin light chain induces smooth muscle contraction	1976	Sobiezek and Small
Protein kinase C requires Ca^{2+}	1979	Takai et al.
Isolation of calmodulin-dependent protein kinase II	1980	Yamauchi and Fujisaw
In Physarium, Ca^{2+} inhibits and not activates actin-myosin-ATP interaction	1980	Kohama et al.
IP_3 releases Ca^{2+} from intracellular Ca stores	1984	Berridge and Irvine

tamine, and oxytocin [66]. Since this period, great advances have been made in the understanding of the regulation of smooth muscle contraction by calcium, and this has been extensively reviewed [18, 44, 59].

In the 1960s, Godfraind and co-workers demonstrated on arterial tissue that the inhibition of Ca^{2+} entry is a mechanism of vasodilatation [31–34, 36]. This discovery was the outcome of earlier studies of Godfraind and Godfraind De

Becker on the role of Ca^{2+} in the pharmacological response to various drugs. In 1960, they studied the influence of the concentration of Na^+ and Ca^{2+} in the physiological solution on the response of isolated smooth muscle to its stimulatory neurotransmitters. They observed that the change in Ca^{2+} concentration did not only change the contractility of the muscle, as could be anticipated by the current theory of muscle contraction, but that the sensitivity of the contractile response to acetylcholine was specifically enhanced by increasing the Ca^{2+} concentration of the perfusion fluid and that this effect was specific for Ca^{2+} when compared with other divalent cations [29, 30]. Thereafter, Godfraind et al. studied the influence of the extracellular concentration of Ca^{2+} on the action of various pharmacological agents, both stimulatory and inhibitory. Their research was focused on drugs classically termed antispasmodics because of their capacity to reduce smooth muscle contraction evoked by various spasmogens. The mechanism of action of antispasmodics could not be accounted for by the receptor theory, which implied that agonists and antagonists compete for the same binding site and that a given concentration of a specific antagonist could inhibit the response to only one given agonist. Godfraind proposed a simple model in order to take into account the action of such drugs that blocked at a same concentration the contractile response to various spasmogens. He made the hypothesis that the interaction of the various agonists with their own receptors activated a common transmembrane mechanism of which Ca^{2+} was the messenger. Structures activated by smooth muscle depolarization that allowed the translocation of Ca^{2+} from outside to inside the cell were suggested to be targets of the blockers. Nowadays, the molecular structure of those calcium channels is identified (see Chapter 2). Among potential calcium entry blockers studied, Godfraind et al. first identified the plant alkaloid papaverine and synthetic chemicals of the phenothiazine and diphenylpiperazine groups, including lidoflazine, used as an antianginal drug [42] and cinnarizine which was at that time considered as antihistaminic [64] and was used as an anti-motion-sickness and antiallergic drug. Lidoflazine and cinnarizine inhibit the contraction of some smooth muscles evoked by several agonists, such as norepinephrine, angiotensin, acetylcholine, and vasopressin [12, 34, 36, 63]. When the action of lidoflazine or of cinnarizine was examined in isolated arteries, a same concentration of one of those inhibitors was able to block the contraction evoked by various agonists, confirming that they could interfere with the common mechanism activated by various spasmogens [33, 34, 36]. The hypothesis that calcium translocation was this common mechanism was indirectly supported by a large body of experimental work [5, 14, 40, 41]. According to the indirect evidence available at that time, the calcium activating the contractile machinery subsequent to agonist stimulation could have been translocated either from the outside to the inside of the cell, or within the cell from an intracellular store. To determine if the antagonism was related to one or the other of those possible mechanisms, the action of diphenylpiperazines on agonist-evoked contraction of arterial smooth muscle in the presence and absence of calcium was examined. In 1969, Godfraind and Kaba [31, 32] showed that cinnarizine displaced to the right the calcium dose-effect curves obtained in depolarized mesenteric arteries. The antagonism was observed for concentrations of cinnarizine as low as 10^{-9} M and was dose-dependent (Fig. 1). Cinnarizine also relaxed depolarized smooth muscle contracted in the presence of Ca^{2+}. They also examined the action of cinnarizine on the contraction evoked by adrenaline and observed that blockade of this contraction was related to extracellular Ca^{2+}, an observation supporting the hypothesis that blockade of calcium entry is a mechanism of drug action [28].

In order to test further this hypothesis, Godfraind and co-workers studied other smooth muscle preparations. They showed that the action of cinnarizine was not related to α-adrenoceptor blockade [32, 33a]. They noted that the inhibition by cinnarizine of the response to adrenaline was more pronounced in small than in large arteries; an observation consistent with their hypothesis that was hardly received at that time (Godfraind et al., 1968). Now it is generally accepted that the contraction of small arteries responsible for the control of

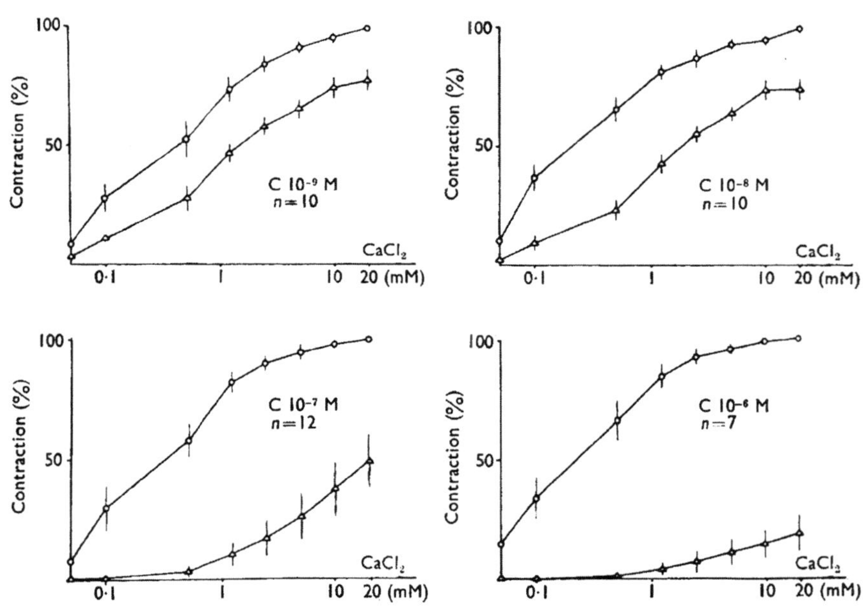

Figure 1. Effect of cinnarizine on contractions evoked by Ca^{2+} in K^+-depolarised rabbit mesenteric arteries. Arterial preparations were pre-incubated in Ca^{2+}-free physiological solution depolarised in Ca^{2+}-free KCl-rich solution, and then further incubated with increasing Ca^{2+} concentrations. Cumulative concentration-effect curves were obtained before (O) and after (Δ) addition of cinnarizine (C) at the concentrations indicated. Responses are expressed in percentage of maximal contraction evoked before addition of cinnarizine. The inhibitory effect of cinnarizine is observed at concentrations as low as 1 nM and resembles the action of antagonists in receptor studies. In view of this similarity, the term 'calcium antagonist' was suggested to describe the action of cinnarizine. From [31] modified.

blood pressure is mainly dependent on extracellular calcium whereas in large arteries, contraction is preferentially related to intracellular calcium release.

Contractions evoked by KCl depolarization (due to calcium translocation from outside to inside the cell) were completely reversed by diphenylpiperazines. When arteries were stimulated with agonists, diphenylpiperazines only blocked the contractions dependent on extracellular calcium, they left unaltered the contractions evoked in the absence of extracellular calcium. This contraction was assumed to be related to release of calcium from intracellular stores [31, 32]. Godfraind and Polster [36] had shown in several arteries, including pig coronary arteries and human pulmonary arteries, depolarized by KCl-rich solution, that by increasing the concentration of calcium in the bathing solution, the inhibitory effect of cinnarizine, lidoflazine, and chlorpromazine on the contractile response was antagonized. To characterize the effect of diphenylpiperazines, they used the term "antagoniste du calcium" (calcium antagonist), a term used coincidentally by Fleckenstein to describe the effects of verapamil and prenylamine on cardiac tissue [17]. Verapamil was described in 1962 by Haas and Hartfelder [38] and classified as a coronary vasodilator, capable of improving the ratio of myocardial oxygen supply to oxygen consumption in anesthetized open chest dogs, this was the time when clinicians strongly believed in the usefulness of coronary vasodilating drugs [57]. Due to its absence of bronchoconstrictive effect [37], it presented a great advantage over propanolol and therefore was of great clinical interest. Verapamil was considered in 1968 by Nayler et al. [51] as interacting with beta-adrenoceptors by a mechanism different from *dl*-propanolol. In the 1960s, Fleckenstein and co-workers [24–27, 46–50] were interested in the study of the utilization of high energy phosphates in relation to muscle contraction and oxygen consumption and of disturbances in high energy phosphate metabolism under the action of catecholamines. In this respect they studied the role of Ca^{2+} in the solution perfusing striated and cardiac muscle. In the course of his studies, Fleckenstein discovered that the action of verapamil and of prenylamine mimicked the effect of calcium withdrawal. Because of this, he proposed that the excitation-contraction uncoupling evoked by prenylamine, verapamil, and its derivative, gallopamil (D600)+ was due to calcium antagonism [26].

The concept of calcium antagonism [23, 35] has been extended to other drugs considered in Chapter 2 and all over this book. They are termed calcium antagonists but also calcium entry blockers, calcium channel blockers (CCBs).

A great deal of experimental work has improved our knowledge on the physiology of calcium [1, 17, 45, 58, 62, 65]. As already mentioned above, calcium under its ionized form (Ca^{2+}) is generally considered as the ubiquitous second messenger. The signaling functions of Ca^{2+} are performed against a background of a tightly controlled Ca^{2+} homeostasis, which maintains the free calcium concentration that is normally held within the narrow range of 20–100 $nmol \cdot l^{-1}$ in a resting cell. Another consequence of this rigid homeostatic control over Ca^{2+} is that this ion has a very low diffusibility in cytoplasm. Distributed throughout the cytoplasm is an extensive array of Ca^{2+}

pumps [8, 9, 11], which rapidly sequester calcium ion, thus restricting its diffusion. In order to overcome the twin problems of an inherent cytotoxicity and low diffusibility, cells have evolved a mechanism of signalling based on presenting Ca^{2+} as brief spikes often organized as regenerative waves [2–4, 6]. This spatiotemporal organization of Ca^{2+} signaling might be related to the properties of the Ca^{2+} channels that regulate the entry of Ca^{2+} into the cytoplasm. Cells have access to two sources of signal Ca^{2+}. First, it enters from the outside; second, it can be released from internal stores. It enters through a variety of plasmalemmal ion channels such as the voltage-operated channels (VOCs), receptor-operated channels (ROCs) or store-operated channels (SOCs), non-selective channels (from TRP family, etc.). Calcium channel blockers (CCBS, also named calcium antagonists, calcium entry blockers) interact with VOCs; these channels will be discussed more extensively later. Which of these sources is used varies somewhat from cell to cell. In the cardiovascular system, calcium entry from the outside plays a major role in regulating muscle function, but, as in most cells, the internal stores also provide signal Ca^{2+}. Those internal stores are located in the endoplasmic reticulum (in muscles, in the sarcoplasmic reticulum), in mitochondria and in nucleus. In endoplasmic reticulum, there are two main types of intracellular Ca^{2+} channels. First, there is the ryanodine receptor (RYR) family comprising three members: RYR1 found in skeletal muscle and certain neurones (e.g., Purkinje cells); RYR2 found in cardiac muscle, brain and some other cells, and; RYR3 found in smooth muscle, brain and other cells. These receptors are sensitive to caffeine, which activates the release of calcium from these stores. Second, the inositol 1,4,5-trisphosphate receptor ($InsP_3R$) family has a number of members. There are four $InsP_3R$ genes, and further diversity results from alternative splicing. This group of receptors may be blocked by heparine. Mitochondria are also calcium regulatory structures. Their function is under intense investigation. It first appeared that they were involved in trancellular calcium waves. Cytosolic Ca^{2+} homeostasis in resting cells is achieved by balancing the leak of Ca^{2+} (entering from the outside or from the stores) by the constant removal of Ca^{2+} using pumps either on the plasma membrane or on the internal stores. These pumps ensure that cytoplasmic $[Ca^{2+}]$ remains low and that the stores are loaded with signal Ca^{2+} signaling molecule. Thus, the concentration of Ca^{2+} ions is under very tight and dynamic control in all major cell compartments (cytoplasm, nucleus, endoplasmic reticulum, mitochondria) [53, 54]. In each compartment, this control is achieved through the interplay of transmembrane entry and extrusion systems (channels, exchangers and transporters) and of buffering systems (Ca^{2+}-binding proteins). Some of these buffers also participate in the further processing of the Ca^{2+} concentration signals. An excellent general review by Brini and Carafoli [8] provides detailed information on intracellular Ca signaling and more specific papers are available on Ca^{2+} stores in the endoplasmic reticulum [10, 60], in the nucleus [7] and in mitochondria [13, 15, 52, 56].

References

1 Berridge MJ. Elementary and global aspects of calcium signalling. *J Exp Biol* 200 (Pt 2): 315–319, 1997

2 Berridge MJ and Irvine RF. Inositol trisphosphate, a novel second messenger in cellular signal transduction. *Nature* 312: 315–321, 1984

3 Berridge MJ, Lipp P and Bootman MD. Signal transduction. The calcium entry pas de deux. *Science* 287: 1604–1605, 2000

4 Berridge MJ, Lipp P and Bootman MD. The versatility and universality of calcium signalling. *Nat Rev Mol Cell Biol* 1: 11–21, 2000

5 Bohr DF. Electrolytes and smooth muscle contraction. *Pharmacol Rev* 16: 85–111, 1964

6 Bootman MD, Lipp P and Berridge MJ. The organisation and functions of local Ca^{2+} signals. *J Cell Sci* 114: 2213–2222, 2001

7 Bootman MD, Thomas D, Tovey SC, Berridge MJ and Lipp P. Nuclear calcium signalling. *Cell Mol Life Sci* 57: 371–378, 2000

8 Brini M and Carafoli E. Calcium signalling: a historical account, recent developments and future perspectives. *Cell Mol Life Sci* 57: 354–370, 2000

9 Brini M, Coletto L, Pierobon N, Kraev N, Guerini D and Carafoli E. A comparative functional analysis of plasma membrane Ca^{2+} pump isoforms in intact cells. *J Biol Chem*, 2003

10 Cancela JM, Van Coppenolle F, Galione A, Tepikin AV and Petersen OH. Transformation of local Ca^{2+} spikes to global Ca^{2+} transients: the combinatorial roles of multiple Ca^{2+} releasing messengers. *Embo J* 21: 909–919, 2002

11 Carafoli E and Brini M. Calcium pumps: structural basis for and mechanism of calcium transmembrane transport. *Curr Opin Chem Biol* 4: 152–161, 2000

12 Cession G, Lecomte J and Van Cauwenberghe H. Action antagoniste de la cinnarizine vis-à-vis de l'angiotensine *in vivo. Compt Rend Soc Biol* 158: 1754–1756, 1964

13 Collins TJ, Lipp P, Berridge MJ and Bootman MD. Mitochondrial Ca^{2+} uptake depends on the spatial and temporal profile of cytosolic Ca^{2+} signals. *J Biol Chem* 276: 26411–26420, 2001

14 Daniel EE. Attempted synthesis of data regarding divalent cations in muscle function. In: *Muscle*, edited by Paul WW, Daniel EE, Kay CM and Monckton G. New York: Pergamon Press, 1965, p. 295–316

15 Duchen MR. Mitochondria and calcium: from cell signaling to cell death. *J Physiol* 529 Pt 1: 57–68, 2000

16 Durbin RP and Jenkinson DH. The calcium-dependence of tension development in depolarized smooth muscle. *J Physiol* 161: 90–96, 1961

17 Ebashi S. From the relaxing factor to troponin. *Biomedical Research* 14: 1–7, 1993

18 Ebashi S. Regulation of muscle contraction. *Proc R Soc Lond B* 207: 259–286, 1980

19 Edman KAP and Schild HO. Calcium and the stimulant and inhibitory effects of adrenaline in depolarized smooth muscle. *J Physiol*: 404–411, 1963

20 Edman KAP and Schild HO. Interaction of acetylcholine, calcium and depolarization in the contraction of smooth muscle. *Nature* 190: 350–352, 1961

21 Edman KAP and Schild HO. The need for calcium in the contractile responses induced by acetylcholine and potassium in the rat uterus. *J Physiol* 161: 424–441, 1962

22 Evans DHL, Schild HO and Thesleff S. Effect of drugs on depolarized plain muscle. *J Physiol* 143: 474–485, 1958

23 Fleckenstein A. *Calcium antagonism in heart and smooth muscle, experimental facts and therapeutic prospects*. New York: John Wiler and Sons, 1983

24 Fleckenstein A. Specific pharmacology of calcium in myocardium, cardiac pacemakers, and vascular smooth muscle. *Annu Rev Pharmacol Toxicol* 17: 149–166, 1977

25 Fleckenstein A, Doring HJ and Kammermeier H. Effect of beta-receptor blocking agents and related substances on the excitation, contraction and energy metabolism of myocardium fibers. *Klin Wochenschr* 46: 343–351, 1968

26 Fleckenstein A, Tritthart H, Flackenstein B, Herbst A and Grun G. A new group of competitive divalent Ca-antagonists (iproveratril, D600, prenylamine) with potent inhibitory effects on electromechanical coupling in mammalian myocardium. *Pflugers Arch* 307: R25, 1969

27 Fleckenstein A, Tritthart H, Fleckenstein B, Herbst A and Grun G. Selective inhibition of myocardial contractility by competitive divalent Ca^{2+} antagonists (iproveratril, D 600, prenylamine). *Naunyn Schmiedebergs Arch Pharmakol* 264: 227–228, 1969

28 Godfraind T. Nouveaux aspects de la pharmacologie du muscle lisse vasculaire. *Prod Probl Pharmac* 26: 117–125, 1971
29 Godfraind T and Godfraind-De Becker A. Activité rythmique de l'intestin provoquée par l'association de la digitoxine et du calcium. *Arch Int Pharmacodyn Ther* 138: 169–174, 1962
30 Godfraind T and Godfraind-De Becker A. Antagonisme de l'action du Cu^{2+}, du Zn^{2+} et du Fe^{3+} vis-à-vis de l'histamine et de l'acétylcholine. *Arch Int Pharmacodyn Ther* 130: 96–119, 1960
31 Godfraind T and Kaba A. Blockade or reversal of the contraction induced by calcium and adrenaline in depolarized arterial smooth muscle. *Br J Pharmacol* 36: 549–560, 1969
32 Godfraind T and Kaba A. Inhibition by cinnarizine and chlorpromazine of the contraction induced by calcium and adrenaline in vascular smooth muscle. *Br J Pharmacol* 35: P354–355, 1969
33 Godfraind T, Kaba A and Polster P. Differences in sensitivity of arterial smooth muscles to inhibition of their contractile response to depolarization by potassium. *Arch Int Pharmacodyn Ther* 172: 235–239, 1968
33a Godfraind T and Kaba A. The role of calcium in the action of drugs on vascular smooth muscle. *Arch Int Pharmacodyn Ther* 196(Suppl.): 35–49, 1972
34 Godfraind T, Kaba A and Polster P. Specific antagonism to the direct and indirect action of angiotensin on the isolated guinea-pig ileum. *Br J Pharmacol Chemother* 28: 93–104, 1966
35 Godfraind T, Miller R and Wibo M. Calcium antagonism and calcium entry blockade. *Pharmacol Rev* 38: 321–416, 1986
36 Godfraind T and Polster P. Comparative study of drugs inhibiting the contractile response of isolated vessels of human and animal origin. *Therapie* 23: 1209–1220, 1968
37 Haas H. Zum wirkungsmechanismus des alpha-isoprpyl-alpha-[(N-methyl-N-homoveratridil)-gamma-aminopropyl]-3,4-dimetoxyphenylacetonitrils, einer substanz mit coronargefässerweiternden eigenschaften. *Arzneim-Forsch* 12: 461–468, 1964
38 Haas H and Hartfelder G. Alpha-isopropylalpha{(N-metyl-N-homoveratriyl).-gamma-aminopropyl}-3,4-dimethoxyphenylacetonitils, einer substanz mit coronargefässerweiternden eigenschaften. *Arzneim-Forsch* 12: 549–558, 1962
39 Heilbrunn LV and Wiercinski FJ. The action of various cations on muscle protoplasm. *J Cell Comp Physiol* 29: 15–32, 1947
40 Hinke JAM. Calcium requirements for noradrenaline and high potassium ion contraction in arterial smooth muscle. In: *Muscle*, edited by Paul WW, Daniel EE, Kay CM and Monckton G. New York: Pergamon Press, 269–284, 1965
41 Hudgins PM and Weiss GB. Differential effects of calcium removal upon vascular smooth muscle contraction induced by norepinephrine, histamine and potassium. *J Pharmacol Exp Ther* 159: 91–97, 1968
42 Jagenau AHM and Schaper WKA. The effectiveness of lidoflazine and other coronary vasodilatators after oral administration in the trained non-anesthethetized dog. *Arzneim-Forsch* 17: 582–587, 1967
43 Kamada T and Kinosita H. Disturbances initiated from naked surface of muscle protoplasm. *Jpn J Zool* 10: 469–493, 1943
44 Karaki H, Ozaki H, Hori M, Mitsui-Saito M, Amano K, Harada K, Miyamoto S, Nakazawa H, Won KJ and Sato K. Calcium movements, distribution, and functions in smooth muscle. *Pharmacol Rev* 49: 157–230, 1997
45 Kendrick-Jones J, Lehman W and Szent-Gyorgyi AG. Regulation in molluscan muscles. *J Mol Biol* 54: 313–326, 1970
46 Kohlhardt M, Bauer B, Krause H and Fleckenstein A. Differentiation of the transmembrane Na and Ca channels in mammalian cardiac fibres by the use of specific inhibitors. *Pflugers Arch* 335: 309–322, 1972
47 Kohlhardt M, Bauer B, Krause H and Fleckenstein A. New selective inhibitors of the transmembrane Ca conductivity in mammalian myocardial fibres. Studies with the voltage clamp technique. *Experientia* 28: 288–289, 1972
48 Kohlhardt M, Bauer B, Krause H and Fleckenstein A. Selective inhibition of the transmembrane Ca conductivity of mammalian myocardial fibres by Ni, Co and Mn ions. *Pflugers Arch* 338: 115–123, 1973
49 Kohlhardt M and Fleckenstein A. Inhibition of the slow inward current by nifedipine in mammalian ventricular myocardium. *Br J Clin Pract Suppl* 8: 3–8, 1980
50 Kohlhardt M and Fleckenstein A. Inhibition of the slow inward current by nifedipine in mammalian ventricular myocardium. *Naunyn Schmiedebergs Arch Pharmacol* 298: 267–272, 1977

51 Nayler WG, McInnes I and Swann JB. Some effects of iproveratril (Isoptin) on the cardiovascular system. *J Pharmacol Exp Ther* 161: 247–251, 1968

52 Park MK, Ashby MC, Erdemli G, Petersen OH and Tepikin AV. Perinuclear, perigranular and subplasmalemmal mitochondria have distinct functions in the regulation of cellular calcium transport. *Embo J* 20: 1863–1874, 2001

53 Petersen OH, Burdakov D and Tepikin AV. Polarity in intracellular calcium signaling. *Bioessays* 21: 851–860, 1999

54 Petersen OH, Tepikin A and Park MK. The endoplasmic reticulum: one continuous or several separate Ca^{2+} stores? *Trends Neurosci* 24: 271–276, 2001

55 Ringer S. A further contribution regarding the influence of the blood on the contraction of the heart. *J Physiol* 4: 29–42, 1883

56 Rizzuto R, Bernardi P and Pozzan T. Mitochondria as all-round players of the calcium game. *J Physiol* 529 Pt 1: 37–47, 2000

57 Schaper WKA. Development of the collateral circulation: History of an idea. *Exp Clin Cardiol* 7: 60–63, 2002

58 Sobieszek A and Small JV. Myosin-linked calcium regulation in vertebrate smooth muscle. *J Mol Biol* 102: 75–92, 1976

59 Somlyo AP and Somlyo AV. Signal transduction and regulation in smooth muscle. *Nature* 372: 231–236, 1994

60 Sorrentino V and Rizzuto R. Molecular genetics of Ca^{2+} stores and intracellular Ca^{2+} signalling. *Trends Pharmacol Sci* 22: 459–464, 2001

61 Stiles PG. On the rhythmic activity of the oesophagus and the influence upon it of various media. *Am J Physiol* 5: 338–357, 1901

62 Takai Y, Kishimoto A, Iwasa Y, Kawahara Y, Mori T and Nishizuka Y. Calcium-dependent activation of a multifunctional protein kinase by membrane phospholipids. *J Biol Chem* 254: 3692–3695, 1979

63 Van Nueten JM, Dresse A and Dony J. Action antagoniste de la cinnarizine vis-à-vis de l'angiotensine *in vitro*. *Compt Rend Soc Biol* 158: 1750, 1964

64 van Proosdij-Hartzema EG and De Jongh DK. A new piperazine compound with antihistaminic effect. *Acta Physiol Pharmacol Neur* 8: 337–342, 1959

65 Yamauchi T and Fujisawa H. Evidence for three distinct forms of calmodulin-dependent protein kinases from rat brain. *FEBS Lett* 116: 141–144, 1980

66 Yukisada N and Ebashi F. Role of calcium in drug action on smooth muscle. *Jpn J Pharmacol* 11: 46–53, 1961

Calcium channel blockers and calcium channels

Eric Ertel* and Théophile Godfraind

* *F. Hoffmann-La Roche Ltd., Postfach, CH-4070 Basel, Switzerland*

Cellular regulation of calcium

In 1883, Ringer showed that to get isolated hearts to contract, it was necessary to have Ca^{2+} ions in the perfusion medium [421]. This was the first demonstration of the critical role of calcium in cellular activity. Remarkably, a hundred years passed before the importance of calcium was recognized in processes other than muscle contraction, and almost as long before the cellular mechanisms responsible for calcium regulation started to be understood. Nowadays, it is acknowledged that calcium is the most ubiquitous intracellular signaling molecule and that the concentration of Ca^{2+} ions is under very tight and dynamic control in all major cell compartments (cytoplasm, nucleus, endoplasmic reticulum, mitochondria). In each compartment, this control is achieved through the interplay of transmembrane entry and extrusion systems (channels, exchangers, and transporters) and of buffering systems (Ca^{2+}-binding proteins). Some of these buffers also participate in the further processing of the Ca^{2+} concentration signals. An excellent general review by Brini and Carafoli [61] provides detailed information on intracellular calcium signaling and more specific papers are available on Ca^{2+} stores in the endoplasmic reticulum [463], in the nucleus [50], and in mitochondria [137, 422].

Specific biological entities through which Ca^{2+} ions enter cells (i.e., Ca^{2+} channels) were not identified until the 1950s [153, 154]. The importance of Ca^{2+} channels in regulating the actions of external calcium became apparent at the end of the 1960s, when critical roles were recognized in the propagation of excitation in cardiac Purkinje fibers [419] and in the release of neurotransmitter at the squid giant synapse [246]. Ca^{2+} channels were subsequently reported in heart [420], smooth and skeletal muscle [28], neurons and endocrine cells [494]. There are three major pathways through which extracellular Ca^{2+} can enter animal cells (Fig. 1): receptor-activated Ca^{2+} channels (RACs), ligand-gated Ca^{2+} channels (LGCs), and voltage-operated Ca^{2+} channels (VOCs). In addition, there is also evidence for more targeted sensory mechanisms of Ca^{2+} entry: mechanically-activated Ca^{2+} channels, pH-activated Ca^{2+} channels, and temperature-activated Ca^{2+} channels. Although the voltage-operated Ca^{2+} channels will be the main subjects of this book, we will start with a short description of the ligand-gated and receptor-activated Ca^{2+} channels.

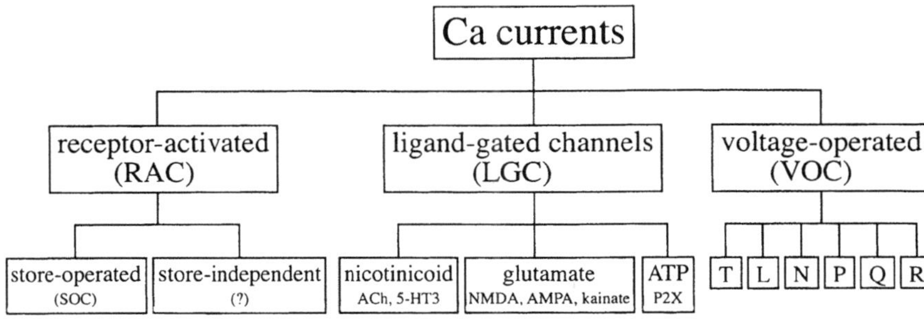

Figure 1. Pathways of Ca^{2+} entry into animal cells.

Ligand-gated Ca^{2+} channels (LGC)

Ligand-gated ion channels (or ionotropic receptors) combine a receptor and an ion channel in the same protein. This complex protein undergoes a conformational change upon the binding of a specific ligand (usually a neurotransmitter), which leads to opening of the intrinsic ion channel. Three superfamilies of ligand-gated ion channels have been described: 1) the nicotinicoid superfamily (receptors for acetylcholine (nicotinic), serotonin (5-HT_3), γ-aminobutyric acid ($GABA_A$, $GABA_C$), or glycine (strychnine-sensitive), plus some invertebrate anionic glutamate receptors); 2) the excitatory glutamate receptor superfamily (NMDA, AMPA, or kainate receptors); and 3) the ATP receptor superfamily (with a single constituting family, P2X).

Structure

Members of the nicotinicoid superfamily assemble as pentameric structures (homomeric or heteromeric) in plasma membranes, with each monomer having the same basic topology (extracellular N-terminal and C-terminal domains, four membrane-spanning segments (TM1–TM4), and a large intracellular loop between TM3 and TM4) (Fig. 2). The N-terminal domains constitute the agonist binding site and the five TM2 segments line the ion channel pore [94, 265]. The structure of the other two superfamilies is not as well established. Present data suggests that members of the excitatory glutamate receptor superfamily assemble as tetrameric structures (homomeric or heteromeric), with each monomer having the same basic topology (extracellular N-terminal and intracellular C-terminal domains, a ligand-binding domain (S1S2), three membrane-spanning segments (TM1, TM3, TM4), and a re-entrant loop M2 between TM1 and TM3) (Fig. 2). This re-entrant loop lines the channel pore and is homologous to the P-loop of voltage-operated cation channels [130, 265, 298]. Finally, members of the ATP receptor superfamily assemble as

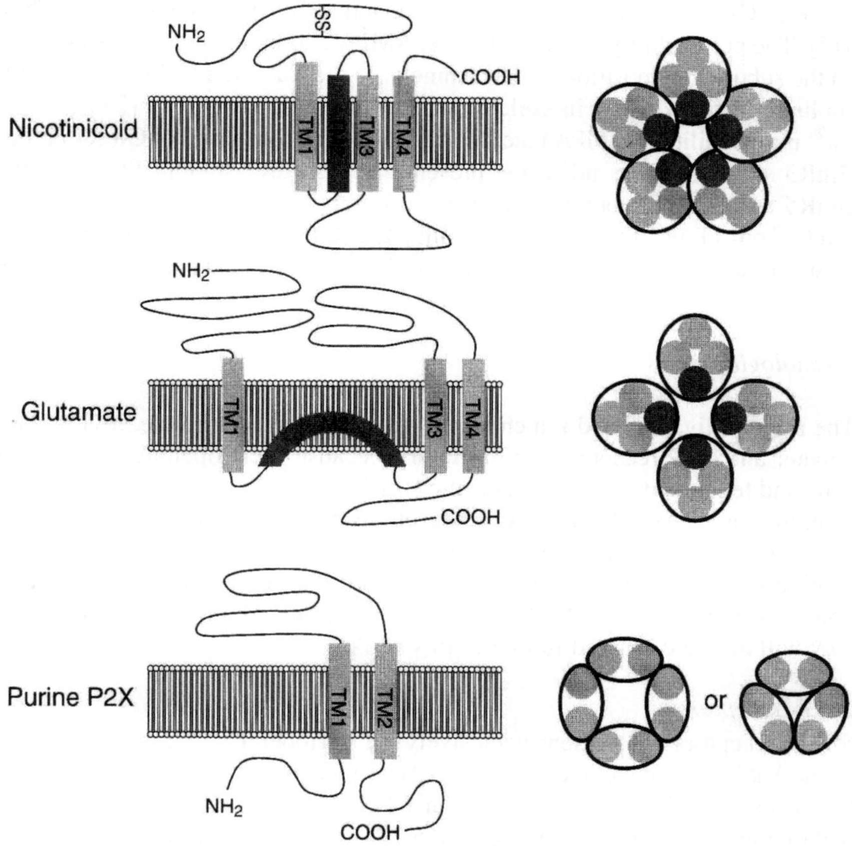

Figure 2. Structure of ligand-gated ion channels.

trimeric or tetrameric structures (homomeric or heteromeric), with each monomer having the same basic topology (intracellular N-terminal and C-terminal domains, two membrane-spanning domains (TM1–TM2), and a large extracellular loop) [138] (Fig. 2).

Ca^{2+} permeability

No ligand-gated ion channel is a Ca^{2+} channel in the strictest sense because they do not conduct Ca^{2+} selectively: the relative permeability of Ca^{2+} *versus* Na^{+} varies from ~0 to ~20 and the fraction of current carried by Ca^{2+} under physiological conditions ranges from ~0% to ~12% [70]. $GABA_A$, $GABA_C$, and glycine receptors are chloride-selective ion channels [94]. P2X, NMDA, and 5-HT_3 receptors are non-selective Ca^{2+}-permeable cation channels although Ca^{2+} can as well, in some cases, inactivate 5-HT_3 receptors [262, 265, 513]. The permeability of acetylcholine, AMPA and kainate receptors depends on the subunit composition of the channels: 1) the Ca^{2+} permeability of acetylcholine receptors is low in skeletal muscle and high in neurons [233]; 2) the Ca^{2+} permeability of AMPA receptors is high when composed of GluR1 and/or GluR3 subunits but is nil in the presence of a GluR2 subunit [314]; 3) the GluR5 and GluR6 subunits of kainate receptors can be edited at the mRNA levels from GluR5(Q) or GluR6(Q) into GluR5(R) or GluR6(R), leading to reduced Ca^{2+} permeability and other significant biophysical changes [46, 103].

Physiological roles

The roles of ligand-gated ion channels are varied. Acetylcholine, 5-HT_3, glutamate, and ATP receptors are excitatory because their opening depolarizes cells and tends to increase cytoplasmic [Ca^{2+}]. $GABA_A$, $GABA_C$, and glycine receptors are generally inhibitory neurotransmitter receptors, since in most cells, opening of chloride channels results in hyperpolarization and/or stabilization of the membrane potential away from the threshold for firing action potentials [262]. Since GABA and glycine receptors are not conducting Ca^{2+}, they will not be discussed further in this book.

5-HT_3 receptors

5-HT_3 receptors are present exclusively on peripheral and central neurons. Remarkably, complete blockade of 5-HT_3 receptors in normal animals or humans seems to produce no particular CNS effects. However, under defined pathological conditions, blockade of 5-HT_3 receptor has very pronounced effects.

Emesis: Probably the clearest role of 5-HT_3 receptors is in the initiation of emesis (chemotherapy-induced, irradiation-induced, or post-operative) and 5-HT_3 receptor antagonists are remarkably active and safe drugs for these indications. The localization of 5-HT_3 receptors in the dorsal vagal complex is consistent with such a role. It was shown that chemotherapy agents (e.g., cisplatin) induce massive release of 5-HT from the enterochromaffin cells of the intestinal mucosa, which stimulates 5-HT_3 receptors on vagal afferents, as well as, more hypothetically, increases the release of 5-HT from neurons of the area postrema and the so-called "emetic center". The synergistic action of central and vagal afferents triggers the emetic reflex.

Anxiety: Clinical data on anxiolytic activity of 5-HT_3 receptor antagonists are more controversial: positive and negative results have been reported from clinical studies in anxiety disorders. Generally, 5-HT_3 receptor antagonists may exhibit a delayed (by days) action on relatively low levels of anxiety. The presence of 5-HT_3 receptors in cortical and limbic region is supportive for a possible role of 5-HT_3 receptors in 'emotional' behavior, but animal data tends to indicate a lack of psychotropic activity of 5-HT_3 receptor antagonists.

Other: Additional potential roles for 5-HT_3 receptors include some participation in cognition, psychosis, fibromyalgia and nociception (particularly in the GI tract), migraine, and moderate drug dependence. For more in-depth reviews, the reader is referred to recent articles [35, 47, 162, 369, 464, 513, 545].

Glutamate receptors

Fifteen different subunits assemble in heteromultimeric complexes to form the various glutamate ionotropic receptors: GluR1–GluR4 form AMPA-type receptors; GluR5–GluR7 and KA1–KA2 form kainate-type receptors; and NR1, NR2A–NR2D and NR3 form NMDA-type receptors. In addition, splice variants have been described for many of these subunits. As with other multi-subunit channels, the subunit composition of the final protein defines its electrophysiological and pharmacological properties. The NMDA-type glutamate receptors are unique among ligand-gated ion channels because their opening actually requires the simultaneous presence of two agonists: glutamate and glycine. The NR1 subunits contain the glycine-binding site and the NR2 subunits contain the glutamate-binding site; the third subunit NR3 may be associated with NR1/NR2 channels to play a regulatory role. Because glycine is thought to be present at near-saturating concentrations in the synaptic cleft, its role in NMDA-receptor function is not understood and glutamate appears to be the physiological ligand.

In the mammalian brain, the glutamate receptors (NMDA, AMPA and possibly kainate) play a critical role in the induction of use-dependent plasticity (long-term potentiation or LTP). Glutamate-evoked post-synaptic potentials are composed of a fast component, mediated mostly by AMPA and possibly kainate receptors, and a slow component, mediated by NMDA receptors. At the resting membrane potential, extracellular Mg^{2+} blocks NMDA receptors, such that LTP induction (mediated by the long-lasting Ca^{2+} entry through NMDA receptors) requires simultaneously the release of glutamate to open the NMDA receptors and a depolarization (due to activation of either AMPA or kainate receptors or other transmitter- or voltage-operated ion channels) to unblock them [262]. The resulting Ca^{2+} influx activates protein kinases and phosphatases, which can trigger long-lasting functional changes, including a sustained enhancement of neurotransmission efficacy. Unfortunately, overactivity of glutamate receptors can also cause "excitotoxicity" and neuronal cell death, which could be involved in ischaemic stroke, epilepsy, or neurodegenerative disorders. Conversely, the underexcitation of NMDA receptors within the brain could produce specific forms of memory dysfunction, up to psychosis and dissociation.

Glutamate receptors are also implicated in the pathophysiology of alcoholism (ethanol blocks NMDA-type receptors [8], which may affect memory), opioid tolerance, and neuropathic pain. Although the physiological roles of kainate receptors are not well understood, AMPA and/or kainate receptors might contribute to pathogenesis of Alzheimer's disease and amyotrophic lateral sclerosis. In-depth evaluations of the molecular biology, electrophysiology, pharmacology, physiology, and pathology of glutamate receptors can be found in recent reviews [41, 46, 103, 116, 130, 169, 171, 261, 262, 270, 298, 314, 356, 375, 428, 532, 548].

Nicotinic receptors

Nicotinic receptors (nAChRs) are key molecules in cholinergic transmission at the neuromuscular junction of striated muscles, at the synapse in the autonomic peripheral ganglia, and in several brain areas. Historically, the 'nicotinic receptive substance' in the neuromuscular junction was the first receptor to be recognized, named, studied electrophysiologically, and characterized biochemically. In addition, the structure of the muscle nAChR has been resolved at 4.6 Å [113], helping to derive a remarkable understanding of the molecular basis of its function. Genetically-manipulated mice have provided model systems to determine the molecular basis for many pharmacological actions of nAChR agonists and the role of nAChR subunits in various disease states [93, 394].

nAChRs are homo- or hetero-pentamers of homologous subunits and various subunit combinations can produce many different nAChR subtypes. These subtypes can be grouped into three general functional classes: muscle subunits (α_1, β_1, γ, δ, ε) that combine in $\alpha_1\alpha_1\beta_1\gamma\delta$ (adult) or $\alpha_1\alpha_1\beta_1\delta\varepsilon$ (embryonic); standard neuronal subunits (α_2–α_6 and β_2–β_4) that form nAChRs in $\alpha\beta$ combinations; and other subunits (α_7–α_{10}) capable of forming homomeric nAChRs (α_7–α_9) or $\alpha\alpha$ combinations (α_9–α_{10}). A formal nomenclature for nAChRs has been proposed [295].

Na^+ and K^+ carry most of the nAChR current and neuromuscular junction nAChRs have a low Ca^{2+} permeability; however, neuronal nAChRs present a fairly large Ca^{2+} permeability. A major difference between Ca^{2+} entry through nAChRs and through VOCs or NMDA receptors is that the former does not require membrane depolarization [233].

It is well-known that ACh and nAChRs are responsible for neuromuscular transmission, where activation of muscle nAChRs provokes the depolarization of the myocytes leading to the activation of dihydropyridine receptors and the release of intracellular Ca^{2+}. In addition, because acetylcholine (ACh) is the principal mediator of synaptic transmission in autonomic ganglia, ACh and nAChRs play a major role in cardiovascular homeostasis through the regulation of the activity of smooth muscle, heart muscle, and exocrine glands [167]. Furthermore, a role of nAChRs in the central control of cardiovascular function has also been demonstrated [159, 443].

The role of nAChRs in the CNS is not well understood. Nicotine can modify behavior, enhance learning, memorization, and vigilance, reduce pain perception and cause dependence, but the mechanisms remain unclear. Many electrophysiological and pharmacological studies demonstrate that nAChR stimulation results predominantly in the presynaptic facilitation of the release of all major neurotransmitters, such as glutamate, GABA, norepinephrine, dopamine, or 5-HT. This occurs following Ca^{2+} entry either directly through the nicotinic channels or indirectly through voltage-operated Ca^{2+} channels. Nevertheless, nAChR activation also produces direct excitatory post-synaptic effects. Although this represents a minor component of the excitatory input, which is overwhelmingly glutamatergic, the broad distribution of cholinergic projections could influence the excitability of wide neuronal circuits. In addition, some nAChR subtypes play a role in synaptic plasticity and development [93, 483]. Among the suggested roles of nAChRs, we can cite:

Neurodegeneration: Epidemiological studies show that tobacco smokers have a reduced incidence of neurodegenerative diseases like Alzheimer's and Parkinson's diseases. Furthermore, the brain tissue of elderly persons demonstrates a consistent loss of nAChRs, which is increased in Alzheimer's disease [362, 388]; this loss is likely to contribute to the overall cognitive deficits associated with aging and Alzheimer's disease [119, 388]. Clinical studies have shown that acute administration of nAChR agonists to Alzheimer's disease patients improves recall but longer clinical trials have failed to show a chronic effect. Agonists of nAChR are also efficacious in animal models of Parkinson's disease where they provide symptomatic relief and decreases in neuronal degeneration.

Nociception: The alkaloid epibatidine, acting via nAChRs, is 200 times more potent than morphine as an analgesic but is toxic probably because of its lack of selectivity among nAChRs. The modulation of the activity of multiple neurotransmitter systems appears to be involved in the analgesic effects of nAChR agonists. Many anesthetic agents inhibit nAChRs and this interaction alters critical brain and ganglionic functions *in vivo*. Although nAChRs do not appear to participate directly in the hypnotic component of anesthesia, they contribute to the analgesia produced by some anesthetic agents [496].

Schizophrenia and depression: Most schizophrenics and many depressives are heavy smokers and tobacco withdrawal results in an exacerbation of the schizophrenic or depressive symptoms. Thus, smoking is viewed as self-medication using nicotine as a therapeutic agent. Nicotine like many antidepressant drugs enhances the release of norepinephrine, dopamine, and serotonin.

Epilepsy: High doses of nicotine can be pro-convulsant and a specific epilepsy syndrome (autosomal dominant nocturnal frontal lobe epilepsy) is associated with mutations in the α_4 nAChR subunit [344, 483].

Cognitive dysfunction and attention disorders: Nicotine use is associated with an improvement in cognitive performance, possibly because activation of nAChRs enhances the release of neurotransmitters involved in focus, attention, execution, learning, and memory. Attention deficit hyperactivity disorder (ADHD) is a fairly common psychiatric disorder. It is a significant risk factor for early cigarette smoking in children and patches of nicotine or a nicotinic agonist (ABT-418) produce significant improvements in adults with ADHD. These lines of evidence suggest that the nicotinic system is important in ADHD.

Tourette's syndrome: This syndrome is characterized by uncontrolled obsessive behavior and spontaneous motor and verbal tics. Nicotine potentiates the efficacy of the neuroleptic haloperidol in animals and clinical trials have shown that it can ameliorate the symptoms of Tourette's syndrome.

Vestibular function: α_9 nAChR subunits are uniquely found in cochlear outer hair cells and α_9 knockout mice present with abnormal vestibular function.

Gastric disorders: Smoking reduces the risk for ulcerative colitis and nicotine patches are efficacious in active disease. This effect is limited in duration and its mechanism is not understood [290].

Two more groups of tissues express functional nAChRs similar to those found in neurons. In the "surface organs", including epithelial cells (in particular bronchial), skin keratinocytes, and endothelial cells (in particular arterial), nAChRs may modulate cell shape and motility, as well as cell proliferation and differentiation. It is thus possible that ACh and nAChRs may have a "local endocrine" role, permitting fast adaptation to new conditions. Finally, nAChRs are also found in the thymus and in lymphocytes; it has been proposed that immune function could be under the control of a non-neuronal lymphocytic cholinergic system [248].

The very complex roles of nAChRs in the function of the nervous system have been discussed in recent reviews [93, 112, 119, 159, 167, 233, 244, 376, 394, 443, 483, 496]. Furthermore, the August 2002 issue of "Current Drug Targets—CNS and Neurological Disorders" is entirely dedicated to nAChRs and covers most of the above-mentioned aspects.

P2X receptors

Like the other LGCs, P2X receptors are built as homo- or hetero-multimers of homologous subunits. Seven different subunits have been cloned and the number of subunits per channel, although not firmly established, is believed to be three or four. Expressed $P2X_1$–$P2X_4$ and $P2X_7$ subunits can form homomultimeric channels in oocytes or in mammalian cell lines; in contrast, recombinant $P2X_5$ subunits produce only small currents and no current has been recorded through homomultimeric $P2X_6$ subunits. However, all subunits except $P2X_7$ can form functional recombinant heteromultimeric receptors and it is clear that many of the naturally occurring P2X receptors are heteromultimers. Nonetheless, there appears to be specificity in the possible associations between subunits since only 11 distinct heteromultimeric assemblies have been demonstrated. Finally, the different P2X subunits are widely but specifically distributed in tissues: $P2X_1$ mRNA is expressed predominantly in smooth muscle, $P2X_4$ and $P2X_6$ mostly in brain, $P2X_3$ only in sensory neurons, and $P2X_7$ mostly in the immune system as well as in retina and cochlea.

Nociception: P2X-mediated ATP signaling plays a critical role in nociception in various tissues. Millimolar ATP is present in most cells and large quantities of ATP may leave the intracellular space following tissue trauma, tumor, inflammation, nerve injury, and vascular or visceral distension. The consequent activation of P2X receptors on sensory afferents is thought to initiate the intense pain sensation occurring under these conditions: indeed, transdermal

ATP causes perceptible pain in humans. This view is further supported by the observations that ATP receptors of subtypes $P2X_1$–$P2X_6$ are present in neural structures involved in nociception and that ATP selectively excites sensory afferents, including mesenteric and vagal afferents, afferents in the pelvic, sinus, and lingual nerves, and nociceptors in the knee. In particular, $P2X_3$ subtypes are selectively expressed by nociceptive sensory neurons in dorsal root ganglia and the abnormal physiology of $P2X_3$-knockout mice has confirmed that $P2X_3$-mediated ATP signaling contributes to pain *in vivo* [110]. In addition, $P2X_7$ receptors are present on immune cells, where they may play a role in pain perception by mediating cytokine release. Indeed, $P2X_7$-deficient mice do not release interleukin-1 from inflammatory cells upon ATP injection [459].

Gastro-intestinal reflex: Functional P2X receptors are present on the nerve endings of afferent fibers in the pelvic nerve in the rat and mouse urinary bladder, where they may play a role in mediating the fullness feeling in response to tissue stretch. Indeed, $P2X_3$-knockout mice have a decreased urine voiding frequency and an increased bladder capacity [110]. Whether this may take place in other species, including humans, is not known.

ATP-mediated synaptic transmission and presynaptic modulation: P2X receptors are found in almost all sympathetic and parasympathetic ganglia and ATP is released from pre-ganglionic nerve fibers: this suggests that ATP may be a ganglionic neurotransmitter. There is also increasing evidence for ATP-mediated synaptic transmission in the central nervous system. In parallel, presynaptic P2X receptors, like other ligand-gated ion channels, appear to produce a range of effects on synaptic transmission, including facilitation and/or inhibition. Interestingly, P2X receptors could, in addition to their role in initiating the pain sensation, participate in the processing of nociceptive stimuli in the spinal cord since ATP released from the terminals of primary afferents may act at presynaptic and/or post-synaptic P2X receptors.

Autonomic neuromuscular transmission: At the neuromuscular junction between sympathetic nerves and the smooth muscle of the guinea-pig vas deferens, ATP acts as a co-transmitter with noradrenaline. ATP, acting on $P2X_1$ receptors, produces a depolarization of the smooth muscle leading to action potentials and a rapid phasic contraction [455]. In contrast, noradrenaline mediates a slow tonic contraction independent of membrane depolarization. The importance of ATP-mediated contraction was confirmed in $P2X_1$-knockout mice, for which contraction of the vas deferens in response to sympathetic nerve stimulation is substantially reduced [345]. A similar ATP-dependent mechanism is found in urogenital, gastrointestinal, and vascular smooth muscle, where a rapid ATP-mediated response is followed by a slow response mediated by another transmitter, such as noradrenaline, acetylcholine, nitric oxide, or a neuropeptide. In gastrointestinal and vascular smooth muscle, an additional hyperpolarization is often observed, which is probably mediated by ATP acting on endothelial P2Y receptors [408].

Heart: Little is known regarding P2X-mediated signaling in cardiomyocytes [517]. $P2X_1$ immunoreactivity is observed at the intercalated disk in rat cardiac tissues; $P2X_1$, $P2X_2$ and $P2X_4$ transcripts are found in rat atria and $P2X_4$ transcript is found in ventricle; and $P2X_5$ was cloned in rat heart. Contrary to the rat, $P2X_3$ transcripts are found in human fetal and adult heart (although it cannot be excluded that transcripts are located in primary sensory afferents innervating these structures). In addition, the levels of $P2X_1$ transcript are increased ~three-fold in rats with congestive heart failure. However, assuming these P2X mRNAs are translated, the role of the P2X receptors is unknown. An extracellular ATP-activated current is found in cardiac cells (frog and mammalian atrial cells including human and mammalian ventricular cells) but its properties are somewhat different from currents recorded through expressed P2X receptors.

Other roles: In humans, a dominant negative mutation of $P2X_1$ gene leads to a severe bleeding disorder due to an impairment of ADP-induced platelet aggregation [371]. In vascular endothelium, shear stress leads to the release of ATP into the blood flow and $P2X_4$ is expressed in vascular endothelium, where it may be involved in shear stress-mediated Ca^{2+} influx [554, 555].

ATP exocytosis and release: ATP can be released by exocytosis like other neurotransmitters, but it can also leak out during cell damage. The existence of an ATP channel has been suggested to enable intracellular ATP to cross the cell membrane, similar to the mitochondrial voltage-dependent anion channel and the Cl channel in cardiac sarcoplasmic reticulum [517].

Many review articles can be consulted that cover the properties and functions of P2X receptors [71, 104, 138, 251, 272, 296, 363, 365, 455, 517].

Receptor-activated Ca^{2+} channels (RAC)

Like ligand-gated ion channels, receptor-activated ion channels open following the binding of an agonist to its receptor; however, in the case of receptor-activated ion channels, the receptor protein is different from the channel protein. Since receptor and channel are distinct proteins, there must exist some transduction mechanism (intracellular messenger, G-protein, depletion of intracellular stores etc.) that connects receptor activation to channel opening. Although the term receptor-activated Ca^{2+} channel (RAC) presumes that a channel selectively conducts Ca^{2+}, this name is often used as well for non-selective cation channels that, under physiological conditions, admit predominantly Na^+ but also sufficient Ca^{2+} to raise cytoplasmic $[Ca^{2+}]$ significantly. Our understanding of the RACs remains very sketchy, in large part because there seems to exist a large number of RAC subtypes and each cell type appears to possess several of these, with different function, mechanism of activation, electrophysiological properties, and structure. For in-depth reviews of receptor-activated Ca^{2+} channels, the reader is referred to many excellent recent articles [142, 220, 286, 405, 571].

Store-operated Ca^{2+} channels (SOC) and I_{CRAC}

Properties

These types of RACs have been characterized in the most detail: they are defined as plasma-membrane Ca^{2+} channels that open in response to a Ca^{2+} concentration decrease inside the endoplasmic reticulum (ER). Physiologically, this concentration decrease is generally the consequence of the sequence (Fig. 3): 1) agonist binding to a cell-surface G-protein-coupled or tyrosine-kinase-coupled receptor; 2) activation of phospholipase C; 3) generation of inositol-1,4,5-trisphophate (IP_3) and diacylglycerol (DAG) from plasma membrane phosphoinositides; 4) activation of Ca^{2+}-permeable IP_3-receptor channels (IP_3Rs) in the ER membrane. However, the decrease can also be induced by pharmacological agents such as thapsigargin, which inhibits the uptake of Ca^{2+} in the ER [498], or EGTA, which lowers cytoplasmic [Ca^{2+}] below the level required for uptake into the ER. Historically, two other major names have been used to describe these channels or the associated Ca entry: "capacitative Ca^{2+} influx" because Ca^{2+} entry follows changes in the Ca^{2+} load in the intracellular stores and "Ca^{2+}-release-activated current" (I_{CRAC}).

The first convincing evidence of Ca^{2+} entry following store depletion came in the early 1980s using Ca^{2+}-sensitive fluorescent dyes [404] but the first detailed electrophysiological characterization of a Ca^{2+} current associated with store depletion (I_{CRAC}) was only published in 1992 using mast cells [224]. I_{CRAC} was shown to be of very small whole-cell amplitude, to be >1,000-fold selective for Ca^{2+} over monovalent cations, and to occur through channels with

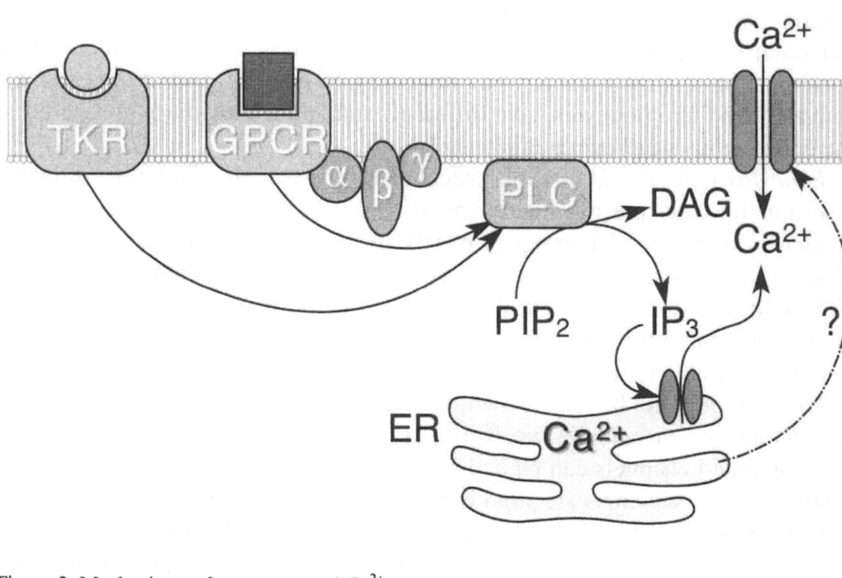

Figure 3. Mechanisms of store-operated Ca^{2+} entry.

extremely low single-channel conductance. The next year, noise analysis of I_{CRAC} in lymphocytes predicted a single-channel Ca^{2+} conductance of ~24 fS [574]; this is > two orders of magnitude below other cation channels and undetectable with the present single-channel recording methodology. However, in the absence of extracellular Ca^{2+}, single-channel Na^+ currents can be measured through I_{CRAC} yielding a single-channel Na^+ conductance of ~40 pS [250]. Based on this data and the Ca^{2+}/Na^+ selectivity of the channels, these authors calculated a revised single-channel Ca^{2+} conductance of 1.6 pS. This value is in good agreement with other measurements of ~1 pS in mouse macrophages and ~3 pS in mouse and rabbit aortic smooth muscle cells. Finally, it is worth noting that, because store-operated Ca^{2+} currents are technically so difficult to measure, a role for SOCs as the most common pathway of store-operated Ca^{2+} entry remains an unproven assumption for many cell types.

Mechanism of activation

There is also no clear understanding of the mechanism(s) underlying the transduction of the filling status of the ER to the opening of the Ca^{2+} entry mechanism (e.g., the SOC). Different groups have proposed three major possibilities.

Diffusible messenger: The first possible mechanism is that store depletion releases a molecule calcium influx factor (CIF) or that diffuses to the plasma membrane and activates I_{CRAC}. Evidence for such a model comes primarily from two forms of experiments: 1) extracellular application or intracellular injection of extracts of activated cells can induce Ca^{2+} entry in naïve cells [414, 503]; and 2) membrane patches of activated cells lose the induced Ca^{2+} current when they are excised from a cell and regain it when they are pushed back into the cell [374]. Nevertheless, in addition to the fact that purification of CIF remains unsuccessful after almost 10 years, there are two problems with the CIF data: 1) contrary to the expectation for a second messenger molecule, CIF appears to be relatively stable when injected into oocytes; and 2) the channels activated by CIF in oocytes have different lanthanum sensitivity compared to the endogenous store-operated channels.

Exocytosis: A second possible mechanism involves the depletion-activated insertion into the plasma membrane of the SOC itself or of an activator. Evidence for this model comes primarily from the observation that inhibitors of secretion or cytoskeleton disruptors can prevent the activation of I_{CRAC} [152, 377, 558]. However, there are also problems with the exocytosis data: 1) not all secretion inhibitors are able to prevent I_{CRAC} activation nor is one cytoskeleton disruptor able to prevent I_{CRAC} activation in all cells [142]; 2) exocytosis is generally thought to be Ca^{2+} dependent whereas store-operated entry is highly activated when cytoplasmic $[Ca^{2+}]$ is strongly buffered to low levels; 3) store-operated channels can be activated in membrane patches [58, 572] suggesting that the channels are already present in the cell membrane; and 4) this model essentially adds an additional step (exocytosis) between store depletion and membrane Ca^{2+} current but does not explain how store depletion and exocytosis are linked (direct coupling or a diffusible messenger remain possible).

Conformational coupling: The third alternative mechanism may have the most support at present and involves a direct protein–protein interaction between an ER protein and the SOCs. This model was originally proposed in analogy to striated muscle cells where Ca^{2+} channels mediate Ca^{2+} release by means of protein–protein interaction of the channels with the calcium stores [231]. In non-excitable cells, the Ca^{2+} content in the ER would alter the configuration of one or more proteins within the store membrane; in turn, these proteins would directly interact with the Ca^{2+} channel in the plasma membrane to control its gating. In most cases, the IP_3 receptor (IP_3R) is suggested as the coupling protein [36]. The best evidence for this model is fairly recent and comes from studies using cloning and expression of a family of proteins (TRP, see below) that are candidates for components of store-operated Ca^{2+} channels. There is general agreement that TRPC3 (and possibly TRPC6 and TRPC7) can be activated in an IP_3- and IP_3R-dependent manner and, although its identity as a SOC component is not established, TRP3 has been used as a model for elucidating the gating of SOCs. In particular: 1) TRPC3 expression is associated with up-regulation of IP_3Rs in HEK293 cells; 2) in freshly-excised inside-out patches, IP_3 increases TRPC3 channel activity while antagonists of IP_3Rs almost completely inhibit it; 3) in extensively-washed patches that do not respond to IP_3, IP_3R-containing microsomes stimulate TRPC3 channel activity in the presence of IP_3 [254]. A similar dependence of endogenous SOCs on IP_3 and its receptor has been shown in A431 cells [572]. These results strongly support an interaction between SOCs and IP_3 receptors as a major mechanism of channel activation. Consistent with this conclusion is the observation that expressed TRPC3 can co-precipitate with IP_3Rs [53, 253]. A missing stone in this demonstration is the fact that physical juxtaposition of SOCs and IP_3Rs has not been demonstrated, contrary to the microscopic evidence of contacts ("feet") between ryanodine receptors and dihydropyridine receptors in skeletal muscle. A missing link could be myosin, which was recently suggested to be involved in SOC opening and/or closing and could couple somewhat distant SOCs and IP_3Rs [21].

Some issues still remain with the conformational coupling model, mainly the fact that, in a cell line from which all IP_3 receptor types were eliminated, Ca^{2+} entry responses are lost to intracellular application of IP_3 and to agonists coupled to phospholipase C but not to thapsigargin [62, 482]. It is also worth noting again that the role of TRP3 as a SOC component is not firmly established such that extrapolating TRP3 data to CRAC channels remains speculative. In particular, TRP3, like most other members of the TRP family, has much lower Ca^{2+} selectivity than usually reported for I_{CRAC}.

Molecular biology

The best current candidates for SOC genes are mammalian homologues of the *Drosophila* trp gene ("trp" stands for "transient receptor potential"). Initially, interest focused on this gene family because TRP has structural homologies with voltage-operated Ca^{2+} channels [393] and its expression leads to enhanced

Ca^{2+} influx after stimulation with thapsigargin [389, 511]. At present, TRP channels represent a large family (20 genes) of non-selective cationic channels, which can be divided in three main families based on sequence homology: TRPC (also "short TRP"), TRPV (also OTRPC) and TRPM (also "long TRP") [109, 338, 339, 520]. Like voltage-operated Ca^{2+} channels, TRP channels belong to the superfamily of 6-transmembrane-spanning-segment cation channels but, like voltage-operated K^+ channels, they require the homomultimeric or heteromultimeric assembly of four gene products from the same family to produce a functional channel. Activation of TRP channels can occur through various mechanisms (Tab. 1) and it will raise cytoplasmic [Ca^{2+}], despite the lack of Ca^{2+}-selectivity of the channels. In particular, TRPC channels are activated through the Receptor/G-protein/Phospholipase cascade, although this can occur at different steps of the cascade, sometimes but not necessarily requiring depletion of the intracellular Ca^{2+} stores. On the other hand, TRPV and TRPM channels are activated by an extreme variety of stimuli.

Remarkably, a large number of mammalian TRP channels appear to be SOCs. Some may be directly coupled to Ca^{2+} stores via interactions with the IP_3 receptor [53] and, in the case of TRPC3, may also be activated through interaction with the ryanodine receptor. For many, the mechanism of activation remains undefined. The search for a Ca^{2+}-selective TRP channel to represent the molecular basis of I_{CRAC} has recently focused on two members of the TRPV family (TRPV5 and TRPV6): these channels display Ca^{2+}-selective permeation [519, 562] and the TRPV6 current possesses some [562] but not all key features of I_{CRAC} [522]. It is also possible that I_{CRAC} represents current(s)

Table 1. Mechanisms of activation of TRP channels

Family	Channel name (alias)	Regulation
TRPC	TRPC1	Receptor-G protein-PLC, store depletion
(or STRPC)	TRPC2	Store depletion
	TRPC3	IP_3/CaM
	TRPC4	Receptor-G protein-PLC, store depletion
	TRPC5	Receptor-G protein-PLC, store depletion
	TRPC6	Diacylglycerol
	TRPC7	Diacylglycerol
TRPC	TRPV1 (VR1)	Heat, capsaicin
(or OTRPC)	TRPV2 (VRL1)	Heat, growth factor
	TRPV4	Osmolarity
	TRPV5 (CaT2)	Low cytoplasmic [Ca^{2+}]
	TRPV6 (CaT1, ECaC)	Low cytoplasmic [Ca^{2+}], store depletion
TRPC	TRPM1 (melanostatin)	
(or LTRPC)	TRPM2 (TRPC7)	ADP-ribose
	TRPM3	
	TRPM4	
	TRPM5 (MTR1)	
	TRPM6	
	TRPM7 (TRP-PLIK)	Endo-channel kinase
	TRPM8 (Trp-p8, CMR1)	Cold, menthol

through heteromultimers of TRP channels, with or without TRPV5/6: most combinations have never been evaluated. Conversely, heteromultimerization of exogenously with endogenously expressed TRP channels may prevent the formation of the "right" channel responsible for I_{CRAC}. Consistent with this idea, bovine adrenal cortical cells express TRP4 protein abundantly and possess I_{CRAC}: both are down-regulated in parallel upon transfection with TRP4 antisense cDNA [392]. Yet, TRPC4 is probably not essential for I_{CRAC} everywhere since it is little or not expressed in other cells (Jurkat lymphocytes and RBL cells) that exhibit much higher I_{CRAC} than adrenal cells. Indeed, in salivary gland cells, TRPC1-antisense but not TRPC4-antisense nucleotides inhibit the appearance of and I_{CRAC}-like current [288]. And one should always keep in mind that TRPC1 and TRPC4 are not Ca^{2+}-selective in expression systems.

In summary, the molecular entity or entities responsible for I_{CRAC} remains the subject of heated debate. It seems somewhat likely that different proteins and/or combinations of proteins are responsible for I_{CRAC} in different cells.

Other RACs

Until recently, investigations of Ca^{2+} entry in non-excitable cells had focused almost exclusively on store-operated Ca^{2+} entry. Yet it is still possible that capacitative Ca^{2+} entry may not represent the most critical route for agonist-activated Ca^{2+} entry since several types of Ca^{2+}-permeable cation channels have been described that are not directly ligand-gated but are nevertheless activated after agonist binding to a receptor, independently of any action on Ca^{2+} stores (reviewed in [20]). Interest in non-capacitative Ca^{2+} entry has revived recently following the observation that TRP channels in heterologous expression systems are often activated upon agonist application or diacylglycerol addition without requiring store depletion (reviewed in [220]). Unfortunately, little information is presently available on the role of TRP channels in native tissues.

Generally, non-store-operated RACs appear to be activated by one of the messengers of the IP_3 signal transduction cascade such as IP_3, inositol 1,3,4,5-tetrakisphosphate (IP_4), Ca^{2+}, G proteins, diacylglycerol (DAG), protein kinase C (PKC), or arachidonic acid (AA). At present, the best-described non-store-operated RAC may be the AA-dependent muscarinic receptor-activated Ca^{2+} entry pathway demonstrated in avian nasal gland and HEK293 cells [446–449]. The corresponding Ca^{2+} current, named I_{ARC} (for arachidonate-regulated Ca^{2+} current), has been described [316] and I_{ARC} and I_{CRAC} were shown to be reciprocally regulated in HEK293 cells [317]. It is quite possible that such a mechanism might co-exist with SOCs in many cell types and may even predominate under physiological conditions. Recently, AA was shown to activate *Drosophila* TRP and TRPL channels [108], suggesting that a mammalian TRP channel may sustain I_{ARC}.

Quite often, the activation of a given cell-surface receptor leads to the opening of multiple RACs as well as other Ca^{2+} channels. For example, in smooth muscle cells, α_{1A}-adrenergic agonists induce the opening of SOCs through depletion of the endoplasmic reticulum, of non-selective RACs through the combined actions of increased cytoplasmic [Ca^{2+}] and a G-protein, and of VOCs (L-type and possibly T-type) through a G-protein → phospholipase → diacylglycerol → protein kinase C cascade [297]. Similarly, vasopressin sequentially stimulates Ca^{2+} inflow in A7r5 smooth muscle cells through non-selective RACs followed by SOCs [73, 335]. The store-independent Ca^{2+} entry component appears to be AA-activated [63] and may be mediated by TRPC6 channels [242].

In summary, the RACs are the most poorly understood of the plasma-membrane Ca^{2+} channels, in large part because there is a large number of RAC subtypes and a given cell may possess several of these subtypes. However, the tissue distribution of the RAC subtypes appears to be more specific than for SOCs: this should allow for a variety of different functions with specific patterns of Ca^{2+} increase.

Voltage-operated Ca^{2+} channels (VOC)

Voltage-operated Ca^{2+} channels, which are the focus of this book, are responsible for mediating Ca^{2+} influx in response to membrane depolarization in neurons and other cell types. Ca^{2+} entry through these channels serves to regulate intracellular processes such as contraction, secretion, neurotransmission, and gene expression in response to action potentials and other membrane potential changes. Although all VOCs are activated by a conformational modification of protein structure induced by a change in membrane potential, these channels can vary considerably in their electrophysiological properties such as voltage-dependencies, activation/inactivation kinetics, sensitivity to extracellular and intracellular ligands, ion selectivity, and single channel properties. Historically, the characterization of voltage-operated Ca^{2+} channels has progressed on two separate fronts: the electrophysiological and pharmacological characterization of voltage-operated Ca^{2+} channel currents and the biochemical and molecular characterization of voltage-operated Ca2+ channel proteins. This has led to the emergence of two separate nomenclatures, the correspondence of which has been difficult to define because many of the features used to associate cloned and native Ca^{2+} channels depend on many factors, such as cellular environment, co-expression of accessory subunits, and modulation by second messengers and G-proteins.

The different electrophysiological and pharmacological properties of native VOCs had led to the description of a number of distinct voltage-operated Ca^{2+} currents, which have been classically classified as L-, N-, T-, P-, Q-, and R-types [249, 465–467]. In addition, the existence of many subtypes was also quite clear.

VOCs that have been characterized biochemically are complex proteins composed of four or five distinct subunits, which are encoded by multiple genes. They belong to a gene superfamily of transmembrane proteins, which also includes voltage-operated K^+ and Na^+ channels. Historically, various names had been given to the corresponding gene products, giving rise to distinct and sometimes confusing nomenclatures. In 1994, a unified nomenclature was proposed based on the most widely accepted system at the time: α_1 subunits were referred to as α_{1S} for the original skeletal muscle isoform and α_{1A} through α_{1E} for those discovered subsequently [42]. Since then, four new α_1 subunits have been identified, which were named α_{1F} through α_{1I}.

Recently, a new nomenclature/classification of voltage-operated Ca^{2+} channels has been proposed [146], similar in form to the widely-accepted classification of voltage-operated K^+ channels [92] as well as the recent classification of voltage-operated Na^+ channels [179]. This new classification (Tab. 2) is derived from the degree of sequence homology/similarity between the genes coding for the various Ca^{2+} channels and it represents an update to, and a reconciliation of, the classification based on electrophysiological properties and drug binding sites and that based on molecular structure.

Table 2. Nomenclature of voltage-operated Ca^{2+} channels

Type	α_1 subunit	Former names	Splice	Former names	Current
$Ca_V1.1$	$\alpha_11.1$	α_{1S}, α_{1Skm}, CaCh1			L
$Ca_V1.2$	$\alpha_11.2$	α_{1C}, rbC, CaCh2	$Ca_V1.2a$ $Ca_V1.2b$ $Ca_V1.2c$	$\alpha_{1C\text{-}a}$ $\alpha_{1C\text{-}b}$ $\alpha_{1C\text{-}c}$	
$Ca_V1.3$	$\alpha_11.3$	α_{1D}, rbD, CaCh3			
$Ca_V1.4$	$\alpha_11.4$	α_{1F}			
$Ca_V2.1$	$\alpha_12.1$	α_{1A}, rbA, CaCh4, BI	$Ca_V2.1a$ $Ca_V2.1b$	BI1 BI2	P/Q
$Ca_V2.2$	$\alpha_12.2$	α_{1B}, rbB, CaCh5, BIII	$Ca_V2.2a$ $Ca_V2.2b$	$\alpha_{1B\text{-}1}$ $\alpha_{1B\text{-}2}$	N
$Ca_V2.3$	$\alpha_12.3$	α_{1E}, rbE, CaCh6, BII	$Ca_V2.3a$ $Ca_V2.3b$	BII BII2	R
$Ca_V3.1$	$\alpha_13.1$	α_{1G}	$Ca_V3.1a$	$Ca_VT.1$	T
$Ca_V3.2$	$\alpha_13.2$	α_{1H}	$Ca_V3.2a$	$Ca_VT.2$	
$Ca_V3.3$	$\alpha_13.3$	α_{1I}	$Ca_V3.3a$	$Ca_VT.3$	

Electrophysiological and pharmacological diversity of voltage-operated Ca^{2+} currents

Formerly, the most commonly used classification of voltage-operated Ca^{2+} channels was actually a classification of the currents flowing through these channels. It is based on a combination of pharmacological properties and electrophysiological characteristics of measured Ca^{2+} current or Ca^{2+} fluxes. So far, this classification recognizes six main categories of voltage-operated Ca^{2+} currents: L (Long-lasting), T (Transient), N (Neither T nor L, or Neuronal), P (Purkinje cells), Q (after P), and R (Remaining, or Resistant, or after Q) (Tab. 3).

L-type Ca^{2+} currents

Most voltage-operated Ca^{2+} current data published before multiple channel types were recognized refers to L-type Ca^{2+} currents. Indeed, these currents are the most commonly encountered in various cell types and often represent the largest current component in "mixed-channel" situations. Since their initial description in the late 1960s [419, 427], L-type Ca^{2+} currents have been thoroughly investigated and several reviews are available [1, 23, 76, 88, 89, 209, 410, 475, 504]. L-type Ca^{2+} currents are most often characterized by their: 1) high-voltage activation (i.e., the cell membrane voltage must be raised quite a bit before the channels open; for this reason they are often called high-voltage-activated or HVA Ca^{2+} currents); 2) slow inactivation (i.e., the channels remain open a long time under maintained depolarization); and 3) block by Ca antagonists such as dihydropyridines (DHPs), phenylalkylamines (PAAs), and benzothiazepines (BTZs). The high affinity of DHPs for the channels responsible for the L-type Ca^{2+} currents is a powerful test to differentiate L-type from non-L-type Ca^{2+} currents. It established the DHPs as the preferred tools for biochemical work and they were used to purify the channel protein underlying the L-type Ca^{2+} currents, initially from skeletal muscle, and to determine its subunit composition and the primary structures of these subunits. Accordingly, the channels responsible for the L-type Ca^{2+} currents are commonly referred to as "dihydropyridine receptors".

L-type Ca^{2+} currents are widely distributed in neuronal tissue, including glia [278], and in non-neuronal tissues, such as cardiac [210, 507], smooth [207, 468], and skeletal muscle [351, 507], endocrine cells [111, 145, 423, 480], oocytes [118], osteoblasts [198], endothelium [51, 52], epithelium [222]. In non-neuronal tissues, they generally constitute the primary, and sometimes the only, pathway for Ca^{2+} entry. In cardiac and smooth muscle cells, L-type Ca^{2+} currents are responsible for the inward movement of Ca^{2+} that initiates contraction. In skeletal muscle, the channel protein underlying the L-type Ca^{2+} current also acts as voltage sensor in excitation-contraction-coupling and it directly couples to Ca^{2+} release channels in the sarcoplasmic reticulum. The functions of L-type Ca^{2+} currents in the nervous system are less well defined but, in addition to some minimal participation in the induction of exocytosis, they include gene expression [17, 44, 127, 128, 348] and induction of some forms of N-methyl-D-aspartate receptor-independent long-term potentiation [239]. Consistent with roles in the slow modulation of neuronal function, the L-type Ca^{2+} currents are mainly found in cell bodies and dendrites [85].

Functionally, the L-type Ca^{2+} current family encompasses several subfamilies with tissue-specific electrophysiological properties. For example, skeletal

Table 3. Electrophysiological and pharmacological properties of Ca^{2+} currents

Property	L-type	N-type	T-type	P-type	Q-type	R-type
Electrophysiology						
Activation threshold	high (–30 to –10 mV)	high (–30 mV)	low (–70 to –50 mV)	medium (–40 mV)	medium (–40 mV)	medium (–40 mV)
Inactivation voltage	high	medium	low	high	high	low
Inactivation rate	slow	moderate	fast	very slow	moderate	fast
Deactivation rate	fast	fast	slow	fast	fast	fast
Ca inactivation	yes	yes	no	yes		no
V-dep inactivation rate	no	no	yes	no	no	no
Conductance (pS)	20–30	12–20	5–9	10–12	16	10–16
Permeation	$Ca^{2+} < Ba^{2+}$	$Ca^{2+} < Ba^{2+}$	$Ca^{2+} = Ba^{2+}$	$Ca^{2+} < Ba^{2+}$	$Ca^{2+} < Ba^{2+}$	$Ca^{2+} \sim Ba^{2+}$
Pharmacology						
Ni^{2+}	low	low	high	low	low	medium to high
Cd^{2+}	high	high	low	high	high	high
DHP agonists	stimulation	slight block	no	slight block	no	slight block
DHP antagonists	high	no	no to medium	no	no/low	no
Verapamil	high					
Diltiazem	high					
Mibefradil	medium	medium	high	low to medium	low to medium	medium
Octanol, amiloride	no/low	no	medium/high			1 mM
Barbiturates	high	medium	no			
ω-CgTx-GVIA	no/low	high	no	no	no	no
ω-CTx-MVIIC	no	high	no	medium	high	no
ω-Aga-IIIA	high	high	no	high	high	high
ω-Aga-IVA	no/low	no/low	no	high	medium	no/low
ω-Aga-IVB	no	no	no	high	high	

muscle L-type Ca^{2+} currents inactivate very slowly, endocrine L-type Ca^{2+} currents inactivate faster, and cardiac L-type Ca^{2+} currents still faster. Atypical L-type Ca^{2+} currents, which do not belong to these subfamilies, have been reported in a variety of preparations including rat dorsal root ganglion neurons [161, 164], rat cerebellar granule cells [165], rat embryonic and post-natal hippocampal neurons [238, 247], and rat adrenal glomerulosa cells [425, 426]. These currents are activated at very negative membrane potentials but they are also sensitive to DHPs. Whether this novel activity is due to a new kind of L-type Ca^{2+} channel or to an unusual modulation of the activity of a known channel is still debated. These questions illustrate the difficulties encountered with a classification based simultaneously on electrophysiology and pharmacology.

T-type Ca^{2+} currents
T-type Ca^{2+} currents were originally described in sensory neurons [78, 79], atrial [26] and ventricular [359] myocytes, and pituitary cells [12] (reviewed in [148, 149, 227]). T-type Ca^{2+} currents are low-voltage-activated (LVA) and they are often referred to as transient Ca^{2+} currents (because they inactivate rapidly) or as slowly-deactivating Ca^{2+} currents. T-type Ca^{2+} currents are also differentiated from other Ca^{2+} currents by the smaller unitary conductance of the underlying channel and the fact that their inactivation rate is voltage-dependent and not Ca-dependent. These currents are less sensitive than L-type to classical Ca antagonists and not at all to ω-CTx-GVIA: in fact, no specific blocker of this current is known. Various pharmacological compounds show some selectivity for T-type Ca^{2+} currents under defined conditions: mibefradil, Ni^{2+}, amiloride, ethosuximide, phenytoin, octanol, flunarizine, sipatrigine, SB-209712, U-92032 [149, 200, 311, 312, 400]. Many volatile anesthetics also block T-type Ca^{2+} currents with some selectivity [75, 500, 553]. In addition, the scorpion toxin kurtoxin blocks T-type Ca^{2+} currents selectively in some preparations ([107], but see [450]) and anandamide has been proposed recently as a potential endogenous blocker [99]. Finally, the classical dihydropyridine antagonists are generally able to block T-type in addition to L-type Ca^{2+} currents with a selectivity ratio ranging from ~2 (oxodipine [174]) to ~500 (nifedipine (473)); the new DHP analog PPK-5 may actually possess selectivity for T-type over L-type Ca^{2+} currents [271] but this needs to be shown in additional preparations.

Presently, mibefradil may be the most selective small molecule blocking T-type Ca^{2+} currents. It has 10–30 fold selectivity for T-type over L-type Ca^{2+} currents in cardiac ([30, 300], but see [402]) and vascular [324] myocytes as well as in endocrine cells [425]. Mibefradil is also selective for T-type over HVA Ca^{2+} currents in some [308, 373] but not all neurons [412, 521].

The lack of a highly specific blocker has slowed the elucidation of the function of T-type Ca^{2+} currents and of the structure of the underlying channel(s). The molecular structure of T-type Ca^{2+} channels was finally described recently (see below), which has considerably sped-up our understanding of the function of T-type Ca^{2+} currents. A remarkable variety of physiological roles have been proposed for T-type Ca^{2+} currents. In the cardiovascular system, these roles include a contribution to the control of vascular tone [22, 114, 149], to the pacemaker depolarization of cardiac cells [189], and to excitation-contraction coupling in the developing heart [256]. In the endocrine system, they include the control of the secretion of aldosterone [111, 282, 293], ANP [285, 534], cortisol [181], and insulin [39, 570]. In the nervous system, they include the maintenance [98, 227, 252, 397, 409, 457, 481] or the inhibition [546] of repetitive firing in neurons as well as a contribution to the initiation of long-term potentiation or depression (LTP/LTD) [431, 528], and to the tolerance and dependence to morphine [131]. A further role for T-type Ca^{2+} currents has been suggested in the capacitation and acrosome reaction of sperm ([18, 235] but see [49]). Finally, developmental roles for T-type Ca^{2+} currents have been proposed based on the correlation between current magnitude or channel expression and 1) cell adhesion [176]; 2) growth [97, 269, 551]; 3) differentiation [34, 186, 216]; 4) cardiac remodeling [150, 151, 226, 432], and 5) oncogenic transformation [100, 302]. Indeed, the expression of the various T-type Ca^{2+} channels is highly regulated during embryogenesis and fetal development as well as during the perinatal period [37, 160, 304, 460, 563].

N-type Ca^{2+} currents

N-type Ca^{2+} currents were originally described in sensory neurons [366] but they are widely distributed in the nervous system (reviewed in [86, 89, 166, 209, 505, 506]). Like L-type Ca^{2+} currents, N-type Ca^{2+} currents are high-voltage-activated but they inactivate faster than L-type. They are generally identified by their pharmacological properties: resistance to DHPs and potent block by ω-CTx-GVIA and ω-CTx-MVIIA, two toxins from the venoms of the marine snails *Conus geographicus* and *Conus magus* [357, 368, 415, 537]. N-type Ca^{2+} currents are exclusively neuronal and they play a major role in mediating neurotransmitter release in the CNS [505] and at the neuromuscular junction [240, 333]. In particular, they are critical to the transmission of specific nociceptive signals [197, 430, 454, 515] and N-type Ca^{2+} antagonists can be effective analgesics [14, 225, 346]. N-type Ca^{2+} channels also play an essential role in the cardiovascular regulation function of the sympathetic nervous system (positive inotropic response, baroreflex response [342]). At the post-synaptic level, N-type Ca^{2+} currents may be responsible for associative long-term depression in the hippocampus [364]. Finally, increases in cytoplasmic $[Ca^{2+}]$ due to N-type Ca^{2+} currents may direct the migration of immature neurons [263] and, in parallel to increases due to L-type Ca^{2+} currents, it may also initiate patterns of gene expression [66].

To initiate neurotransmitter release, voltage-operated Ca^{2+} currents must produce a high transient cytoplasmic $[Ca^{2+}]$ (20–400 μM). Since cytoplasmic $[Ca^{2+}]$ decreases very rapidly away from the entry site, such high levels probably occur only extremely close to the Ca^{2+} channels. Thus, the Ca^{2+} sensor responsible for initiating neurotransmitter release must remain close to the

Ca^{2+} channels at all times and an actual physical link is quite likely between release mechanism and Ca^{2+} channels. A group of proteins (SNARE proteins or Soluble N-ethylmaleimide-sensitive factor Attachment protein REceptor), including the synaptic vesicle protein VAMP/synaptobrevin and the plasma membrane proteins syntaxin and SNAP-25, mediates the membrane docking and the fusion of exocytotic vesicles. An additional synaptic vesicle protein, synaptotagmin, binds Ca^{2+} and interacts with syntaxin in a Ca^{2+}-dependent manner. Synaptotagmin is generally believed to represent the Ca^{2+} sensor for neurotransmitter release [38, 85, 86, 332, 499] although the possibility has also been suggested that the Ca^{2+} channel itself represents the Ca^{2+} sensor [15, 16]. A direct interaction between the SNARE proteins and a cytoplasmic domain of N-type Ca^{2+} channels appears fundamental for efficient neurotransmission. Interestingly, two widely-expressed N-type Ca^{2+} channels variants lack this interaction site, which suggests that they may have physiological roles distinct from neurotransmitter release [243].

P-type Ca^{2+} currents

P-type Ca^{2+} currents were originally described in cerebellar Purkinje cells [289] where they are particularly predominant. They were subsequently identified in various central [213] and peripheral neurons [399, 415] and in chromaffin cells [13]. They have rarely been described outside the nervous system, with the notable exception of vascular smooth muscle [194]. P-type Ca^{2+} currents are moderately HVA and they inactivate slowly [319]. They differ from L-type and N-type Ca^{2+} currents by their resistance to DHPs and ω-CTx-GVIA and their sensitivity to the toxins ω-Aga-IVA and ω-CTx-MVIIC, respectively from the venoms of the funnel web spider *Agelenopsis aperta* and the marine snail *Conus magus* [321, 322, 411].

Like N-type Ca^{2+} currents, P-type Ca^{2+} currents are involved in neuronal transmission [508]; in particular, they appear to regulate the release of excitatory amino acids, catecholamines, and GABA. The channels underlying P-type Ca^{2+} currents also interact with SNARE proteins [85] and Ca^{2+} entry through these channels (and/or Q-type, see below) activates the expression of the SNARE protein syntaxin-1A, which may provide a positive feedback mechanism for exocytosis [484]. The role of P-type Ca^{2+} currents in specific neural functions remains very speculative. Observations of the pathophysiology of abnormal P-type Ca^{2+} currents in humans and transgenic mice suggest, not unexpectedly, that these currents are critical for normal cerebellar and cortical function: defective currents lead to migraine and/or ataxia [241, 398, 469]. Patients with Lambert-Eaton myasthenic syndrome produce autoimmune antibodies directed against the channels underlying the P-type Ca^{2+} currents (and/or Q-type, see below); these antibodies reduce the release of acetylcholine from nerve terminals in the neuromuscular junction [144, 487].

Functional diversity among P-type Ca^{2+} currents was recently suggested by the identification in rat cerebellar granule cells of a novel current subtype (G1). This current displays the characteristic pharmacology of P-type Ca^{2+} currents but has unusual electrophysiological characteristics: it is slowly inactivated during depolarizing pulses and completely inactivated at voltages where steady state inactivation of P-type Ca^{2+} currents in Purkinje cells is negligible [501].

Q-type Ca^{2+} currents

Q-type Ca^{2+} currents were originally described in cerebellar granule cells [411, 435, 568] and hippocampal neurons [536]. In ligand-binding studies, the Ca^{2+} channels likely to correspond to these currents have also been called O-type Ca^{2+} channels [3]. Q-type Ca^{2+} currents appear to be exclusively neuronal, they are moderate to HVA, and they exhibit inactivation kinetics similar to those of N-type Ca^{2+} currents [319]. Their pharmacology is very similar to that of P-type Ca^{2+} currents: they are resistant to DHPs and ω-CTx-GVIA and sensitive to ω-Aga-IVA and ω-CTx-MVIIC [411]. Q-type Ca^{2+} currents are slightly less sensitive to ω-Aga-IVA than P-type Ca^{2+} currents and possibly slightly more sensitive to ω-CTx-MVIIC. In hippocampal neurons, Q-type Ca^{2+} currents play a predominant role in glutamatergic synaptic transmission [497]. It is very difficult to distinguish the individual functions of Q-type and P-type Ca^{2+} currents because of their high similarity: in most cases, the functions attributed to P-type Ca^{2+} currents could be those of Q-type Ca^{2+} currents as well.

R-type Ca^{2+} currents

R-type Ca^{2+} currents were originally described in cerebellar granule cells [411, 568] as the remaining or resistant current after blocking other Ca^{2+} current types with drugs and toxins. Based on this definition by default, it is not surprising that R-type Ca^{2+} currents in different cells possess a wide variety of distinct electrophysiological properties [502]. It is quite likely that multiple channel types are responsible for R-type Ca^{2+} currents, in different cells or even in the same cell [501]. Indeed, in transgenic mice lacking one the putative Ca^{2+} channel proteins underlying R-type Ca^{2+} currents, only a small fraction of the wild-type R-type Ca^{2+} currents is lost [541]. Similarly, depending on the cellular preparation, the compound SNX-482 blocks R-type Ca^{2+} currents entirely, partially, or not at all. It is even possible that channel proteins that normally underlie L-, T-, N-, P-, or Q-type Ca^{2+} currents, but have been unusually processed or regulated, can sometimes carry R-type Ca^{2+} currents.

In many cases (but not all), R-type Ca^{2+} currents are low- to moderate-voltage-activated and they inactivate faster than L- or N-type Ca^{2+} currents [319]. Therefore, R-type Ca^{2+} currents often resemble T-type Ca^{2+} currents and distinguishing the two current types can be difficult [56] although not impossible [412]. By and large, R-type Ca^{2+} currents have been mostly described in neurons although there is good evidence that they are also found in glia [101] and sperm [535]. Like N-, P-, and Q-type Ca^{2+} currents, one of their major roles in neurons is to contribute to the Ca^{2+} entry necessary for transmitter release. For instance, R-type Ca^{2+} currents evoke transmitter release at rat central synapses [549] and, for example, they contribute to the fast excitatory synaptic transmission in rat hippocampus [177]. Neuroendocrine secretion may also involve R-type Ca^{2+} currents: the secretion of oxytocin [527] and of insulin [382, 383] may be preferentially regulated by R-type Ca^{2+} currents.

Many reports have also suggested that R-type Ca^{2+} currents may exist in non-neuronal cells. However, in most cases, it remains difficult to ascertain whether the recorded currents are definitely R-type or rather T-type Ca^{2+} currents. In rat atrial myocytes, it is likely that part of the described T-type Ca^{2+} currents may really be R-type Ca^{2+} currents [396]. In contrast, in vascular smooth muscle, part or most of the suggested R-type Ca^{2+} currents may really be T-type Ca^{2+} currents [45, 343].

Conclusion

The weakness of the above classification is the lack of clear-cut dividing lines between classes. The activation of Ca^{2+} currents spans the entire range from "low" voltage to "high" voltage with no clear dividing line. Most pharmacological tools are not entirely specific, with the exception of the N-type Ca^{2+} current blockers ω-CTx-GVIA and ω-CTx-MVIIA. DHPs block T-type Ca^{2+} currents with slightly lower potency than L-type; mibefradil blocks all VOCs; ω-Aga-IVA and ω-CTx-MVIIC block N-, P-, and Q-type Ca^{2+} currents; SNX-482 blocks a fraction of the R-type Ca^{2+} currents. This classification is being overwhelmed by the unexpected diversity of Ca^{2+} currents and it cannot be extended to fit the characteristics of new current subtypes. Furthermore, the properties of any one class of currents may vary with the species, the tissue and the experimental conditions.

Molecular diversity of voltage-operated Ca^{2+} channels

In parallel to the description of the properties of the voltage-operated Ca^{2+} currents, many laboratories have worked on the characterization of the underlying proteins, the voltage-operated Ca^{2+} channels. The channel responsible for a dihydropyridine-sensitive L-type Ca^{2+} current was initially purified from the T-tubule system of the skeletal muscle, where it is particularly abundant. It is a complex protein composed of four distinct subunits, α_1, β, $\alpha_2\delta$, and γ, encoded by four distinct genes [143, 236, 429, 491] (α_2 and δ are derived from the same gene with the product cleaved into two peptides linked by a disulfide bond [121]). Subsequently, the channels underlying the N-, P-, Q-, and non-skeletal L-type Ca^{2+} currents were also found to be multi-subunit complexes composed of elements homologous to those of the skeletal muscle channel (Fig. 4). An exception may be the γ-subunit, which may be present only in muscle L-type Ca^{2+} channels [5, 310, 485, 544] although recently-described subunits may be associated with neuronal HVA Ca^{2+} channels [283]. The subunit composition of T-type Ca^{2+} channels remains very controversial: there is no convincing evidence for a β-subunit; a γ-subunit may be associated with

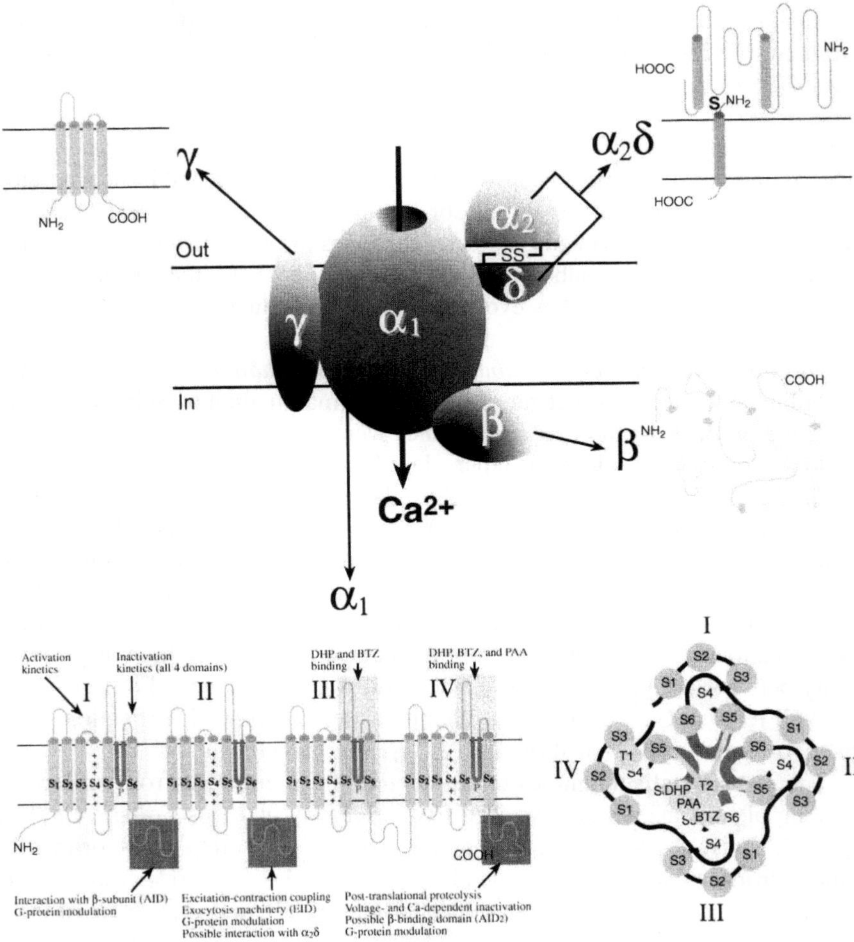

Figure 4. Structure of the voltage-operated Ca^{2+} channels. The channel protein is composed of multiple subunits: the obligatory α1-subunit comprises the Ca^{2+} pathway and the β-, α2δ-, γ- accessory subunits play modulatory roles. The folding patterns of the subunits are shown as predicted from the amino-acid sequences. The α1-subunit is constituted of four homologous domains (I–IV), each of which contains six α-helical transmembrane segments (S1–S6). The S4 segment is rich in positively-charged amino-acids and it is believed to serve as the voltage sensor. The peptide chain between S5 and S6 (H5 or P-loop) lines the channel pore and constitutes the Ca^{2+} selectivity filter. The binding sites for dihydropyridines (DHP), phenylalkylamines (PAA), benzothiazepines (BTZ), gating-modifier toxins (T1), and pore-blocking toxins (T2) are shown in the lower right panel.

functional channels and modify their electrophysiological properties [185, 257]; and an $\alpha_2\delta$-subunit may be involved in channel expression and/or membrane insertion but may or may not be associated with functional channels [135, 175]. The stoichiometry of the components of the Ca^{2+} channel complex has generally been viewed as zero or one accessory subunit (of each type) per α_1-subunit, although this has been challenged [495]. General aspects of the structure of voltage-operated Ca^{2+} channels have been reviewed in [1, 76, 89, 440, 475, 485].

The α_1-subunit

The α_1-subunit is the largest constituent of the final protein and it incorporates the conduction pore, the voltage sensor, and many modulatory sites. Thus, the diversity of voltage-operated Ca^{2+} currents arises primarily from the existence of multiple forms of α_1-subunits. High homology between the various cloned α_1-subunits suggests that they evolved from a single ancestral gene.

Correspondence between α_1-subunits and native channels: A gene family including at least ten distinct genes encodes the mammalian α_1-subunits. In the past, the products of the first seven genes were most often referred to as α_{1S} and α_{1A} through α_{1F} although other classifications were also used (Tab. 2). After the cloning of the genes encoding the α_1-subunits of the low-voltage-activated Ca^{2+} channels (α_{1G}, α_{1H}, α_{1I}), a new nomenclature/classification of voltage-operated Ca^{2+} channels was proposed [146], similar in form to the widely-accepted classification of voltage-operated K^+ channels [92] as well as the recent classification of voltage-operated Na^+ channels [179]. This new classification (Tab. 2) is derived from the degree of sequence homology/similarity between the genes coding for the various Ca^{2+} channels. From here on, we will refer to Ca^{2+} channel α_1-subunits using this new classification, with the corresponding historical $\alpha_{1S,A,B,C,D,E,F,G,H,I}$ in parenthesis.

Three structural subfamilies of α_1-subunits have emerged from molecular cloning of mammalian cDNAs. The first subfamily includes $Ca_V1.1$, $Ca_V1.2$, $Ca_V1.3$, and $Ca_V1.4$ (α_{1S}, α_{1C}, α_{1D}, and α_{1F}). $Ca_V1.1$ (α_{1S}) was originally cloned from rabbit skeletal muscle [143, 491], $Ca_V1.2$ (α_{1C}) from rabbit heart [318, 453] and lung [40] and rat aorta and brain [260], and $Ca_V1.3$ (α_{1D}) from human brain [538] and pancreas [441]. Functional expression and immunoprecipitation studies have demonstrated that these genes encode DHP-sensitive L-type Ca^{2+} channels. The mRNA for $Ca_V1.4$ (α_{1F}) has been found in human, mouse and rat retina, the cDNA appears specific to retinal libraries, and immunoreactivity has been shown in rat retina; however, $Ca_V1.4$ (α_{1F}) has not yet been functionally expressed [29, 340, 352, 477].

The second α_1-subfamily includes $Ca_V2.1$, $Ca_V2.2$, and $Ca_V2.3$ (α_{1A}, α_{1B}, and α_{1E}). So far, these genes appear to encode Ca^{2+} channels that are localized mostly in the nervous system and that lack the characteristic DHP-sensitivity of L-type Ca^{2+} channels. While expression of $Ca_V2.2$ (α_{1B}) clearly produces a ω-CTx-GVIA-sensitive N-type Ca^{2+} channel [67, 136, 172, 537], it seems that $Ca_V2.1$ (α_{1A}) encodes both P-type and Q-type Ca^{2+} channels. This is generally thought to occur through alternative splicing [55, 341, 435, 456, 472, 505, 568]. However cloning of $Ca_V2.1$ (α_{1A}) from single cerebellar Purkinje cells (where P-type Ca^{2+} currents predominate and Q-type Ca^{2+} currents are minimal) yielded three splice variants that all expressed into Q-type Ca^{2+} channels; this suggests that "some specific environmental modifications such as post-translational processing or modulation by putative proteins associated with the channels may be necessary to generate the native P-type current" [461]. The $Ca_V2.3$ (α_{1E}) gene is the most recent addition to the "neuronal" (non-L) channel family [358]. Its expression is widespread in mammalian neurons [462, 539] and it is also found in specific non-neuronal tissues [325]. Its assignment to one of the native Ca^{2+} currents has been problematic. $Ca_V2.3$ (α_{1E}) has been proposed to encode a T-type Ca^{2+} channel, because of its negative potentials for activation and inactivation, its sensitivity to Ni^{2+} [462], and its permeation characteristics [56, 134, 474]. However, the current produced by expression of $Ca_V2.3$ (α_{1E}) differs from the "classical" T-type Ca^{2+} current in its slower inactivation rate, its single-channel conductance (5–9 pS for T-type and 14 pS for $Ca_V2.3$ (α_{1E})), its high sensitivity to Cd^{2+}, and its insensitivity to octanol and amiloride. On the other hand, the human and rat $Ca_V2.3$ (α_{1E}) currents share a number of characteristics with R-type Ca^{2+} currents [141, 411, 539], which are sensitive to both Ni^{2+} and Cd^{2+} but not to DHPs and ω-CTx-GVIA. There is a striking resemblance between currents through $Ca_V2.3$ (α_{1E}) expressed in HEK293 cells and R-type Ca^{2+} currents with respect to voltage dependence, rates of activation and inactivation, and the relative size of Ba^{2+} and Ca^{2+} currents [411, 539].

The third α_1-subfamily includes $Ca_V3.1$, $Ca_V3.2$, and $Ca_V3.3$ (α_{1G}, α_{1H}, and α_{1I}). $Ca_V3.1$ (α_{1G}) was originally cloned from rat brain and homologues were found in human and mouse [259, 313, 329, 386], $Ca_V3.2$ (α_{1H}) from human heart [115], from a human medullary thyroid carcinoma cell line [540], from rat brain [313], and from a rat insulin-secreting cell line [570], and $Ca_V3.3$ (α_{1I}) from rat [279, 313] and human brain [180, 330, 336]. Functional expression studies have demonstrated that these genes encode low-voltage-activated T-type Ca^{2+} channels.

From structure to biophysical properties: Although the three-dimensional structure of the L-type Ca^{2+} channel from rabbit skeletal muscle has been visualized with electron cryomicroscopy at 30-Å resolution [442], most of the structural information has been provided by studies combining molecular biology and electrophysiology. The α_1-subunit is a large (165–260 kDa) transmembrane protein with 4 repeated units of homology (I–IV) (Fig. 4). Each repeat contributes a quarter of the wall of the channel pore and contains six α-helical membrane-spanning segments (S1–S6) [491]. These transmembrane segments are highly conserved among the various α_1 isoforms as well as across species [228, 260, 318, 341, 384] and α_1-isoforms differ essentially in the extramembranous regions. When expressed in *Xenopus* oocytes, individual $Ca_V1.2$ (α_{1C}), $Ca_V2.3$ (α_{1E}), or $Ca_V3.x$ ($\alpha_{1G,H,I}$) subunits are sufficient to form functional voltage-operated Ca^{2+} channels [40, 279, 318, 386, 539, 570]. This appears not to be true for $Ca_V1.1$ (α_{1S}) [416], $Ca_V1.3$ (α_{1D}) [538], $Ca_V2.1$ (α_{1A}) [341, 495], and $Ca_V2.2$ (α_{1B}) [537], for which successful functional expression has required additional subunits.

Using a combination of antibody mapping and site-directed mutagenesis, recent studies have identified regions that are important for β-subunit binding, voltage-dependent activation and inactivation, ion selectivity, regulation by protein phosphorylation, N-glycosylation, or GTP-binding proteins (G-proteins), and modulation by drugs and toxins (Fig. 4).

Domain I, particularly IS3 and the IS3–IS4 extracellular loop, determines whether an L-type Ca^{2+} channel has slow (skeletal muscle-like) or rapid (cardiac-like) activation [349, 489, 490].

The Alpha-Interaction-Domain (AID) is an 18-amino-acid region of the I–II cytoplasmic loop of the α_1-subunit and it represents the major determinant of β-subunit binding. Mutations in this region remove any interaction between the two subunits [77, 125, 126, 401, 567] and a fusion protein that contains the AID binds β-subunits with high affinity [543]. The corresponding region in the β-subunit (BID) has also been mapped [124]. More controversial, a second AID has also been suggested at the carboxy-terminus, such that a single α_1-subunit may bind two β-subunits [495]. In contrast, the amino acid sequence of all three cloned $Ca_V3.x$ ($\alpha_{1G,H,I}$) subunits lacks the AID domain and elimination of the four known β-subunits with antisense oligonucleotides does not affect the size or voltage-dependence of native T-type Ca^{2+} currents [277, 284]: this suggests that β-subunits do not interact with $Ca_V3.x$ ($\alpha_{1G,H,I}$) subunits.

The four transmembrane segments S6 and their adjacent extracellular and cytoplasmic loops are responsible for the inactivation kinetics [205, 566]. In the intracellular I–II linker, $Ca_V2.1$ (α_{1A}) includes the sequence QQIER whereas $Ca_V1.2$ (α_{1C}) has QQLEE. The replacement of arginine to glutamate in $Ca_V2.1$ (α_{1A}) slows inactivation and shifts its voltage-dependence to more positive voltages; the opposite replacement in $Ca_V1.2$ (α_{1C}) has the opposite effect [206]. The IIIS6 segment is also important for the rapid inactivation of $Ca_V3.1$ (α_{1G}) [303].

The three different classes of voltage-operated Ca^{2+} channels vary in their modulation by G-proteins. On the one hand, all Ca^{2+} channel types appear to be modulated to some degree by phosphorylation consecutive to the activation of protein kinases or phosphatases by G-protein-coupled receptors [133, 282, 379, 391, 536, 550]. On the other hand, G-proteins are generally considered to modulate directly the activity of $Ca_V2.x$ ($\alpha_{1A,B,E}$) channels only. At least three different regions of the α_1-subunit seem involved in this interaction. First, as mentioned above, in the intracellular I–II linker, $Ca_V2.1$ (α_{1A}) includes the sequence QQIER whereas $Ca_V1.2$ (α_{1C}) has QQLEE. The replacement of isoleucine to leucine in $Ca_V2.1$ (α_{1A}) produces a channel with very reduced interaction with G-proteins, similar to $Ca_V1.2$ (α_{1C}) [206]. Second, the intracellular I–II linker and the carboxy-terminus in of $Ca_V2.2$ (α_{1B}) must both be replaced by their $Ca_V2.1$ (α_{1A}) counterparts to transfer the modulatory behaviors of the two channels [567]. Even among $Ca_V1.x$ ($\alpha_{1S,C,DF}$) channels, structural differences in the carboxy-terminus of the α_1-subunit could account for differential association with intracellular proteins and regulation by phosphorylation [202, 203]. Third, the intracellular II–III linker has been called an 'effector interaction domain' [206] because it plays a role in coupling $Ca_V2.x$ channels ($\alpha_{1A,B,E}$) to receptors and G proteins [24, 488]. For example, the II–III linker of $Ca_V2.2$ (α_{1B}) [444, 445, 561] and that of $Ca_V2.1$ (α_{1A}) [417, 418] interact with the SNARE proteins involved in the exocytosis of neurotransmitter vesicles in neurons. Deletions in this "synprint" site in $Ca_V2.1$ (α_{1A}) reduced the effectiveness of P-type Ca^{2+} currents in initiating synaptic transmission whereas insertion of the synprint site from $Ca_V2.1$ (α_{1A}) or $Ca_V2.2$ (α_{1B}) into $Ca_V1.2$ (α_{1C}) established synaptic transmission initiated by L-type Ca^{2+} currents [331]. However, the physiological function of natural splice variants of $Ca_V2.2$ (α_{1B}) lacking the synprint site remains unknown [243]. The II–III linker plays an analogous role in $Ca_V1.1$ (α_{1S}), where it interacts with the ryanodine-sensitive Ca^{2+} channel in the sarcoplasmic reticulum and constitutes an important determinant of skeletal excitation-contraction coupling [24, 488]. These examples illustrate the link between the structure of the α_1-subunit and type-specific regulatory properties of voltage-operated Ca^{2+} channels.

It is notable that the intracellular I–II linker includes pieces of the β-subunit interaction domain (AID), the G-protein interaction domain, and regions critical to channel inactivation: this is consistent with the observed interplay between inactivation, the actions of β-subunits, and those of G-proteins [567].

$Ca_V1.x$ ($\alpha_{1S,C,D,F}$), $Ca_V2.x$ ($\alpha_{1A,B,E}$), and $Ca_V3.x$ ($\alpha_{1G,H,I}$) channels have notably different gating properties, which could be associated with variations in the putative four S4 voltage-sensors. Although the S4's are highly conserved between voltage-operated Ca^{2+} channels, there are noticeable differences between the three subfamilies [341, 384, 471]. In particular, $Ca_V3.x$ ($\alpha_{1G,H,I}$) channels carry more negative charges in this region than the other α_1-subunits: this likely relates to the lower voltage of activation of T-type Ca^{2+} channels.

Permeation properties vary considerably among voltage-operated Ca^{2+} channels. Structurally, the regions linking the S5 and S6 segments of each repeat (also called the H5 segments or the SS1–SS2 or P-loop regions) appear to contribute to the formation of the ion conduction pore [188, 201]. In this region, $Ca_V2.3$ (α_{1E}) stands apart from the other high-voltage-activated Ca^{2+} channels, which may relate to its specific permeation properties: in contrast to the other HVA α_1-subunits, $Ca_V2.3$ (α_{1E}) conducts larger currents with Ca^{2+} than with Ba^{2+}. Furthermore, the net charge of the P-region of $Ca_V2.3$ (α_{1E}, −16) is less than those of $Ca_V2.2$ (α_{1B}, −22) and $Ca_V2.1$ (α_{1A}, −26), which may explain the smaller conductance of $Ca_V2.3$ (α_{1E}, 12 pS) compared to $Ca_V2.2$ (α_{1B}, 14 pS) and $Ca_V2.1$ (α_{1A}, 16 pS) [524]. Not surprisingly, $Ca_V3.x$ ($\alpha_{1G,H,I}$) channels are even more distinct: instead of the highly-conserved glutamates found in all four pore regions of the other voltage-operated Ca^{2+} channels, all three cloned $Ca_V3.x$ ($\alpha_{1G,H,I}$) channels have glutamate residues in the pore regions of repeats I and II but aspartate residues in repeats III and IV. This may relate to the lack of selectivity for Ba^{2+} over Ca^{2+} and the relatively low unitary conductance of $Ca_V3.1$ (α_{1G}, 7.5 pS [386]), $Ca_V3.2$ (α_{1H}, 5.3 pS [115] or

9.1 pS [540]) and $Ca_V3.1$ (α_{1I}, 1 1.0 pS [279, 337]). Indeed, $Ca_V1.2$ (α_{1C}) has a larger effective pore size (diameter ~6.2 Å) than $Ca_V3.x$ (diameter ~5.1 Å), while $Ca_V2.3$ (α_{1E}) is intermediate [82].

Feedback regulation of Ca^{2+} channels by Ca^{2+} ("Ca-inactivation") is another property linked to structural differences in α_1-subunits. Thus, Ca^{2+} channels based on $Ca_V1.2$ (α_{1C}) or $Ca_V2.3$ (α_{1E}) differ in that only $Ca_V1.2$ (α_{1C}) produces channels that are inhibited by Ca^{2+} flowing inside the cell through the channel [354, 436]. A portion of the carboxy-terminus, which contains an EF-hand motif, is essential for Ca^{2+} channel block by Ca^{2+} [458, 569] such that transfer of the $Ca_V1.2$ (α_{1C}) EF-hand region to $Ca_V2.3$ (α_{1E}) transfers Ca^{2+}-inactivation [122]. Additional regions downstream the EF-hand are also important for Ca^{2+}-inactivation [458, 573]. In particular, alternative splicing of $Ca_V1.2$ (α_{1C}) in the second quarter of the C-terminal tail eliminates Ca^{2+}-inactivation and the important regions have been narrowed to four critical stretches (I1572–G1576, L1600–V1604, Asn1582–E1583 and I1624–Lys1639). The last motif comprises a calmodulin (CaM)-binding consensus sequence (IQxxFRKxxxRx) and $Ca_V1.2$ (α_{1C}) appears to act as a CaM-binding protein with CaM regulating channel activity in response to Ca^{2+} influx. Indeed, deletion of eight amino-acids within the CaM-binding sequence removes Ca^{2+}-inactivation [573] and a non-functional CaM mutant suppresses Ca^{2+}-inactivation [390, 406]. Consistent with the role of CaM and the CaM-binding sequence in Ca^{2+}-inactivation, $Ca_V3.x$ ($\alpha_{1G,H,I}$) channels, which exhibit no Ca^{2+}-inactivation, possess no CaM-binding sequence [279] and CaM activation appears to have no direct effect on $Ca_V3.2$ (α_{1H}) [547].

Finally, the α_1-subunits contain binding sites for dihydropyridines (DHPs), phenylalkylamines (PAAs), and benzothiazepines (BTZs), at least in $Ca_V1.1$, $Ca_V1.2$, and $Ca_V1.3$ ($\alpha_{1S,C,D}$) [229]. Data on $Ca_V1.4$ (α_{1F}) is not available at present. In order to define the channel regions involved in drug binding, research groups have used three general methods, namely: 1) the evaluation of drug-induced inhibition of Ca^{2+} current using permanently-charged drug analogs, which can only act, in principle, from the membrane side that they were applied to; 2) the photoaffinity labeling of the channel protein using radiolabeled drug analogs that covalently bind to nearby amino-acids after exposure to light; and 3) the analysis of drug-induced inhibition of Ca^{2+} current using chimeric and mutant α_1-subunits. These studies revealed that the three chemically-unrelated classes of Ca^{2+} antagonists bind to the same region of the channel (Fig. 4), which is formed by transmembrane segments IIIS5, IIIS6 and IVS6, in very close proximity to the central pore-forming regions [90, 204, 266, 328, 452, 493, 530]. Drugs from different classes can bind simultaneously: this explains the non-competitive stimulation or inhibition of binding that is observed between any two drugs [31, 59]. However, drugs from different classes also share parts of their binding sites: this explains the apparent steric interaction that is sometimes observed [476]. The close proximity to the channel pore and the Ca^{2+}-selectivity filter also clarifies the observed reciprocal allosteric interaction between DHPs and Ca^{2+} present at the selectivity filter

[327]. In conclusion, there does not exist separate drug-binding domains as initially proposed [178] but a so-called "multi-subsite-domain" [326].

Further studies have narrowed down the critical amino acids responsible for DHP, PAA, and BTZ sensitivity [219, 326]. For DHP, two residues in IIIS5, seven in IIIS6, and four in IVS6 are the most critical. Four of those 13 residues are conserved in non-L-type channels but are not sufficient for high-affinity DHP sensitivity. For PAA, four residues in IIIS6, four in IVS6, and the "selectivity glutamate" of each of the P-loops of repeats III and IV are critical to PAA binding. The IIIS6 residues, and the glutamates, are conserved in non-L-type channels. For BTZ, the site is less well defined: the same IVS6 residues responsible for PAA affinity appear important as well as two residues in IIIS6 [267] and some additional residues in the IVS5-IVS6 linker [204]. As a final note of caution, it should not be assumed that these regions are the only sites of interaction between the channel and the drug: although these represent the major determinants of drug binding, additional domains have been implicated in specific cases [276].

The four $Ca_V1.x$ (α_{1S}, α_{1C}, α_{1D}, α_{1F}) channels are very similar in the binding regions whereas the $Ca_V2.x$ (α_{1A}, α_{1B}, α_{1E}) and $Ca_V3.x$ (α_{1G}, α_{1H}, α_{1I}) channels present some major differences. When the proposed binding domain of $Ca_V1.1$ and $Ca_V1.2$ (α_{1S}, α_{1C}) was inserted in place of the non-binding domains of the DHP, PAA, BTZ-insensitive channel $Ca_V2.1$ (α_{1A}), a DHP, PAA, BTZ-sensitive channel was created [184]. After this chimera demonstrated that specific portions of L-type channels could transfer DHP sensitivity to non-L-type channels, further studies confirmed that DHP sensitivity could be transferred to $Ca_V2.1$ (α_{1A}) or $Ca_V2.3$ (α_{1E}) by introducing the nine non-conserved L-type amino-acid residues in IIIS5, IIIS6, and IVS6 [234, 452].

The binding sites of the other Ca^{2+} channel blockers (toxins, mibefradil, etc.) have not been precisely defined as yet. The only data regarding the binding of ω-Aga-IVA showed that the affinity of the expressed $Ca_V2.1$ (α_{1A}) channel for ω-Aga-IVA is affected by the deletion or the insertion of two amino-acid residues in the IVS3–IVS4 linker [55, 193] or the conversion of a nearby glutamate to lysine [542] (Fig. 4). For ω-CTx-GVIA, mutations in the S5-P linkers affect the kinetics and reversibility of toxin block, with major effects associated with the IIIS5–IIIP linker (Fig. 4); this is consistent with a direct pore-blocking mechanism [140, 158]. Qualitatively similar results were obtained with ω-CTx-MVIIA suggesting that common molecular determinants underlie block by these two toxins [158]. Generally, large peptide toxins inhibit current by blocking the channel pore (pore-blocking toxins, site T2), although ω-grammotoxin-SIA, and ω-Aga-IVA appear to act by shifting the voltage dependence of the channels from a remote binding site (gating-modifying toxins, site T1) [309].

Alternative splicing: There is considerably more structural heterogeneity encountered *in vivo* than can be accounted for by ten different α_1 genes. A molecular basis for this heterogeneity comes from alternative splicing [60] or post-translational editing [4]. Alternative splicing has been observed for all α_1-subunits and is particularly noticeable in the amino- and carboxy-termini, IS6 and adjacent I–II loop, IIS6, IIIS2, IVS3 and adjacent IVS3–IVS4 loop. The structural differences found in the splice variants result in altered biophysical, physiological, and pharmacological properties. For example, different $Ca_V1.2$ (α_{1C}) splice variants in heart and smooth muscle could be associated with specific pharmacological properties of these tissues, such as the higher sensitivity of smooth muscle to DHPs [533]. Similarly, $Ca_V1.2$ (α_{1C}) splice variants in the carboxy-terminus are differently affected by hypoxia [155]. Finally, four $Ca_V1.2$ (α_{1C}) splice variants are expressed in human ventricular myocardium and their relative levels change with the appearance of heart failure [557]. Examples of alternative splicing can be found for $Ca_V1.1$ (α_{1S}, [387]), $Ca_V1.2$ (α_{1C}, [155, 533, 557]), $Ca_V1.3$ (α_{1D}, [264]), $Ca_V1.4$ (α_{1F}, [57]), $Ca_V2.1$ (α_{1A}, [268]), $Ca_V2.2$ (α_{1B}, [372]), $Ca_V2.3$ (α_{1E}, [437]), $Ca_V3.1$ (α_{1G}, [96]), $Ca_V3.2$ (α_{1H}, [235]), $Ca_V3.3$ (α_{1I}, [313, 347]).

Evolutionary perspective: The concept of species classification according to evolutionary history can be attributed to Darwin [120]. A similar classification of related proteins, based on amino-acid sequence similarities and presented as evolutionary trees, has the advantage of being easily updated with new sequences. Moreover, it provides a definitive identification of a protein by its sequence.

Voltage-sensitive Ca^{2+} channels belong to a superfamily of ion channels, which includes the voltage-sensitive Na^+ and K^+ channels as well as the cyclic-nucleotide-gated non-selective cation channels (CNG channels). In contrast to the α_1-subunits of Na^+ and Ca^{2+} channels, which comprise four homologous domains of six transmembrane stretches, the α-subunits of K^+ and CNG channels contain a single such domain and the functional channels appear to be built around tetramers of these α-subunits. Furthermore, each of the four domains of the Ca^{2+} channels α_1-subunits has significant sequence homology with the α-subunits of K^+ and CNG channels [87]. The nature of the single-domain ancestor of these four channel types is controversial [168, 478, 479]. While Na^+ channels have been found so far only in multicellular organisms, Ca^{2+} and K^+ channels are present in simpler organisms such as protozoa [211]. It is therefore hypothesized that two intragenic duplications in a single-domain ancestral channel gave rise to a primordial four-domain Ca^{2+} channel, which gave rise later to a primordial Na^+ channel by further divergence following gene duplication [212]. Several gene duplication events also explain the diversity of the Ca^{2+} channel family as well as that of the Na^+, K^+, and CNG channels.

In agreement with the pharmacological classification, the phylogenetic analysis distinguishes three subfamilies of α_1-subunits, with clearly separate limbs, comprising $Ca_V1.x$ (α_{1S}, α_{1C}, α_{1D}, α_{1F}), $Ca_V2.x$ (α_{1A}, α_{1B}, α_{1E}), and $Ca_V3.x$ (α_{1G}, α_{1H}, α_{1I}) (Fig. 5). The division of Ca^{2+} channels into L-, N- and T-types probably occurred prior to the emergence of the first chordates. In

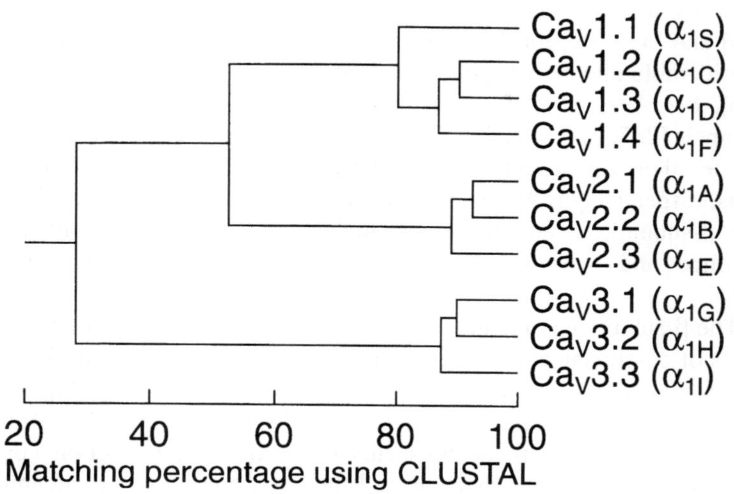

Figure 5. Phylogeny of voltage-gated Ca^{2+} channel α_1-subunits. Only the membrane spanning segments and the pore loops (~350 amino acids) are compared. First, all sequence pairs are compared, which clearly defines three families with intra-family homologies above 80% (Ca$_V$1.x, Ca$_V$2.x, Ca$_V$3.x). Then, a consensus sequence is defined for each family and these three sequences are compared to one another, with inter-family homologies of ~52% (Ca$_V$1.x and Ca$_V$2.x) and 28% (Ca$_V$3x and Ca$_V$1/2.x). Matches were defined using CLUSTAL.

addition to mammals, Ca^{2+} channel types have been reported in the marine ray *Discopyge ommata* [223], in *Aplysia* [139], and in *Drosophila* [378] and the few known invertebrate Ca^{2+} channel sequences segregate into L-, N- and T-types. In contrast, further subdivision of these three subfamilies likely occurred after the emergence of the vertebrates: whereas the invertebrate Ca^{2+} channels cannot be preferentially associated to any of the seven mammalian subtypes, a *Cyprinus carpio* Ca^{2+} channel α_1-subunit shows a higher homology to the mammalian Ca$_V$1.1 (α_{1S}, [183]). The divergence between the carp subunit and the mammalian Ca$_V$1.1 (α_{1S}) corresponds to the divergence between fish and mammals, i.e., to the apparition of amphibians, approximately 300 million years ago. The cloning of Ca^{2+} channels in other animal species will be necessary to date more precisely the apparition of the subtypes.

Other subunits (β, $\alpha_2\delta$, γ)

The diversity of voltage-operated Ca^{2+} channels also arises from the genetic diversity of secondary subunits and the existence of splice variants of these subunits, which modulate to various extents the electrophysiological and pharmacological properties of the complete channels.

β-subunit: Like the α_1-subunit, the β-subunit is derived from a multigene family; cDNA cloning and genomic localization have established the existence of

at least four genes expressed in overlapping sets of tissues [80, 81, 218, 230, 429] and [43, 102] for detailed reviews). β-subunit diversity also arises from considerable alternative splicing and post-translational modification [43, 102, 486]. Members of all four classes of β-subunits may combine in neuronal channels [287, 294, 395, 439, 514, 523]. Skeletal muscle and cardiac channels, on the other hand, seem to be exclusively associated with β1a- and β2a-subunits, respectively [294]. The secondary and tertiary structure of the cytoplasmic β-subunits is not firmly established: the proteins contain a series of α-helices and β-sheets that appear to organize in five separate domains [192, 526].

The β-subunit can modulate both the kinetics and voltage-dependent properties of α_1-subunits and different β-subunits appear to have different quantitative and qualitative effects in various species (reviewed in [526]). β-subunits also alter the pharmacology of the α_1-subunits, in particular high-affinity DHP binding [292, 361]. A β-subunit seems to be required for functional expression of some neuronal Ca^{2+} channels and the co-expression of β-subunits modulates the level of expression of most other recombinant α_1-subunits [230, 385, 537, 538]. Finally, β-subunits appear to facilitate coupling of the voltage sensor to pore-opening [353, 355] and they play important roles in the regulation by G-proteins [54]. In summary, the β-subunit regulates the activity of the α_1-subunit and further contributes to the functional diversity of Ca^{2+} channels [526].

$\alpha_2\delta$-subunit: The $\alpha_2\delta$-subunit is encoded by four separate genes and there is also evidence for tissue-specific alternative splicing [11, 67, 258, 407, 538]. The $\alpha_2\delta3$-subunit is expressed exclusively in brain whereas the $\alpha_2\delta1$-, $\alpha_2\delta2$-, and $\alpha_2\delta4$-subunits are found in several tissues [258, 407]. The $\alpha_2\delta$-subunit is translated as a 175 kDa protein that is cleaved post-translationally into disulfide-linked α_2- and δ-portions [121, 237]. The δ-portion anchors the $\alpha_2\delta$-subunit to the membrane via a single transmembrane segment [187]. Co-expression of $\alpha_2\delta$-subunits with α1-subunits increases current density, shifts the voltage dependence of channel activation and inactivation in a hyperpolarizing direction, and accelerates current decay (reviewed in [156, 217, 258, 526]). The extracellular α_2-portion is responsible for channel stimulation [187] and the δ-portion mediates the effects on activation and inactivation [157]. The magnitudes of these various effects depend on the type of expressed α1-subunit and on the additional presence of β-subunits [258].

γ-subunit: Until recently, it was believed that there existed a single γ-subunit, possibly associated only with skeletal muscle $Ca_V1.1$ channels [117, 163, 170]. However, in the last five years, γ-subunit genes have blossomed, bringing the present number to eight distinct γ-subunits [69, 106, 257, 283]. Generally, the results of co-expression studies with α_1-, β-, $\alpha_2\delta$-, and γ-subunits show that the γ-subunit increases the current magnitude, shifts the voltage dependencies of activation and inactivation to more negative potentials, and accelerates activation and inactivation. A recent study with transgenic mice lacking the $\gamma 1$-subunit showed that the inactivation of the skeletal muscle Ca^{2+} currents was slowed and shifted to more positive potentials, as expected, but that the current magnitude was increased [170].

Ca^{2+} channel drugs and their binding sites

Classification

In 1992, a list of criteria was approved for the identification of distinct drug binding sites on Ca^{2+} channels by the IUPHAR Committee on Receptor Nomenclature and Drug Classification [466, 516]. It includes: 1) the demonstration of a stereoselective binding site supported by drug interaction studies (competition with other drugs, non-competitive interactions with other sites, reversal of inhibitory effects by channel activators); 2) demonstration of the electrophysiological effects of the drug and selectivity of action compared to other sites; 3) determination of the affinity for the type and subtype of ion channel. These criteria have identified different classes of Ca antagonists (Tab. 4).

Class 1 includes agents selective for L-type ($Ca_V1.x$: α_{1S}, α_{1C}, α_{1D}, α_{1F}) Ca^{2+} channels, such as dihydropyridines (DHP), phenylalkylamines, and benzothiazepines, which have distinct binding sites on the α_1-subunit. This class could be extended to include new drugs potentially acting on a novel site on the L-type Ca^{2+} channel (Class 1b). By far the largest group of Ca antagonists is made up of the DHPs: these agents are remarkably efficacious therapeutically and various pharmaceutical companies have characterized to different levels more than 50 such compounds. The structural variety is astonishing and appears to lead to significant therapeutic specificities (Tab. 5).

Class 2 regroups the compounds interacting selectively with other voltage-dependent Ca^{2+} channels. Mibefradil belongs to Class 2 in view of its selectivity for T-type ($Ca_V3.x$: α_{1G}, α_{1H}, α_{1I}) over high-voltage-activated Ca^{2+} channels. Selective blockers of T-type Ca^{2+} currents are scarce. Although many compounds have been reported to block these currents (amiloride, ethosuximide, phenytoin, octanol, flunarizine, bepridil, cinnarizine, sipatrigine, amiodarone, penfluridol, fluspirilene, pimozide, tetrandrine, SB-209712, some DHPs, many volatile anesthetics, the scorpion toxin kurtoxin), block is often cell- or species-dependent, it requires a relatively high concentration, and it is generally nonselective (often, it is concomitant to or even weaker than block of Na^+ channels). Consequently, these drugs belong to Class 3, "non-selective channel modulators". A few other compounds may belong in Class 2 (anandamide, the DHP analog PPK-5) but additional studies are needed to confirm this preliminary assignment. Hybrid molecules (usually derived from DHPs) that cumulate Ca antagonism with another function ($\alpha 1/\beta 1$ adrenoceptor block, thromboxane synthase inhibition) are also found in Class 3 (Class 3b).

Table 4. Classification of drugs binding to voltage-operated Ca^{2+} channels. Underlined are the compounds with structures shown at right

Family name	Representative compounds	Representative structure
Class 1: Drugs binding selectively to the L-type Ca^{2+} channel		
Class 1a: Defined binding site		
Phenylalkylamine	verapamil gallopamil, anipamil, devapamil tiapamil, falipamil, ludopamil	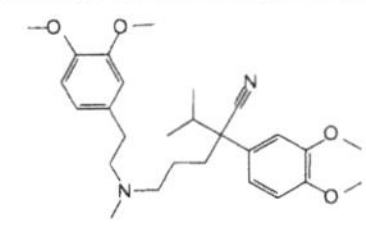
Dihydropyridine	nifedipine amlodipine, felodipine, isradipine, nimodipine, nicardipine, nisoldipine, benidipine, nilvadipine, nitrendipine, lacidipine, elgodipine, mepirodipine	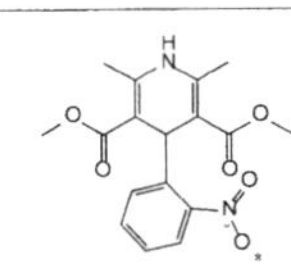
Benzothiazepine (*: analogs)	diltiazem clentiazem, naltiazem* benzazepinones* benzothiazepinones*	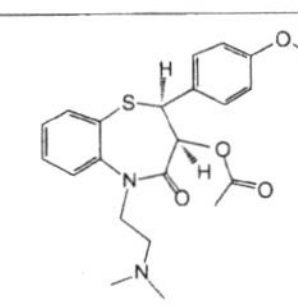
Class 1b: Undefined, potentially novel binding site		
Indolizinsulfone	fantofarone (SR33557)	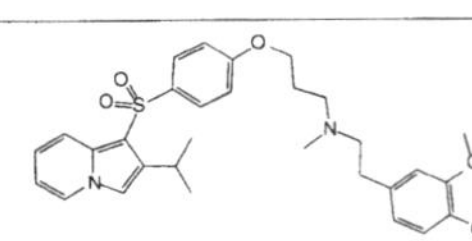
Benzothiazine	semotiadil (SD-3211) HOE-166	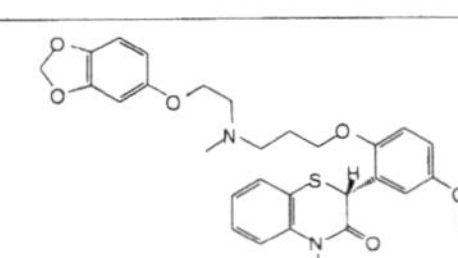
Ethynylbenzene-alkanamine	McN-6186 McN-5691	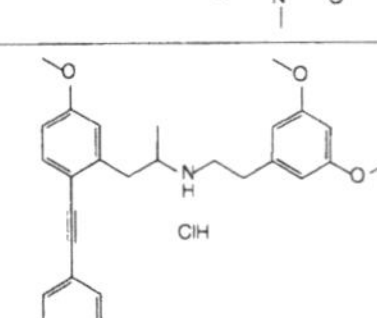
Morpholine	pinaverium bromide	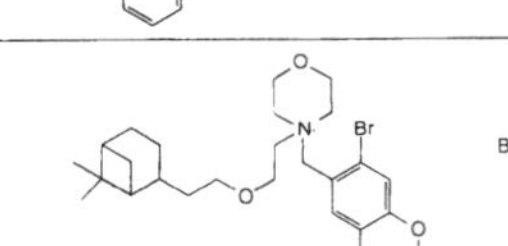
Phosphonate	fostedil	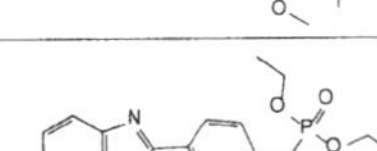
Class 1c: Natural toxins blocking selectively L-type Ca^{2+} channels		

(Continued on next page)

Table 4. (Continued)

Family name	Representative compounds	Representative structure
Class 2: Drugs binding selectively to non-L-type Ca^{2+} channels		
Class 2a: Defined binding site		
Class 2b: Undefined, potentially novel binding site		
Tetralol derivative	mibefradil	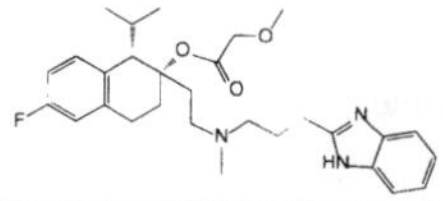
Miscellaneous	anandamide PPK-5	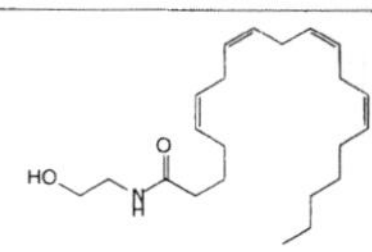
Class 2c: Natural toxins blocking selectively non-L-type Ca^{2+} channels		
	ω-CTx-GVIA ω-CTx-MVIIA ω-Aga-IVA	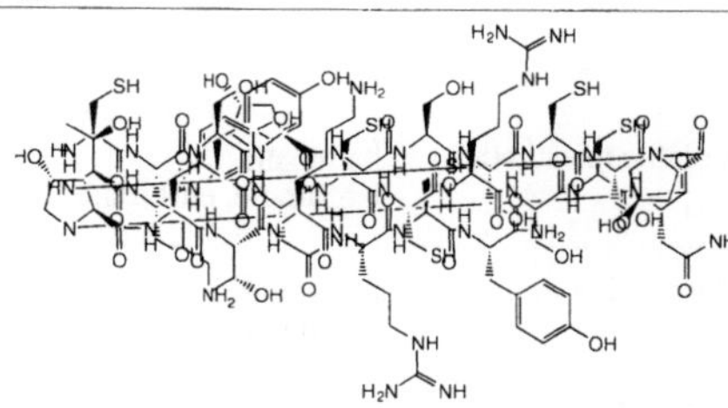
Class 3: Non selective Ca^{2+} channel modulators		
Class 3a: Miscellaneous		
Benzylisoquinoline	tetrandrine	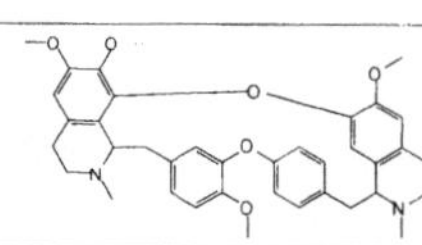
	papaverine daurisoline cularine, diproteverine	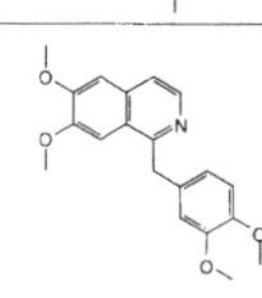
Diphenylalkylamine	bepridil	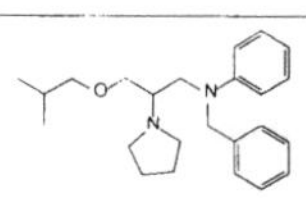
	cinnarizine	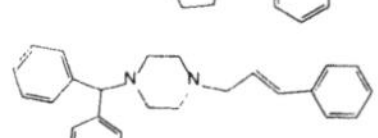
	flunarizine fendiline	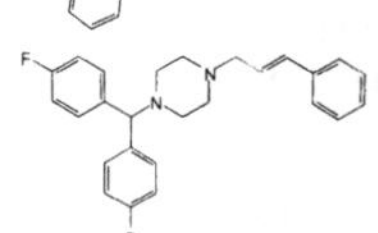

(Continued on next page)

Table 4. (Continued)

Family name	Representative compounds	Representative structure
Class 3a: Miscellaneous (Continued)		
Imidazole	E-4080	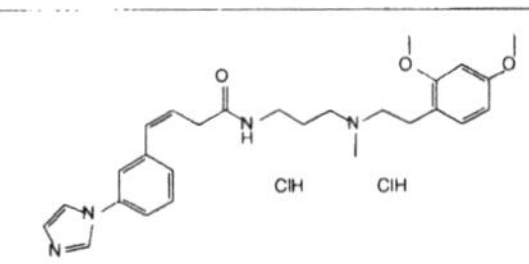
Pyrazine	amiloride dichlorobenzamil	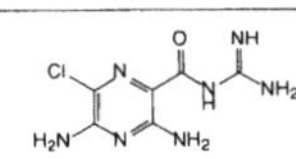
Ergot alkaloid	nicergoline	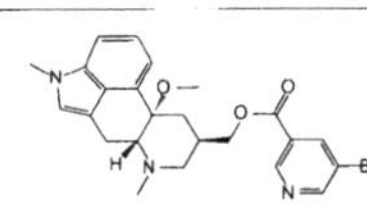
Quinuclidine	CP-96345	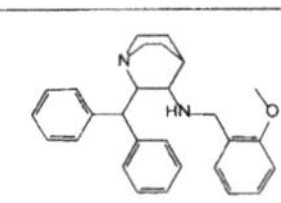
Volatile anesthetics	halothane isoflurane, enflurane	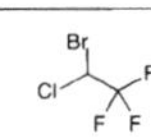
Phenylalkylamine	emopamil levemopamil	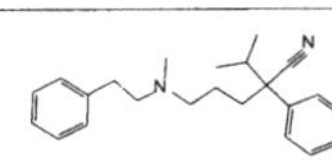
Diphenylbutyl-piperidine	pimozide	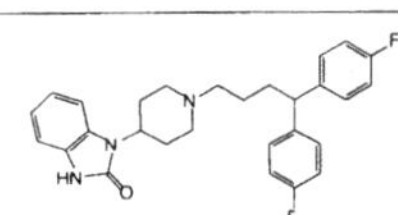
	fluspirilene	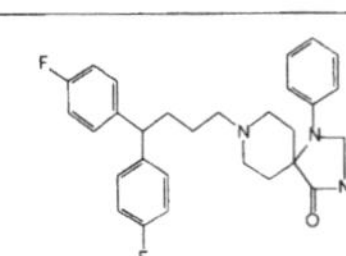
	penfluridol	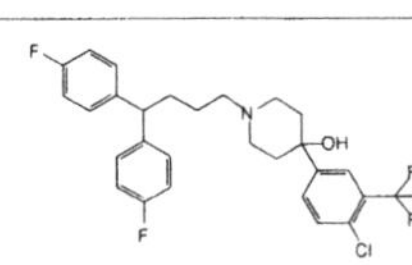
Lactamimide	MDL 12330A MDL-12334A	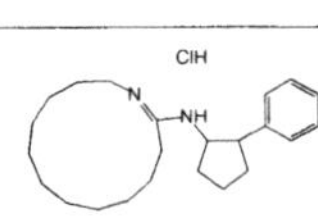
Arylalkyl-sulfonamide	WY-46622 WY-47324	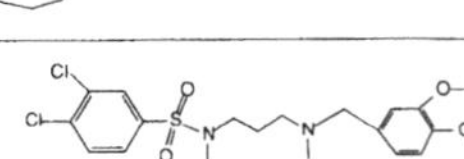

(Continued on next page)

Table 4. (Continued)

Family name	Representative compounds	Representative structure
Class 3a: Miscellaneous (Continued)		
Miscellaneous	amiodarone	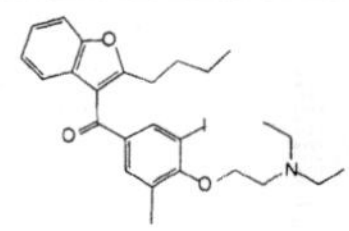
	phenytoin	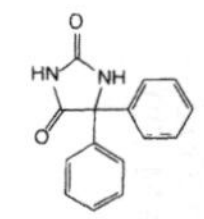
	prajmalium	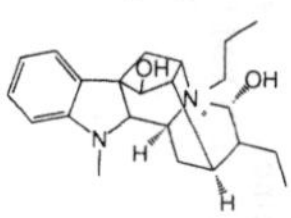
	ethosuximide	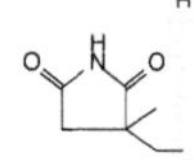
	octanol	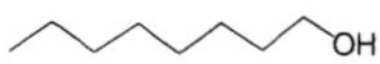
	sipatrigine	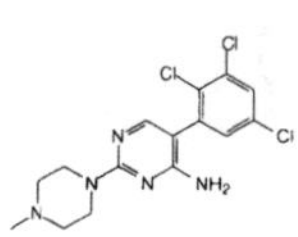
	SB-209712	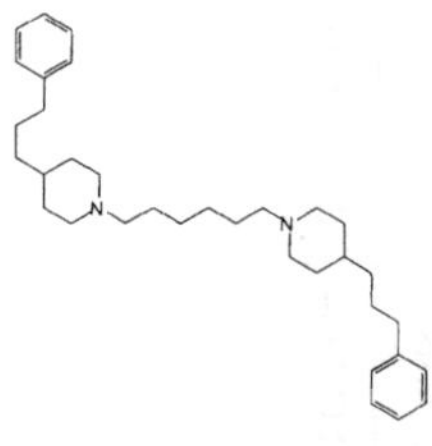
	some dihydropyridines	
Class 3b: Hybrid molecules derived from DHPs		
	niguldipine	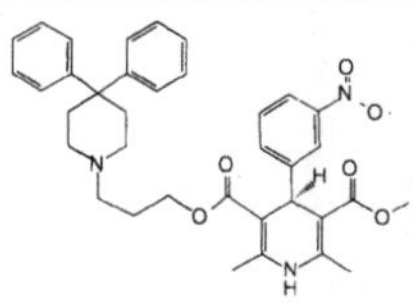
	naftopidil	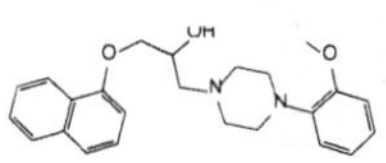
	franidipine, AE0047, NKY-722, YM 16151-1, WY 27,569	
Class 3c: Natural toxins blocking Ca^{2+} channels non-selectively		
	kurtoxin, ω-Aga-IIIA	

Table 5. Structural diversity of dihydropyridine Ca antagonists

Amlodipine UK-48340 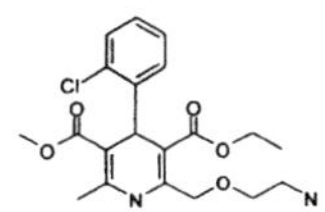 [123, 564]	Aranidipine MPC-1304 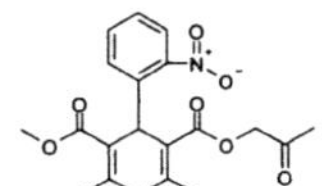 [305, 434]	Azelnidipine CS-905 RS-9054 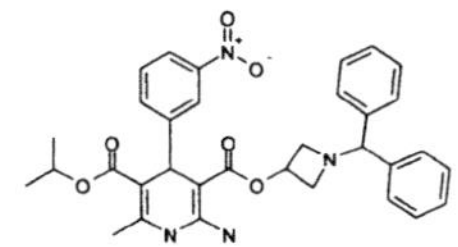 [273, 552]	Barnidipine EU-730 Mepirodipine YM-09730-5 YM-730 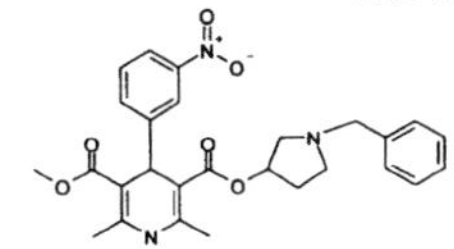 [299, 531]	Benidipine KW-3049 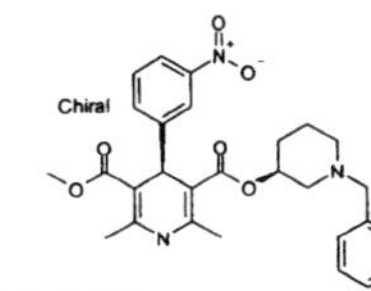 [173, 350]
Cilnidipine FRC-8653 Cinaldipine 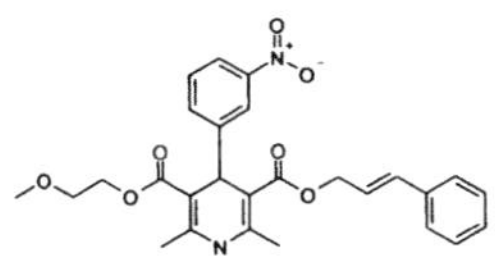 [291, 320]	Clevidipine 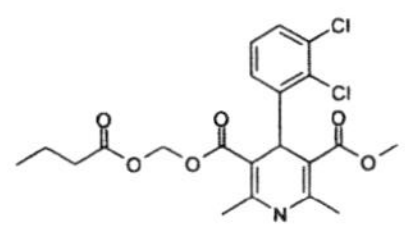 [560, 565]	Cronidipine LF-2.0254 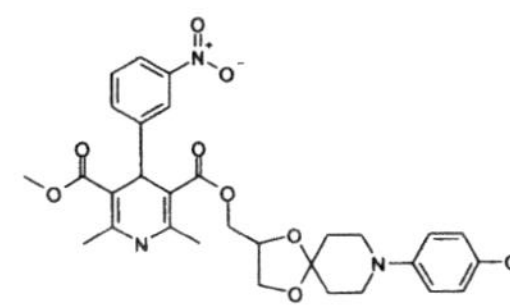 [403]	Darodipine PY-108068 Dazodipine 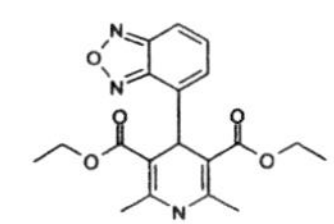 [105, 221]	Dexniguldipine B859-35 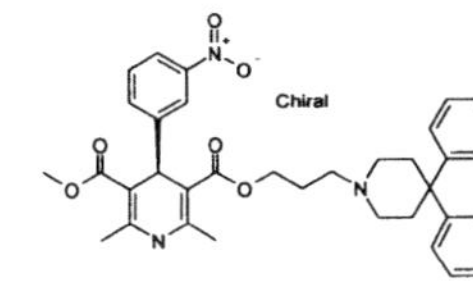 [190, 510]
Dibudipine 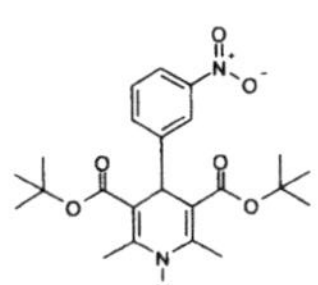 [323]	Diperdipine YS-201 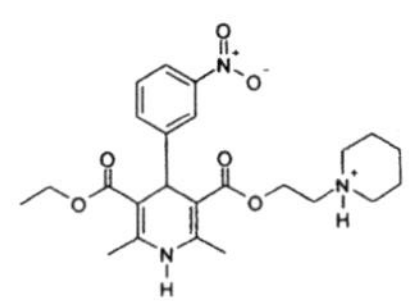 [129]	Efonidipine NZ-105 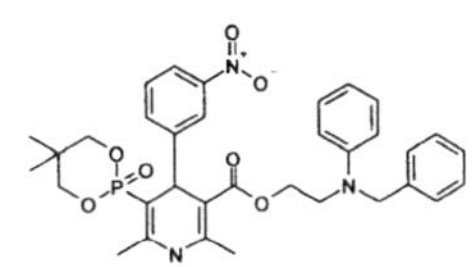 [195, 492]	Elgodipine IQB-875 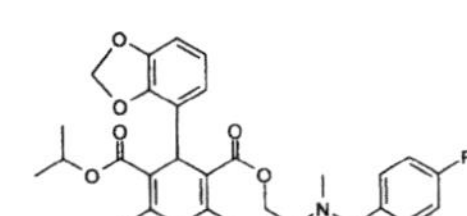 [174, 451]	Elnadipine 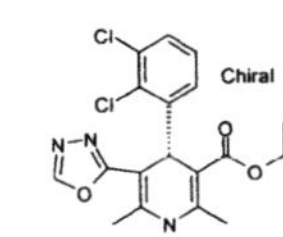 [301]

(Continued on next page)

Table 5. (Continued)

Felodipine CGH-869 H-154/82 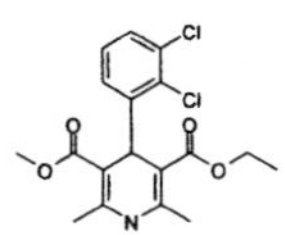 [173, 370]	Flordipine REV-2609 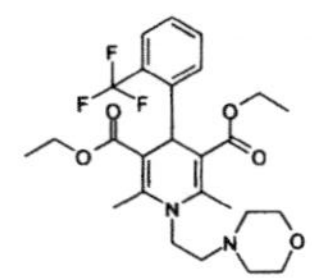 [182, 306]	Fluodipine 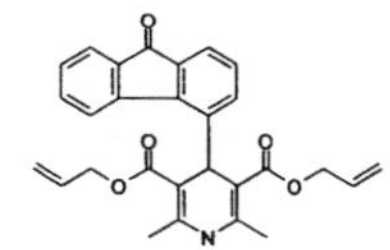 [68]	Furnidipine CRE-319 Furaldipine 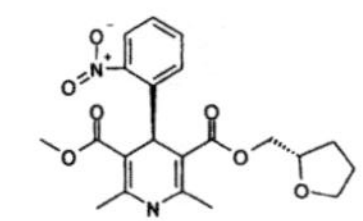 [7]	Iganidipine NKY-722 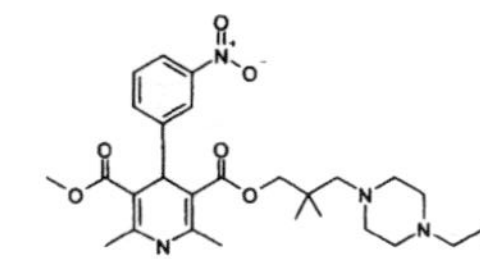 [525, 529]
Isradipine PN-200110 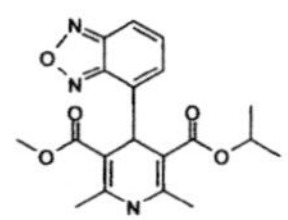 [32, 65]	Lacidipine GR-43659X GX-1048 SN-305 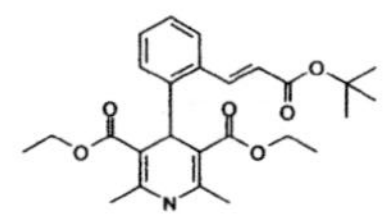 [123, 564]	Lemildipine NB-818 NPK-1886 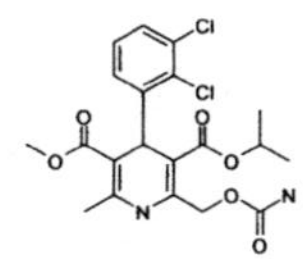 [199]	Lercanidipine Rec-15/2375 Masnidipine TJN-324 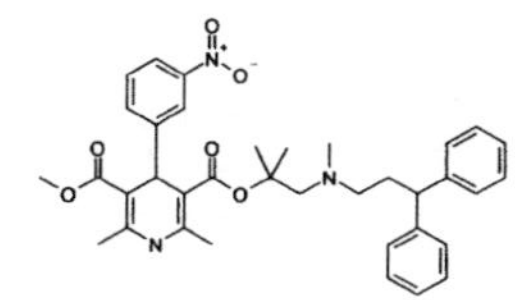 [512, 564]	Manidipine CV-4093 Franidipine 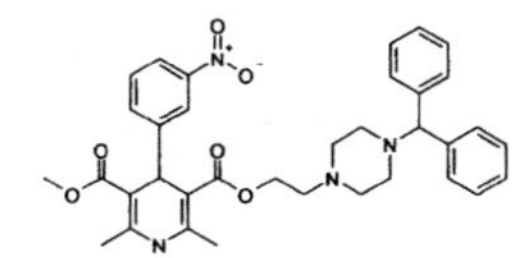 [83, 95]
Mebudipine 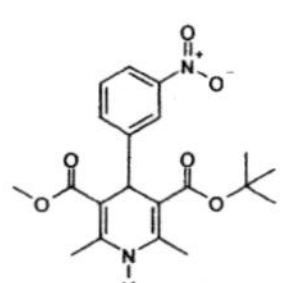 [323]	Mesudipine 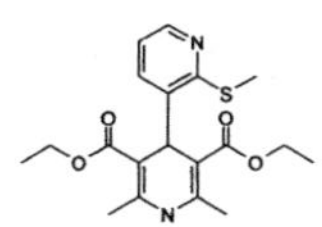 [334]	Nicardipine RS-69216 TN-901 YC-93 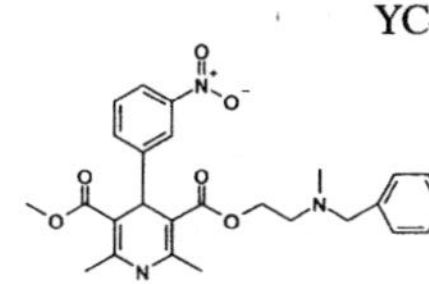 [173, 245]	Nifedipine BayA-1040 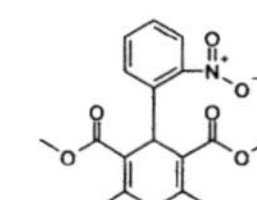 [64, 173]	Niguldipine B859-34 B844-39 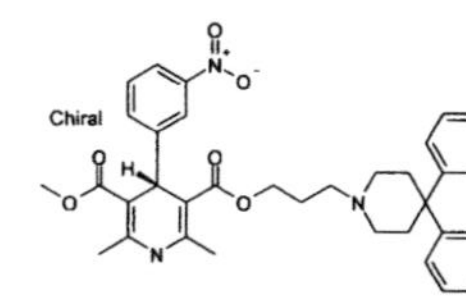 [48, 190]

(Continued on next page)

Table 5. (Continued)

Niludipine BayA-7168 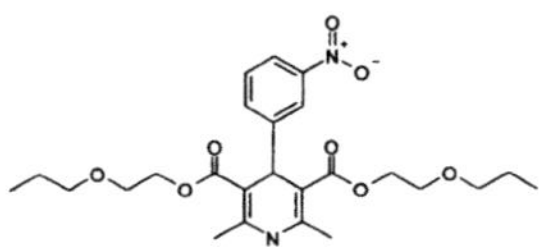 [196, 559]	Nilvadipine CL-287389 Nivadipine FK-235 FK-34235 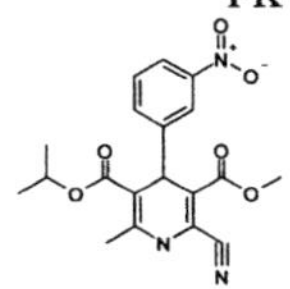 [232, 367]	Nimodipine BayE-9736 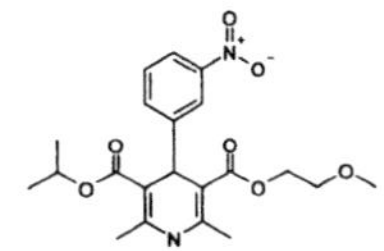 [6, 91]	Nisoldipine BayK-5552 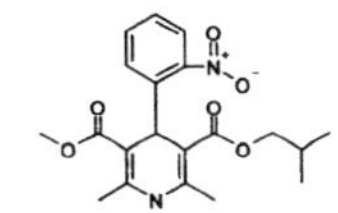 [214, 380]	Nitrendipine BayE-5009 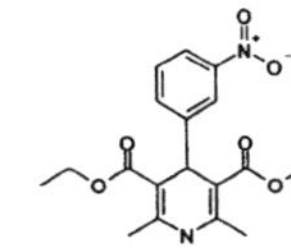 [26, 438]
Olradipine S-11568 Pranedipine S-12968 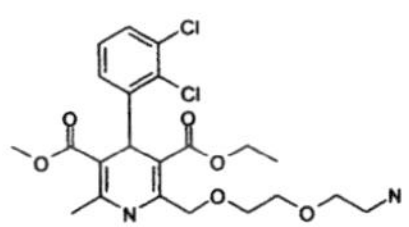 [132, 413]	Oxodipine IQB-837V 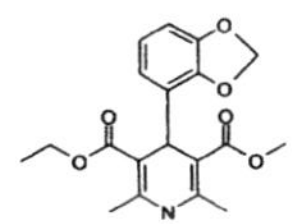 [9, 174]	Palonidipine TC-81 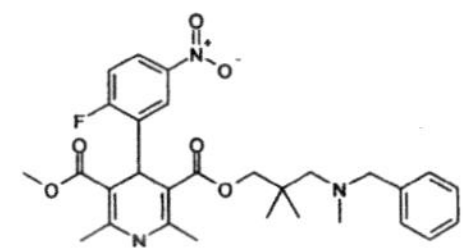 [255]	Pranidipine OPC-13340 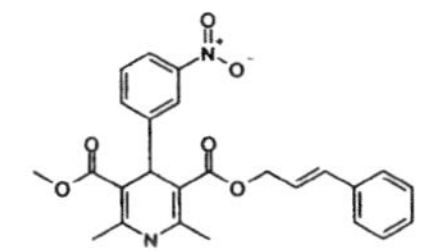 [215, 424]	Riodipine PP-1466 Ryodipine, Foridon(e) 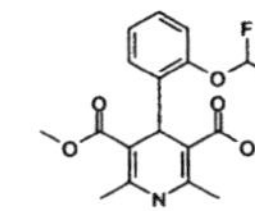 [10, 518]
Sagandipine 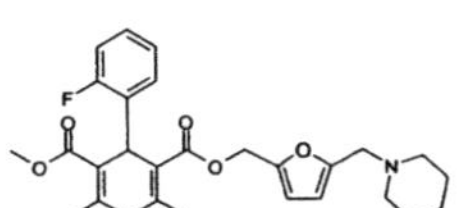	Sornidipine MCF-1113 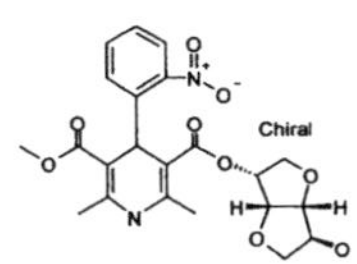 [281]	Teludipine GR-53992B Taludipine GX-1296B 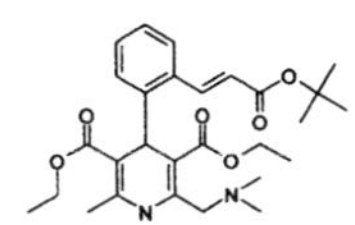 [315]	Tiamdipine BBR 1961 (analog: BBR 2160) 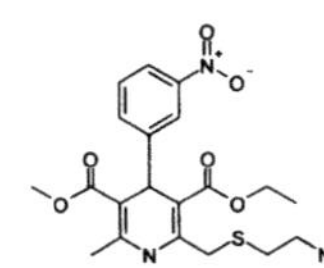 [19, 274]	Vatanidipine AE-0047 Watanidipine GJ-0956 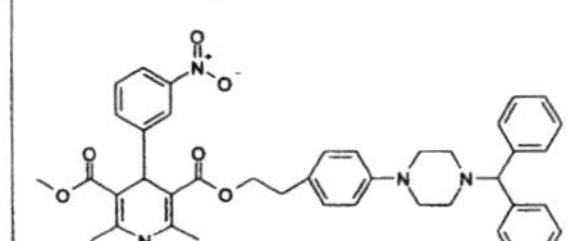 [360, 556]

For each compound: top left: common name(s); top right: development code(s); bottom left: literature citation(s). Some compounds have been extensively studied and reported upon, in which case an attempt was made to select one *in vitro* electrophysiology reference and one clinical reference. However, for some compounds, only one or two published references can be found (none in the case of sagandipine).

Mechanisms of block

Many major drugs exert their therapeutic effect by inhibiting currents through voltage-operated ion channels. In particular, local anesthetics, Class I antiarrhythmics, and some anticonvulsants block Na^+ channels, Class III antiarrhythmics block K^+ channels, and antihypertensives, antianginals, Class IV antiarrhythmics, anti-epileptics, and some analgesics block Ca^{2+} channels. Although their binding site is often present in many different tissues, most of these compounds have a remarkably good therapeutic index and are relatively tissue-specific in their action. Interestingly, many of these drugs have similar mechanisms of action, such that drug binding is strongly modulated by the pattern of electrical activity associated with the target channel and is most potent for patterns associated with pathological conditions. The most widely held hypothesis suggests that this happens because nearly all the therapeutically-useful blockers of voltage-gated ion channels have an allosteric interaction with the gating mechanism of the target channel, such that drug binding is greatly favored by specific conformations of the channel. The following section is based in large part on an earlier article [147].

The best-studied example of voltage-dependent modulation of an ion channel by a drug is the block of voltage-operated Na^+ channels by local anesthetics [72, 84]. A simple theoretical framework, the "modulated receptor theory" (MRT), has been developed, which describes well many aspects of this interaction [211]. The MRT proposes that drug receptors on an ion channel have multiple conformational states that are associated with the multiple voltage-dependent states of the conductance pathway and that differ in affinity and rate constants for drug binding (Fig. 6). Under control conditions, the main aspects of Na^+ channels gating can be described as: 1) under quiescent conditions, the channels are mostly in the resting (R) state; 2) upon depolarization of the cells, the channels move rapidly to the open (O) state; 3) after opening, the channels

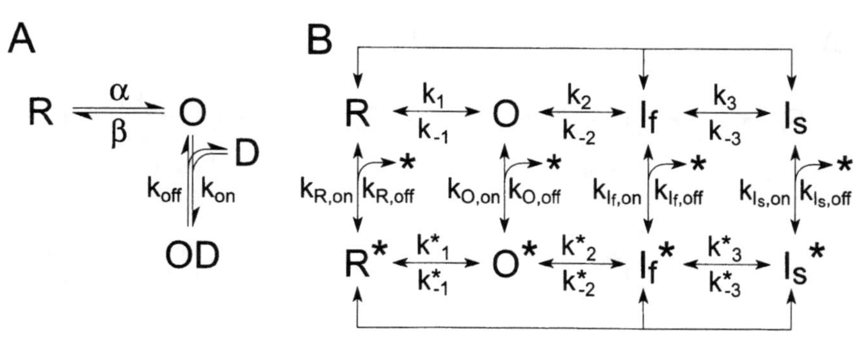

Figure 6. Modulated receptor theory for drug action on voltage-gated ion channels. A: According to voltage, the drug-free channel (top) switches between multiple states (R: resting; O: open; If: fast inactivated; Is: slow inactivated). B: The drug (*) binds to these conformations with distinct rate constants. The drug-bound channel (bottom) then switches between the different states with rate constants distinct from those of the drug-free channel.

inactivate rapidly to the non-conducting "fast inactivated" state (I_f); and 4) prolonged depolarization causes many Na^+ channels to enter a further non-conducting "slow inactivated" state (I_s), the recovery from which requires prolonged hyperpolarization. A drug can bind to these different states with distinct rate constants and the drug-bound channel can switch between the same four states with rate constants distinct from those of the drug-free channel. Whether the drug-bound "open" channel is conducting or not depends on the drug and channel studied.

The "guarded receptor" theory has been presented as an alternative to the MRT to explain the action of local anesthetics on Na^+ channels. This model postulates that channel gating does not change the binding affinity of the drug but rather that it removes a barrier to the access of the drug [470]. In fact, this model can be considered an extreme case of the MRT, where the on-rate of drug for some conformations of the channel is zero. Two subtypes of the guarded receptor theory need to be considered. In the first, the drug only binds to some conformation(s) of the channel and it needs to unbind before the channel can gate into conformations with no affinity for drug (foot-in-the-door model, Fig. 7A). In the second subtype, the drug can only access its binding site when the channel is in some defined conformation(s); however, the drug does not need to unbind for the channel to gate into conformations where unbound drug cannot access the binding site (trapped drug model, Fig. 7B).

By design, the MRT, or the guarded receptor theory, accounts for the time and voltage dependencies of Na^+ channel block by local anesthetics. If a pattern of electrical activity increases the fraction of time that the channel spends in the high affinity state, then it also increases drug binding and channel block. In addition, the model accounts for the concentration dependence of block, in that the rate and amount of block increase with drug concentration as expected by the law of mass action and a 1:1 binding reaction [27]. Finally, the model

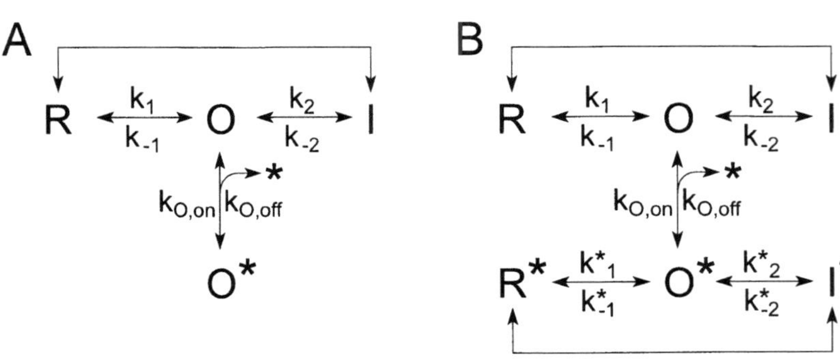

Figure 7. Guarded receptor theory for drug action on voltage-gated ion channels. A: Foot-in-the-door version. The drug (*) binds only to the open conformation and the channel cannot leave this conformation until the drug unbinds. B: Trapped drug version. The drug binds and unbinds only to and from the open conformation but the channel can change to other conformations while the drug remains bound. For simplicity, only one inactivated state is shown.

is very popular because it provides a relatively simple physical model of the effects of drugs as well as a means to quantify drug binding for structure/activity studies [27]. Using the MRT, many predictions can be made about the modification of gating currents by voltage-dependent drugs and many of these have been verified. Finally, this model agrees well with the observed action of Na^+ channel drugs on enzymatically or pharmacologically modified channels.

The MRT can also account for most aspects of the time and voltage dependencies of block of L-type Ca^{2+} currents by therapeutically useful Ca^{2+} antagonists, typified by nifedipine, verapamil, and diltiazem. The block of voltage-operated Ca^{2+} channels by gallopamil (also known as methoxyverapamil or D600) is similar to that of Na^+ channels by tertiary amines, in that the drug exists in both neutral and cationic forms and the cationic drug enters open channels from the intracellular side to produce block [208, 280, 307]. The block of Ca^{2+} channels by DHPs is analogous to that of Na^+ channels by neutral local anesthetics, except that the binding affinity is $\approx$10,000-fold greater for DHPs. The voltage dependence of the block of Ca^{2+} channels by DHPs was first elucidated in cardiac myocytes, where it was interpreted as due to the preferential binding of drug to inactivated channels [25, 433, 509]. Since then, a number of studies have enhanced our understanding of the mechanism of voltage-dependent block by DHPs (as well as PAAs and BTZs) but a number of open questions still remain.

In general, for DHPs, PAAs, and BTZs, there is good agreement that the inactivated state(s) of the channels provide high-affinity binding whereas the resting state has much lower affinity. However, there is still some debate whether binding of the drug to open channels occurs with similar or lower affinity than to inactivated channels. Thus, it is possible that the conformational change that enhances drug binding is associated with channel opening; whether the channel subsequently inactivates has little effect on drug affinity. In that case, when inactivation develops relatively rapidly (cardiac myocytes), drug binds primarily to the inactivated state but, when inactivation develops more slowly (smooth muscle, neurons, neuroendocrine cells), binding to the open state becomes more important.

In addition, whether the modulated receptor or the guarded receptor model is the most accurate is not clear and may depend on the drug and the channel that is tested. For diltiazem, the guarded receptor may be best [74]. For mibefradil, the foot-in-the-door model may also be correct for $Ca_V2.1$ (α_{1A}) channels [2] and the trapped drug model for $Ca_V1.2$ (α_{1C}) and $Ca_V2.3$ (α_{1E}) channels [33] but the modulated receptor model is needed for $Ca_V3.2$ (α_{1H}) channels [381]. For isradipine and $Ca_V1.2$ (α_{1C}), there may actually be two distinct binding sites, one being access through the open channel (guarded receptor) and the other providing high affinity binding to the inactivated channel (modulated receptor) [191, 275]. In what may be a related issue, DHP activation of $Ca_V1.x$ ($\alpha_{1S,C,D}$, maybe α_{1F}) channels may also require a different binding site from the one responsible for DHP block.

References

1 Abernethy DR and Soldatov NM. Structure-functional diversity of human L-type Ca^{2+} channel: perspectives for new pharmacological targets. *J Pharmacol Exp Ther* 300: 724–728, 2002
2 Aczel S, Kurka B and Hering S. Mechanism of voltage- and use-dependent block of class A Ca^{2+} channels by mibefradil. *Br J Pharmacol* 125: 447–454, 1998
3 Adams ME, Myers RA, Imperial JS and Olivera BM. Toxityping rat brain calcium channels with omega-toxins from spider and cone snail venoms. *Biochemistry* 32: 12566–12570, 1993
4 Adler BK and Hajduk SL. Mechanisms and origins of RNA editing. *Curr Opin Genet Dev* 4: 316–322, 1994
5 Ahlijanian MK, Westenbroek RE and Catterall WA. Subunit structure and localization of dihydropyridine-sensitive calcium channels in mammalian brain, spinal cord, and retina. *Neuron* 4: 819–832, 1990
6 Ahmed N, Nasman P and Wahlgren NG. Effect of intravenous nimodipine on blood pressure and outcome after acute stroke. *Stroke* 31: 1250–1255, 2000
7 Alajarin R, Vaquero JJ, Alvarez-Builla J, Pastor M, Sunkel C, Fau de Casa-Juana M, Priego J, Statkow PR, Sanz-Aparicio J and Fonseca I. Synthesis, structure, and pharmacological evaluation of the stereoisomers of furnidipine. *J Med Chem* 38: 2830–2841, 1995
8 Allgaier C. Ethanol sensitivity of NMDA receptors. *Neurochem Int* 41: 377–382, 2002
9 Alloui A, Talmant JM and Duchene-Marullaz P. Cardiovascular profile of oxodipine, a novel dihydropyridine calcium channel blocker, in anesthetized open-chest dogs: a comparison with nitrendipine. *Arch Int Pharmacodyn Ther* 313: 63–75, 1991
10 Andreeva TN. Foridone and other calcium antagonists in the treatment of essential hypertension. *Cor Vasa* 32: 45–55, 1990
11 Angelotti T and Hofmann F. Tissue-specific expression of splice variants of the mouse voltage-gated calcium channel alpha2/delta subunit. *FEBS Lett* 397: 331–337, 1996
12 Armstrong CM and Matteson DR. Two distinct populations of calcium channels in a clonal line of pituitary cells. *Science* 227: 65–67, 1985
13 Artalejo CR, Adams ME and Fox AP. Three types of Ca^{2+} channel trigger secretion with different efficacies in chromaffin cells. *Nature* 367: 72–76, 1994
14 Atanassoff PG, Hartmannsgruber MW, Thrasher J, Wermeling D, Longton W, Gaeta R, Singh T, Mayo M, McGuire D and Luther RR. Ziconotide, a new N-type calcium channel blocker, administered intrathecally for acute postoperative pain. *Reg Anesth Pain Med* 25: 274–278, 2000
15 Atlas D. Functional and physical coupling of voltage-sensitive calcium channels with exocytotic proteins: ramifications for the secretion mechanism. *J Neurochem* 77: 972–985, 2001
16 Atlas D, Wiser O and Trus M. The voltage-gated Ca^{2+} channel is the Ca^{2+} sensor of fast neurotransmitter release. *Cell Mol Neurobiol* 21: 717–731, 2001
17 Bading H, Ginty DD and Greenberg ME. Regulation of gene expression in hippocampal neurons by distinct calcium signaling pathways. *Science* 260: 181–186, 1993
18 Bai J and Shi Y. Inhibition of T-type Ca^{2+} currents in mouse spermatogenic cells by gossypol, an antifertility compound. *Eur J Pharmacol* 440: 1–6, 2002
19 Barbieri M, Cerbai E, Masini I, Porciatti F, Visentin S and Mugelli A. Effect of BBR 2160 on ICa recorded from guinea-pig isolated myocytes. *Pharmacol Res* 22 Suppl 3: 121–122, 1990
20 Barritt GJ. Receptor-activated Ca^{2+} inflow in animal cells: a variety of pathways tailored to meet different intracellular Ca^{2+} signaling requirements. *Biochem J* 337 (Pt 2): 153–169, 1999
21 Bauer NN and Stevens T. Putative role for a myosin motor in store-operated calcium entry. *Cell Biochem Biophys* 37: 53–70, 2002
22 Baylis C, Qiu C and Engels K. Comparison of L-type and mixed L- and T-type calcium channel blockers on kidney injury caused by deoxycorticosterone-salt hypertension in rats. *Am J Kidney Dis* 38: 1292–1297, 2001
23 Bean BP. Classes of calcium channels in vertebrate cells. *Annu Rev Physiol* 51: 367–384, 1989
24 Bean BP. Multiple types of calcium channels in heart muscle and neurons. Modulation by drugs and neurotransmitters. *Ann NY Acad Sci* 560: 334–345, 1989
25 Bean BP. Nitrendipine block of cardiac calcium channels: high-affinity binding to the inactivated state. *Proc Natl Acad Sci USA* 81: 6388–6392, 1984
26 Bean BP. Two kinds of calcium channels in canine atrial cells. Differences in kinetics, selectivity, and pharmacology. *J Gen Physiol* 86: 1–30, 1985
27 Bean BP, Cohen CJ and Tsien RW. Lidocaine block of cardiac sodium channels. *J Gen Physiol*

81: 613–642, 1983
28 Beaty GN and Stefani E. Calcium dependent electrical activity in twitch muscle fibres of the frog. *Proc R Soc Lond B Biol Sci* 194: 141–150, 1976
29 Bech-Hansen NT, Naylor MJ, Maybaum TA, Pearce WG, Koop B, Fishman GA, Mets M, Musarella MA and Boycott KM. Loss-of-function mutations in a calcium-channel alpha1-subunit gene in Xp11.23 cause incomplete X-linked congenital stationary night blindness. *Nat Genet* 19: 264–267, 1998
30 Bénardeau A and Ertel EA. Selective block of myocardial T-type calcium channels by mibefradil: A comparison with the 1,4-dihydropyridine amlodipine. In: *Low-voltage-activated T-type Ca channels*, edited by Tsien RW, Clozel J-P and Nargeot J. Chester, UK: Adis International, 1998, p. 386–394
31 Berger W, Prinz H, Striessnig J, Kang HC, Haugland R and Glossmann H. Complex molecular mechanism for dihydropyridine binding to L-type Ca^{2+}-channels as revealed by fluorescence resonance energy transfer. *Biochemistry* 33: 11875–11883, 1994
32 Berjukow S and Hering S. Voltage-dependent acceleration of Ca(v)1.2 channel current decay by (+)- and (–)-isradipine. *Br J Pharmacol* 133: 959–966, 2001
33 Bernatchez G, Sauve R and Parent L. State-dependent inhibition of inactivation-deficient Ca(V)1.2 and Ca(V)2.3 channels by mibefradil. *J Membr Biol* 184: 143–159, 2001
34 Bernheim L and Bader CR. Human myoblast differentiation: Ca^{2+} channels are activated by K(+) channels. *News Physiol Sci* 17: 22–26, 2002
35 Berrada D and Lembo T. Novel therapies in the treatment of irritable bowel syndrome. *Expert Opin Investig Drugs* 12: 635–645, 2003
36 Berridge MJ. Capacitative calcium entry. *Biochem J* 312 (Pt 1): 1–11, 1995
37 Berthier C, Monteil A, Lory P and Strube C. Alpha(1H) mRNA in single skeletal muscle fibres accounts for T-type calcium current transient expression during fetal development in mice. *J Physiol* 539: 681–691, 2002
38 Bezprozvanny I, Zhong P, Scheller RH and Tsien RW. Molecular determinants of the functional interaction between syntaxin and N-type Ca^{2+} channel gating. *Proc Natl Acad Sci USA* 97: 13943–13948, 2000
39 Bhattacharjee A, Whitehurst RM, Jr, Zhang M, Wang L and Li M. T-type calcium channels facilitate insulin secretion by enhancing general excitability in the insulin-secreting beta-cell line, INS-1. *Endocrinology* 138: 3735–3740, 1997
40 Biel M, Ruth P, Bosse E, Hullin R, Stuhmer W, Flockerzi V and Hofmann F. Primary structure and functional expression of a high voltage activated calcium channel from rabbit lung. *FEBS Lett* 269: 409–412, 1990
41 Bigge CF. Ionotropic glutamate receptors. *Curr Opin Chem Biol* 3: 441–447, 1999
42 Birnbaumer L, Campbell KP, Catterall WA, Harpold MM, Hofmann F, Horne WA, Mori Y, Schwartz A, Snutch TP, Tanabe T et al. The naming of voltage-gated calcium channels. *Neuron* 13: 505–506, 1994
43 Birnbaumer L, Qin N, Olcese R, Tareilus E, Platano D, Costantin J and Stefani E. Structures and functions of calcium channel beta subunits. *J Bioenerg Biomembr* 30: 357–375, 1998
44 Bito H, Deisseroth K and Tsien RW. Ca^{2+}-dependent regulation in neuronal gene expression. *Curr Opin Neurobiol* 7: 419–429, 1997
45 Bkaily G, Naik R, Jaalouk D, Jacques D, Economos D, D'Orleans-Juste P and Pothier P. Endothelin-1 and insulin activate the steady-state voltage dependent R-type Ca^{2+} channel in aortic smooth muscle cells via a pertussis toxin and cholera toxin sensitive G-protein. *Mol Cell Biochem* 183: 39–47, 1998
46 Bleakman D. Kainate receptor pharmacology and physiology. *Cell Mol Life Sci* 56: 558–566, 1999
47 Bloom FE and Morales M. The central 5-HT3 receptor in CNS disorders. *Neurochem Res* 23: 653–659, 1998
48 Boer R, Grassegger A, Schudt C and Glossmann H. (+)-Niguldipine binds with very high affinity to Ca^{2+} channels and to a subtype of alpha 1-adrenoceptors. *Eur J Pharmacol* 172: 131–145, 1989
49 Bonaccorsi L, Forti G and Baldi E. Low-voltage-activated calcium channels are not involved in capacitation and biological response to progesterone in human sperm. *Int J Androl* 24: 341–351, 2001
50 Bootman MD, Thomas D, Tovey SC, Berridge MJ and Lipp P. Nuclear calcium signaling. *Cell Mol Life Sci* 57: 371–378, 2000

51 Bossu JL, Elhamdani A and Feltz A. Voltage-dependent calcium entry in confluent bovine capillary endothelial cells. *FEBS Lett* 299: 239–242, 1992
52 Bossu JL, Elhamdani A, Feltz A, Tanzi F, Aunis D and Thierse D. Voltage-gated Ca entry in isolated bovine capillary endothelial cells: evidence of a new type of BAY K 8644-sensitive channel. *Pflugers Arch* 420: 200–207, 1992
53 Boulay G, Brown DM, Qin N, Jiang M, Dietrich A, Zhu MX, Chen Z, Birnbaumer M, Mikoshiba K and Birnbaumer L. Modulation of Ca^{2+} entry by polypeptides of the inositol 1,4, 5-trisphosphate receptor (IP3R) that bind transient receptor potential (TRP): evidence for roles of TRP and IP3R in store depletion-activated Ca^{2+} entry. *Proc Natl Acad Sci USA* 96: 14955–14960, 1999
54 Bourinet E, Soong TW, Stea A and Snutch TP. Determinants of the G protein-dependent opioid modulation of neuronal calcium channels. *Proc Natl Acad Sci USA* 93: 1486–1491, 1996
55 Bourinet E, Soong TW, Sutton K, Slaymaker S, Mathews E, Monteil A, Zamponi GW, Nargeot J and Snutch TP. Splicing of alpha 1A subunit gene generates phenotypic variants of P- and Q-type calcium channels. *Nat Neurosci* 2: 407–415, 1999
56 Bourinet E, Zamponi GW, Stea A, Soong TW, Lewis BA, Jones LP, Yue DT and Snutch TP. The alpha 1E calcium channel exhibits permeation properties similar to low-voltage-activated calcium channels. *J Neurosci* 16: 4983–4993, 1996
57 Boycott KM, Maybaum TA, Naylor MJ, Weleber RG, Robitaille J, Miyake Y, Bergen AA, Pierpont ME, Pearce WG and Bech-Hansen NT. A summary of 20 CACNA1F mutations identified in 36 families with incomplete X-linked congenital stationary night blindness, and characterization of splice variants. *Hum Genet* 108: 91–97, 2001
58 Braun FJ, Broad LM, Armstrong DL and Putney JW, Jr, Stable activation of single Ca^{2+} release-activated Ca^{2+} channels in divalent cation-free solutions. *J Biol Chem* 276: 1063–1070, 2001
59 Brauns T, Prinz H, Kimball SD, Haugland RP, Striessnig J and Glossmann H. L-type calcium channels: binding domains for dihydropyridines and benzothiazepines are located in close proximity to each other. *Biochemistry* 36: 3625–3631, 1997
60 Breitbart RE, Andreadis A and Nadal-Ginard B. Alternative splicing: a ubiquitous mechanism for the generation of multiple protein isoforms from single genes. *Annu Rev Biochem* 56: 467–495, 1987
61 Brini M and Carafoli E. Calcium signaling: a historical account, recent developments and future perspectives. *Cell Mol Life Sci* 57: 354–370, 2000
62 Broad LM, Braun FJ, Lievremont JP, Bird GS, Kurosaki T and Putney JW, Jr, Role of the phospholipase C-inositol 1,4,5-trisphosphate pathway in calcium release-activated calcium current and capacitative calcium entry. *J Biol Chem* 276: 15945–15952, 2001
63 Broad LM, Cannon TR and Taylor CW. A non-capacitative pathway activated by arachidonic acid is the major Ca^{2+} entry mechanism in rat A7r5 smooth muscle cells stimulated with low concentrations of vasopressin. *J Physiol* 517 (Pt 1): 121–134, 1999
64 Brogden RN and McTavish D. Nifedipine gastrointestinal therapeutic system (GITS). A review of its pharmacodynamic and pharmacokinetic properties and therapeutic efficacy in hypertension and angina pectoris. *Drugs* 50: 495–512, 1995
65 Brogden RN and Sorkin EM. Isradipine. An update of its pharmacodynamic and pharmacokinetic properties and therapeutic efficacy in the treatment of mild to moderate hypertension. *Drugs* 49: 618–649, 1995
66 Brosenitsch TA and Katz DM. Physiological patterns of electrical stimulation can induce neuronal gene expression by activating N-type calcium channels. *J Neurosci* 21: 2571–2579, 2001
67 Brust PF, Simerson S, McCue AF, Deal CR, Schoonmaker S, Williams ME, Velicelebi G, Johnson EC, Harpold MM and Ellis SB. Human neuronal voltage-dependent calcium channels: studies on subunit structure and role in channel assembly. *Neuropharmacology* 32: 1089–1102, 1993
68 Budriesi R, Aicardi G, Campana G, Spampinato S, Zaza A, Bisi A, Rampa A, Valenti P and Chiarini A. Selective cardiodepressant activity of fluodipine, a fluorenone-1,4-dihydropyridine derivative. *Eur J Pharmacol* 359: 161–170, 1998
69 Burgess DL, Davis CF, Gefrides LA and Noebels JL. Identification of three novel Ca^{2+} channel gamma subunit genes reveals molecular diversification by tandem and chromosome duplication. *Genome Res* 9: 1204–1213, 1999
70 Burnashev N. Calcium permeability of ligand-gated channels. *Cell Calcium* 24: 325–332, 1998
71 Burnstock G. P2X receptors in sensory neurones. *Br J Anaesth* 84: 476–488, 2000
72 Butterworth JFt and Strichartz GR. Molecular mechanisms of local anesthesia: a review. *Anesthesiology* 72: 711–734, 1990

73 Byron K and Taylor CW. Vasopressin stimulation of Ca^{2+} mobilization, two bivalent cation entry pathways and Ca^{2+} efflux in A7r5 rat smooth muscle cells. *J Physiol* 485 (Pt 2): 455–468, 1995
74 Cai D, Mulle JG and Yue DT. Inhibition of recombinant Ca^{2+} channels by benzothiazepines and phenylalkylamines: class-specific pharmacology and underlying molecular determinants. *Mol Pharmacol* 51: 872–881, 1997
75 Camara AK, Begic Z, Kwok WM and Bosnjak ZJ. Differential modulation of the cardiac L- and T-type calcium channel currents by isoflurane. *Anesthesiology* 95: 515–524, 2001
76 Campbell KP, Leung AT and Sharp AH. The biochemistry and molecular biology of the dihydropyridine-sensitive calcium channel. *Trends Neurosci* 11: 425–430, 1988
77 Campbell V, Berrow NS, Fitzgerald EM, Brickley K and Dolphin AC. Inhibition of the interaction of G protein G(o) with calcium channels by the calcium channel beta-subunit in rat neurones. *J Physiol* 485 (Pt 2): 365–372, 1995
78 Carbone E and Lux HD. A low voltage-activated calcium conductance in embryonic chick sensory neurons. *Biophys J* 46: 413–418, 1984
79 Carbone E and Lux HD. A low voltage-activated, fully inactivating Ca channel in vertebrate sensory neurones. *Nature* 310: 501–502, 1984
80 Castellano A, Wei X, Birnbaumer L and Perez-Reyes E. Cloning and expression of a neuronal calcium channel beta subunit. *J Biol Chem* 268: 12359–12366, 1993
81 Castellano A, Wei X, Birnbaumer L and Perez-Reyes E. Cloning and expression of a third calcium channel beta subunit. *J Biol Chem* 268: 3450–3455, 1993
82 Cataldi M, Perez-Reyes E and Tsien RW. Differences in apparent pore sizes of low and high voltage-activated Ca^{2+} channels. *J Biol Chem* 277: 45969–45976, 2002
83 Cataldi M, Taglialatela M, Palagiano F, Secondo A, de Caprariis P, Amoroso S, di Renzo G and Annunziato L. Effects of manidipine and nitrendipine enantiomers on the plateau phase of K^+-induced intracellular Ca^{2+} increase in GH3 cells. *Eur J Pharmacol* 376: 169–178, 1999
84 Catterall WA. Common modes of drug action on Na^+ channels: local anesthetics, antiarrhythmics and anticonvulsants. *Trends Pharmacol Sci* 8: 57–65, 1987
85 Catterall WA. Interactions of presynaptic Ca^{2+} channels and snare proteins in neurotransmitter release. *Ann NY Acad Sci* 868: 144–159, 1999
86 Catterall WA. Structure and function of neuronal Ca^{2+} channels and their role in neurotransmitter release. *Cell Calcium* 24: 307–323, 1998
87 Catterall WA. Structure and function of voltage-gated ion channels. *Annu Rev Biochem* 64: 493–531, 1995
88 Catterall WA. Structure and function of voltage-gated sodium and calcium channels. *Curr Opin Neurobiol* 1: 5–13, 1991
89 Catterall WA. Structure and regulation of voltage-gated Ca^{2+} channels. *Annu Rev Cell Dev Biol* 16: 521–555, 2000
90 Catterall WA and Striessnig J. Receptor sites for Ca^{2+} channel antagonists. *Trends Pharmacol Sci* 13: 256–262, 1992
91 Cerbai E, Giotti A and Mugelli A. Characteristics of L-type calcium channel blockade by lacidipine in guinea-pig ventricular myocytes. *Br J Pharmacol* 120: 667–675, 1997
92 Chandy KG and Gutman GA. Nomenclature for mammalian potassium channel genes. *Trends Pharmacol Sci* 14: 434, 1993
93 Changeux J and Edelstein SJ. Allosteric mechanisms in normal and pathological nicotinic acetylcholine receptors. *Curr Opin Neurobiol* 11: 369–377, 2001
94 Chebib M and Johnston GA. GABA-Activated ligand gated ion channels: medicinal chemistry and molecular biology. *J Med Chem* 43: 1427–1447, 2000
95 Cheer SM and McClellan K. Manidipine: a review of its use in hypertension. *Drugs* 61: 1777–1799, 2001
96 Chemin J, Monteil A, Bourinet E, Nargeot J and Lory P. Alternatively spliced alpha(1G) (Ca(V)3.1) intracellular loops promote specific T-type Ca^{2+} channel gating properties. *Biophys J* 80: 1238–1250, 2001
97 Chemin J, Monteil A, Briquaire C, Richard S, Perez-Reyes E, Nargeot J and Lory P. Overexpression of T-type calcium channels in HEK-293 cells increases intracellular calcium without affecting cellular proliferation. *FEBS Lett* 478: 166–172, 2000
98 Chemin J, Monteil A, Perez-Reyes E, Bourinet E, Nargeot J and Lory P. Specific contribution of human T-type calcium channel isotypes (alpha(1G), alpha(1H) and alpha(1I)) to neuronal excitability. *J Physiol* 540: 3–14, 2002

99 Chemin J, Monteil A, Perez-Reyes E, Nargeot J and Lory P. Direct inhibition of T-type calcium channels by the endogenous cannabinoid anandamide. *Embo J* 20: 7033–7040, 2001
100 Chen CF, Corbley MJ, Roberts TM and Hess P. Voltage-sensitive calcium channels in normal and transformed 3 T3 fibroblasts. *Science* 239: 1024–1026, 1988
101 Chen S, Ren YQ, Bing R and Hillman DE. Alpha 1E subunit of the R-type calcium channel is associated with myelinogenesis. *J Neurocytol* 29: 719–728, 2000
102 Chien AJ and Hosey MM. Post-translational modifications of beta subunits of voltage-dependent calcium channels. *J Bioenerg Biomembr* 30: 377–386, 1998
103 Chittajallu R, Braithwaite SP, Clarke VR and Henley JM. Kainate receptors: subunits, synaptic localization and function. *Trends Pharmacol Sci* 20: 26–35, 1999
104 Chizh BA and Illes P. P2X receptors and nociception. *Pharmacol Rev* 53: 553–568, 2000
105 Chrysant SG, Chrysant C, Trus J and Hitchcock A. Monotherapy of hypertension with darodipine: a new calcium-channel blocker. *Clin Cardiol* 11: 467–472, 1988
106 Chu PJ, Robertson HM and Best PM. Calcium channel gamma subunits provide insights into the evolution of this gene family. *Gene* 280: 37–48, 2001
107 Chuang RS, Jaffe H, Cribbs L, Perez-Reyes E and Swartz KJ. Inhibition of T-type voltage-gated calcium channels by a new scorpion toxin. *Nat Neurosci* 1: 668–674, 1998
108 Chyb S, Raghu P and Hardie RC. Polyunsaturated fatty acids activate the *Drosophila* light-sensitive channels TRP and TRPL. *Nature* 397: 255–259, 1999
109 Clapham DE, Runnels LW and Strubing C. The TRP ion channel family. *Nat Rev Neurosci* 2: 387–396, 2001
110 Cockayne DA, Hamilton SG, Zhu QM, Dunn PM, Zhong Y, Novakovic S, Malmberg AB, Cain G, Berson A, Kassotakis L et al. Urinary bladder hyporeflexia and reduced pain-related behaviour in P2X3-deficient mice. *Nature* 407: 1011–1015, 2000
111 Cohen CJ, McCarthy RT, Barrett PQ and Rasmussen H. Ca channels in adrenal glomerulosa cells: K^+ and angiotensin II increase T-type Ca channel current. *Proc Natl Acad Sci USA* 85: 2412–2416, 1988
112 Conti-Fine BM, Navaneetham D, Lei S and Maus AD. Neuronal nicotinic receptors in non-neuronal cells: new mediators of tobacco toxicity? *Eur J Pharmacol* 393: 279–294, 2000
113 Corringer PJ, Le Novere N and Changeux JP. Nicotinic receptors at the amino acid level. *Annu Rev Pharmacol Toxicol* 40: 431–458, 2000
114 Cribbs LL. Vascular smooth muscle calcium channels: could "T" be a target? *Circ Res* 89: 560–562, 2001
115 Cribbs LL, Lee JH, Yang J, Satin J, Zhang Y, Daud A, Barclay J, Williamson MP, Fox M, Rees M and Perez-Reyes E. Cloning and characterization of alpha1H from human heart, a member of the T-type Ca^{2+} channel gene family. *Circ Res* 83: 103–109, 1998
116 Cull-Candy S, Brickley S and Farrant M. NMDA receptor subunits: diversity, development and disease. *Curr Opin Neurobiol* 11: 327–335, 2001
117 Curtis BM and Catterall WA. Purification of the calcium antagonist receptor of the voltage-sensitive calcium channel from skeletal muscle transverse tubules. *Biochemistry* 23: 2113–2118, 1984
118 Dale B, Talevi R and DeFelice LJ. L-type Ca^{2+} currents in ascidian eggs. *Exp Cell Res* 192: 302–306, 1991
119 Dani JA. Overview of nicotinic receptors and their roles in the central nervous system. *Biol Psychiatry* 49: 166–174, 2001
120 Darwin CR. *On the origin of species by means of natural selection*. London,: J. Murray, 1859
121 De Jongh KS, Warner C and Catterall WA. Subunits of purified calcium channels. Alpha 2 and delta are encoded by the same gene. *J Biol Chem* 265: 14738–14741, 1990
122 de Leon M, Wang Y, Jones L, Perez-Reyes E, Wei X, Soong TW, Snutch TP and Yue DT. Essential Ca^{2+}-binding motif for Ca^{2+}-sensitive inactivation of L-type Ca^{2+} channels. *Science* 270: 1502–1506, 1995
123 De Paoli P, Cerbai E, Koidl B, Kirchengast M, Sartiani L and Mugelli A. Selectivity of different calcium antagonists on T- and L-type calcium currents in guinea-pig ventricular myocytes. *Pharmacol Res* 46: 491–497, 2002
124 De Waard M, Pragnell M and Campbell KP. Ca^{2+} channel regulation by a conserved beta subunit domain. *Neuron* 13: 495–503, 1994
125 De Waard M, Scott VE, Pragnell M and Campbell KP. Identification of critical amino acids involved in alpha1-beta interaction in voltage-dependent Ca^{2+} channels. *FEBS Lett* 380: 272–276, 1996

126 De Waard M, Witcher DR, Pragnell M, Liu H and Campbell KP. Properties of the alpha 1-beta anchoring site in voltage-dependent Ca^{2+} channels. *J Biol Chem* 270: 12056–12064, 1995
127 Deisseroth K, Bito H and Tsien RW. Signaling from synapse to nucleus: postsynaptic CREB phosphorylation during multiple forms of hippocampal synaptic plasticity. *Neuron* 16: 89–101, 1996
128 Deisseroth K and Tsien RW. Dynamic multiphosphorylation passwords for activity-dependent gene expression. *Neuron* 34: 179–182, 2002
129 Di Donato M, Maioli M, Venturi F, Burgisser C, Fantini F, Biamino G and Marchionni N. Acute hemodynamic effects of intravenous diperdipine, a new dihydropyridine derivative, in coronary heart disease. *Am Heart J* 121: 776–781, 1991
130 Dingledine R and Conn PJ. Peripheral glutamate receptors: molecular biology and role in taste sensation. *J Nutr* 130: 1039S–1042S, 2000
131 Dogrul A, Zagli U and Tulunay FC. The role of T-type calcium channels in morphine analgesia, development of antinociceptive tolerance and dependence to morphine, and morphine abstinence syndrome. *Life Sci* 71: 725–734, 2002
132 Dolle F, Hinnen F, Valette H, Fuseau C, Duval R, Peglion JL and Crouzel C. Synthesis of two optically active calcium channel antagonists labelled with carbon-11 for *in vivo* cardiac PET imaging. *Bioorg Med Chem* 5: 749–764, 1997
133 Dolphin AC. The G.L. Brown Prize Lecture. Voltage-dependent calcium channels and their modulation by neurotransmitters and G proteins. *Exp Physiol* 80: 1–36, 1995
134 Dolphin AC. Properties and modulation of T currents in dorsal root ganglia and ND7-23 cells: comparison with α_{1E} currents expressed in COS-7 cells. In: *Low-voltage-activated T-type Ca channels*, edited by Tsien RW, Clozel J-P and Nargeot J. Chester, UK: Adis International, 1998, p. 269–278
135 Dolphin AC, Wyatt CN, Richards J, Beattie RE, Craig P, Lee JH, Cribbs LL, Volsen SG and Perez-Reyes E. The effect of alpha2-delta and other accessory subunits on expression and properties of the calcium channel alpha1G. *J Physiol* 519 Pt 1: 35–45, 1999
136 Dubel SJ, Starr TV, Hell J, Ahlijanian MK, Enyeart JJ, Catterall WA and Snutch TP. Molecular cloning of the alpha-1 subunit of an omega-conotoxin-sensitive calcium channel. *Proc Natl Acad Sci USA* 89: 5058–5062, 1992
137 Duchen MR. Mitochondria and calcium: from cell signaling to cell death. *J Physiol* 529 Pt 1: 57–68, 2000
138 Dunn PM, Zhong Y and Burnstock G. P2X receptors in peripheral neurons. *Prog Neurobiol* 65: 107–134, 2001
139 Edmonds B, Klein M, Dale N and Kandel ER. Contributions of two types of calcium channels to synaptic transmission and plasticity. *Science* 250: 1142–1147, 1990
140 Ellinor PT, Zhang JF, Horne WA and Tsien RW. Structural determinants of the blockade of N-type calcium channels by a peptide neurotoxin. *Nature* 372: 272–275, 1994
141 Ellinor PT, Zhang JF, Randall AD, Zhou M, Schwarz TL, Tsien RW and Horne WA. Functional expression of a rapidly inactivating neuronal calcium channel. *Nature* 363: 455–458, 1993
142 Elliott AC. Recent developments in non-excitable cell calcium entry. *Cell Calcium* 30: 73–93, 2001
143 Ellis SB, Williams ME, Ways NR, Brenner R, Sharp AH, Leung AT, Campbell KP, McKenna E, Koch WJ, Hui A et al. Sequence and expression of mRNAs encoding the alpha 1 and alpha 2 subunits of a DHP-sensitive calcium channel. *Science* 241: 1661–1664, 1988
144 Elmqvist D and Lambert EH. Detailed analysis of neuromuscular transmission in a patient with the myasthenic syndrome sometimes associated with bronchogenic carcinoma. *Mayo Clin Proc* 43: 689–713, 1968
145 Enyeart JJ, Biagi B and Day RN. Opposing actions of Bay K 8644 enantiomers on calcium current, prolactin secretion, and synthesis in pituitary cells. *Mol Endocrinol* 4: 727–735, 1990
146 Ertel EA, Campbell KP, Harpold MM, Hofmann F, Mori Y, Perez-Reyes E, Schwartz A, Snutch TP, Tanabe T, Birnbaumer L et al. Nomenclature of voltage-gated calcium channels. *Neuron* 25: 533–535, 2000
147 Ertel EA and Cohen CJ. Voltage-dependent interactions: the influence and significance of membrane potential on drug-receptor interactions. *Drug Dev Res* 33: 203–213, 1994
148 Ertel SI and Ertel EA. Low-voltage-activated T-type Ca^{2+} channels. *Trends Pharmacol Sci* 18: 37–42, 1997
149 Ertel SI, Ertel EA and Clozel JP. T-type Ca^{2+} channels and pharmacological blockade: potential pathophysiological relevance. *Cardiovasc Drugs Ther* 11: 723–739, 1997

150 Fareh S, Benardeau A and Nattel S. Differential efficacy of L- and T-type calcium channel blockers in preventing tachycardia-induced atrial remodeling in dogs. *Cardiovasc Res* 49: 762–770, 2001
151 Fareh S, Benardeau A, Thibault B and Nattel S. The T-type Ca^{2+} channel blocker mibefradil prevents the development of a substrate for atrial fibrillation by tachycardia-induced atrial remodeling in dogs. *Circulation* 100: 2191–2197, 1999
152 Fasolato C, Hoth M and Penner R. A GTP-dependent step in the activation mechanism of capacitative calcium influx. *J Biol Chem* 268: 20737–20740, 1993
153 Fatt P and Ginsborg BL. The ionic requirements for the production of action potentials in crustacean muscle fibres. *J Physiol (Lond)* 142: 516–543, 1958
154 Fatt P and Katz B. The electrical properties of crustacean muscle fibres. *J Physiol (Lond)* 121: 374–389, 1953
155 Fearon IM, Varadi G, Koch S, Isaacsohn I, Ball SG and Peers C. Splice variants reveal the region involved in oxygen sensing by recombinant human L-type Ca^{2+} channels. *Circ Res* 87: 537–539, 2000
156 Felix R. Voltage-dependent Ca^{2+} channel alpha2delta auxiliary subunit: structure, function and regulation. *Receptors Channels* 6: 351–362, 1999
157 Felix R, Gurnett CA, De Waard M and Campbell KP. Dissection of functional domains of the voltage-dependent Ca^{2+} channel alpha2delta subunit. *J Neurosci* 17: 6884–6891, 1997
158 Feng ZP, Hamid J, Doering C, Bosey GM, Snutch TP and Zamponi GW. Residue Gly1326 of the N-type calcium channel alpha 1B subunit controls reversibility of omega-conotoxin GVIA and MVIIA block. *J Biol Chem* 276: 15728–15735, 2001
159 Ferreira M, Singh A, Dretchen KL, Kellar KJ and Gillis RA. Brainstem nicotinic receptor subtypes that influence intragastric and arterial blood pressures. *J Pharmacol Exp Ther* 294: 230–238, 2000
160 Ferron L, Capuano V, Deroubaix E, Coulombe A and Renaud JF. Functional and Molecular Characterization of a T-type Ca^{2+} Channel During Fetal and Postnatal Rat Heart Development. *J Mol Cell Cardiol* 34: 533–546, 2002
161 Ferroni A, Galli A and Mazzanti M. Functional role of low-voltage-activated dihydropyridine-sensitive Ca channels during the action potential in adult rat sensory neurones. *Pflugers Arch* 431: 954–963, 1996
162 Fletcher S and Barnes NM. Desperately seeking subunits: are native 5-HT3 receptors really homomeric complexes? *Trends Pharmacol Sci* 19: 212–215, 1998
163 Flockerzi V, Oeken HJ, Hofmann F, Pelzer D, Cavalie A and Trautwein W. Purified dihydropyridine-binding site from skeletal muscle t-tubules is a functional calcium channel. *Nature* 323: 66–68, 1986
164 Formenti A, Arrigoni E and Mancia M. Low-voltage activated calcium channels are differently affected by nimodipine. *Neuroreport* 5: 145–147, 1993
165 Forti L and Pietrobon D. Functional diversity of L-type calcium channels in rat cerebellar neurons. *Neuron* 10: 437–450, 1993
166 Fox AP, Nowycky MC and Tsien RW. Kinetic and pharmacological properties distinguishing three types of calcium currents in chick sensory neurones. *J Physiol* 394: 149–172, 1987
167 Franceschini D, Orr-Urtreger A, Yu W, Mackey LY, Bond RA, Armstrong D, Patrick JW, Beaudet al. and De Biasi M. Altered baroreflex responses in alpha7 deficient mice. *Behav Brain Res* 113: 3–10, 2000
168 Franciolini F and Petris A. Evolution of ionic channels of biological membranes. *Mol Biol Evol* 6: 503–513, 1989
169 Franciosi S. AMPA receptors: potential implications in development and disease. *Cell Mol Life Sci* 58: 921–930, 2001
170 Freise D, Held B, Wissenbach U, Pfeifer A, Trost C, Himmerkus N, Schweig U, Freichel M, Biel M, Hofmann F et al. Absence of the gamma subunit of the skeletal muscle dihydropyridine receptor increases L-type Ca^{2+} currents and alters channel inactivation properties. *J Biol Chem* 275: 14476–14481, 2000
171 Frerking M and Nicoll RA. Synaptic kainate receptors. *Curr Opin Neurobiol* 10: 342–351, 2000
172 Fujita Y, Mynlieff M, Dirksen RT, Kim MS, Niidome T, Nakai J, Friedrich T, Iwabe N, Miyata T, Furuichi T et al. Primary structure and functional expression of the omega-conotoxin-sensitive N-type calcium channel from rabbit brain. *Neuron* 10: 585–598, 1993
173 Furukawa T, Yamakawa T, Midera T, Sagawa T, Mori Y and Nukada T. Selectivities of dihydropyridine derivatives in blocking Ca^{2+} channel subtypes expressed in *Xenopus* oocytes. *J*

Pharmacol Exp Ther 291: 464–473, 1999
174 Galan L, Talavera K, Vassort G and Alvarez JL. Characteristics of Ca^{2+} channel blockade by oxodipine and elgodipine in rat cardiomyocytes. *Eur J Pharmacol* 357: 93–105, 1998
175 Gao B, Sekido Y, Maximov A, Saad M, Forgacs E, Latif F, Wei MH, Lerman M, Lee JH, Perez-Reyes E et al. Functional properties of a new voltage-dependent calcium channel alpha(2)delta auxiliary subunit gene (CACNA2D2). *J Biol Chem* 275: 12237–12242, 2000
176 Garber SS, Hoshi T and Aldrich RW. Regulation of ionic currents in pheochromocytoma cells by nerve growth factor and dexamethasone. *J Neurosci* 9: 3976–3987, 1989
177 Gasparini S, Kasyanov AM, Pietrobon D, Voronin LL and Cherubini E. Presynaptic R-type calcium channels contribute to fast excitatory synaptic transmission in the rat hippocampus. *J Neurosci* 21: 8715–8721, 2001
178 Glossmann H, Ferry DR, Goll A, Striessnig J and Zernig G. Calcium channels and calcium channel drugs: recent biochemical and biophysical findings. *Arzneimittelforschung* 35: 1917–1935, 1985
179 Goldin AL, Barchi RL, Caldwell JH, Hofmann F, Howe JR, Hunter JC, Kallen RG, Mandel G, Meisler MH, Netter YB et al. Nomenclature of voltage-gated sodium channels. *Neuron* 28: 365–368, 2000
180 Gomora JC, Murbartian J, Arias JM, Lee JH and Perez-Reyes E. Cloning and expression of the human T-type channel Ca(v)3.3: Insights into prepulse facilitation. *Biophys J* 83: 229–241, 2002
181 Gomora JC, Xu L, Enyeart JA and Enyeart JJ. Effect of mibefradil on voltage-dependent gating and kinetics of T-type Ca^{2+} channels in cortisol-secreting cells. *J Pharmacol Exp Ther* 292: 96–103, 2000
182 Gordon EH, Wong SC and Klaustermeyer WB. Comparison of nifedipine with a new calcium channel blocker, flordipine, in exercise-induced asthma. *J Asthma* 24: 261–265, 1987
183 Grabner M, Friedrich K, Knaus HG, Striessnig J, Scheffauer F, Staudinger R, Koch WJ, Schwartz A and Glossmann H. Calcium channels from *Cyprinus carpio* skeletal muscle. *Proc Natl Acad Sci USA* 88: 727–731, 1991
184 Grabner M, Wang Z, Hering S, Striessnig J and Glossmann H. Transfer of 1,4-dihydropyridine sensitivity from L-type to class A (BI) calcium channels. *Neuron* 16: 207–218, 1996
185 Green PJ, Warre R, Hayes PD, McNaughton NC, Medhurst AD, Pangalos M, Duckworth DM and Randall AD. Kinetic modification of the alpha(1I) subunit-mediated T-type Ca^{2+} channel by a human neuronal Ca^{2+} channel gamma subunit. *J Physiol* 533: 467–478, 2001
186 Gu X and Spitzer NC. Low-threshold Ca^{2+} current and its role in spontaneous elevations of intracellular Ca^{2+} in developing *Xenopus* neurons. *J Neurosci* 13: 4936–4948, 1993
187 Gurnett CA, De Waard M and Campbell KP. Dual function of the voltage-dependent Ca^{2+} channel alpha 2 delta subunit in current stimulation and subunit interaction. *Neuron* 16: 431–440, 1996
188 Guy HR and Conti F. Pursuing the structure and function of voltage-gated channels. *Trends Neurosci* 13: 201–206, 1990
189 Hagiwara N, Irisawa H and Kameyama M. Contribution of two types of calcium currents to the pacemaker potentials of rabbit sino-atrial node cells. *J Physiol* 395: 233–253, 1988
190 Handrock R and Herzig S. Stereoselectivity of Ca^{2+} channel block by dihydropyridines: no modulation by the voltage protocol. *Eur J Pharmacol* 309: 317–321, 1996
191 Handrock R, Rao-Schymanski R, Klugbauer N, Hofmann F and Herzig S. Dihydropyridine enantiomers block recombinant L-type Ca^{2+} channels by two different mechanisms. *J Physiol* 521 Pt 1: 31–42, 1999
192 Hanlon MR, Berrow NS, Dolphin AC and Wallace BA. Modelling of a voltage-dependent Ca^{2+} channel beta subunit as a basis for understanding its functional properties. *FEBS Lett* 445: 366–370, 1999
193 Hans M, Urrutia A, Deal C, Brust PF, Stauderman K, Ellis SB, Harpold MM, Johnson EC and Williams ME. Structural elements in domain IV that influence biophysical and pharmacological properties of human alpha1A-containing high-voltage-activated calcium channels. *Biophys J* 76: 1384–1400, 1999
194 Hansen PB, Jensen BL, Andreasen D, Friis UG and Skott O. Vascular smooth muscle cells express the alpha(1A) subunit of a P-/Q-type voltage-dependent Ca^{2+} Channel, and It is functionally important in renal afferent arterioles. *Circ Res* 87: 896–902, 2000
195 Harada K, Nomura M, Nishikado A, Uehara K, Nakaya Y and Ito S. Clinical efficacy of efonidipine hydrochloride, a T-type calcium channel inhibitor, on sympathetic activities. *Circ J* 67: 139–145, 2003

196 Hashimoto K, Takeda K, Katano Y, Nakagawa Y, Tsukada T, Hashimoto T, Shimamoto N, Sakai K, Otorii T and Imai S. Effects of niludipine (Bay a 7168) on the cardiovascular system with a note on its calcium-antagonistic effects. *Arzneimittelforschung* 29: 1368–1373, 1979

197 Hatakeyama S, Wakamori M, Ino M, Miyamoto N, Takahashi E, Yoshinaga T, Sawada K, Imoto K, Tanaka I, Yoshizawa T et al. Differential nociceptive responses in mice lacking the alpha(1B) subunit of N-type Ca^{2+} channels. *Neuroreport* 12: 2423–2427, 2001

198 Hattori T, Maehashi H, Miyazawa T and Naito M. Potentiation by stannous chloride of calcium entry into osteoblastic MC3T3-E1 cells through voltage-dependent L-type calcium channels. *Cell Calcium* 30: 67–72, 2001

199 Hattori Y, Fukao M, Houzen H, Qi F, Yamada Y and Kanno M. *In vitro* assessment for vascular selectivity of a new dihydropyridine derivative, NB-818. *Eur J Pharmacol* 301: 99–106, 1996

200 Heady TN, Gomora JC, Macdonald TL and Perez-Reyes E. Molecular pharmacology of T-type Ca^{2+} channels. *Jpn J Pharmacol* 85: 339–350, 2001

201 Heinemann SH, Terlau H, Stuhmer W, Imoto K and Numa S. Calcium channel characteristics conferred on the sodium channel by single mutations. *Nature* 356: 441–443, 1992

202 Hell JW, Westenbroek RE, Elliott EM and Catterall WA. Differential phosphorylation, localization, and function of distinct alpha 1 subunits of neuronal calcium channels. Two size forms for class B, C, and D alpha 1 subunits with different COOH-termini. *Ann NY Acad Sci* 747: 282–293, 1994

203 Hell JW, Yokoyama CT, Wong ST, Warner C, Snutch TP and Catterall WA. Differential phosphorylation of two size forms of the neuronal class C L-type calcium channel alpha 1 subunit. *J Biol Chem* 268: 19451–19457, 1993

204 Hering S, Aczel S, Grabner M, Doring F, Berjukow S, Mitterdorfer J, Sinnegger MJ, Striessnig J, Degtiar VE et al. Transfer of high sensitivity for benzothiazepines from L-type to class A (BI) calcium channels. *J Biol Chem* 271: 24471–24475, 1996

205 Hering S, Aczel S, Kraus RL, Berjukow S, Striessnig J and Timin EN. Molecular mechanism of use-dependent calcium channel block by phenylalkylamines: role of inactivation. *Proc Natl Acad Sci USA* 94: 13323–13328, 1997

206 Herlitze S, Hockerman GH, Scheuer T and Catterall WA. Molecular determinants of inactivation and G protein modulation in the intracellular loop connecting domains I and II of the calcium channel alpha1A subunit. *Proc Natl Acad Sci USA* 94: 1512–1516, 1997

207 Hermsmeyer K, Sturek M, Marvin W, Mason R and Puga A. Vascular muscle calcium channel modulation in hypertension. *J Cardiovasc Pharmacol* 14 Suppl 6: S45–48, 1989

208 Hescheler J, Pelzer D, Trube G and Trautwein W. Does the organic calcium channel blocker D600 act from inside or outside on the cardiac cell membrane? *Pflugers Arch* 393: 287–291, 1982

209 Hess P. Calcium channels in vertebrate cells. *Annu Rev Neurosci* 13: 337–356, 1990

210 Hess P, Lansman JB, Nilius B and Tsien RW. Calcium channel types in cardiac myocytes: modulation by dihydropyridines and beta-adrenergic stimulation. *J Cardiovasc Pharmacol* 8 Suppl 9: S11–21, 1986

211 Hille B. *Ionic channels of excitable membranes*. Sunderland, Mass.: Sinauer Associates, 1992

212 Hille B. The Sharpey-Schafer Lecture. Ionic channels: evolutionary origins and modern roles. *Q J Exp Physiol* 74: 785–804, 1989

213 Hillman D, Chen S, Aung TT, Cherksey B, Sugimori M and Llinas RR. Localization of P-type calcium channels in the central nervous system. *Proc Natl Acad Sci USA* 88: 7076–7080, 1991

214 Himmel HM, Stengel W and Ravens U. Selectivity of blocking of low- *versus* high-voltage activated calcium currents by the dihydropyridine derivatives Bay E5759 and Bay A4339 in neuroblastoma—glioma NG 108-15 cells. *Pharmacol Res* 44: 113–116, 2001

215 Hirano T, Mori T, Kido M, Toide K, Ohura M, Fujiki H, Orito K, Yoshida K, Ikezono K, Sumida T et al. Differential properties of the optical-isomers of pranidipine, a 1,4-dihydropyridine calcium channel modulator. *Fundam Clin Pharmacol* 13: 650–655, 1999

216 Hirooka K, Bertolesi GE, Kelly ME, Denovan-Wright EM, Sun X, Hamid J, Zamponi GW, Juhasz AE, Haynes LW and Barnes S. T-type calcium channel alpha1G and alpha1H subunits in human retinoblastoma cells and their loss after differentiation. *J Neurophysiol* 88: 196–205, 2002

217 Hobom M, Dai S, Marais E, Lacinova L, Hofmann F and Klugbauer N. Neuronal distribution and functional characterization of the calcium channel alpha2delta-2 subunit. *Eur J Neurosci* 12: 1217–1226, 2000

218 Hofmann F, Biel M and Flockerzi V. Molecular basis for Ca^{2+} channel diversity. *Annu Rev Neurosci* 17: 399–418, 1994

219 Hofmann F, Lacinova L and Klugbauer N. Voltage-dependent calcium channels: from structure

to function. *Rev Physiol Biochem Pharmacol* 139: 33–87, 1999
220 Hofmann T, Schaefer M, Schultz G and Gudermann T. Transient receptor potential channels as molecular substrates of receptor-mediated cation entry. *J Mol Med* 78: 14–25, 2000
221 Holck M and Osterrieder W. Inhibition of myocardial Ca^{2+} channels by three dihydropyridines with different structural features: potential-dependent blockade by Ro 18-3981. *Br J Pharmacol* 91: 61–67, 1987
222 Homaidan FR, Donowitz M, Weiland GA and Sharp GW. Two calcium channels in basolateral membranes of rabbit ileal epithelial cells. *Am J Physiol* 257: G86–93, 1989
223 Horne WA, Ellinor PT, Inman I, Zhou M, Tsien RW and Schwarz TL. Molecular diversity of Ca^{2+} channel alpha 1 subunits from the marine ray *Discopyge ommata*. *Proc Natl Acad Sci USA* 90: 3787–3791, 1993
224 Hoth M and Penner R. Depletion of intracellular calcium stores activates a calcium current in mast cells. *Nature* 355: 353–356, 1992
225 Hu LY, Ryder TR, Rafferty MF, Taylor CP, Feng MR, Kuo BS, Lotarski SM, Miljanich GP, Millerman E, Siebers KM and Szoke BG. The discovery of [1-(4-dimethylamino-benzyl)-piperidin-4-yl]-[4-(3,3-dimethylbutyl)-phen yl]-(3-methyl-but-2-enyl)-amine, an N-type Ca+2 channel blocker with oral activity for analgesia. *Bioorg Med Chem* 8: 1203–1212, 2000
226 Huang B, Qin D, Deng L, Boutjdir M and N E-S. Reexpression of T-type Ca^{2+} channel gene and current in post-infarction remodeled rat left ventricle. *Cardiovasc Res* 46: 442–449, 2000
227 Huguenard JR. Low-threshold calcium currents in central nervous system neurons. *Annu Rev Physiol* 58: 329–348, 1996
228 Hui A, Ellinor PT, Krizanova O, Wang JJ, Diebold RJ and Schwartz A. Molecular cloning of multiple subtypes of a novel rat brain isoform of the alpha 1 subunit of the voltage-dependent calcium channel. *Neuron* 7: 35–44, 1991
229 Hullin R, Biel M, Flockerzi V and Hofmann F. Tissue-specific expression of calcium channels. *Trends Cardiovasc Med* 3: 48–53, 1993
230 Hullin R, Singer-Lahat D, Freichel M, Biel M, Dascal N, Hofmann F and Flockerzi V. Calcium channel beta subunit heterogeneity: functional expression of cloned cDNA from heart, aorta and brain. *Embo J* 11: 885–890, 1992
231 Irvine RF. 'Quantal' Ca^{2+} release and the control of Ca^{2+} entry by inositol phosphates—a possible mechanism. *FEBS Lett* 263: 5–9, 1990
232 Ishibashi H, Murai Y and Akaike N. Effect of nilvadipine on the voltage-dependent Ca^{2+} channels in rat hippocampal CA1 pyramidal neurons. *Brain Res* 813: 121–127, 1998
233 Itier V and Bertrand D. Neuronal nicotinic receptors: from protein structure to function. *FEBS Lett* 504: 118–125, 2001
234 Ito H, Klugbauer N and Hofmann F. Transfer of the high affinity dihydropyridine sensitivity from L-type To non-L-type calcium channel. *Mol Pharmacol* 52: 735–740, 1997
235 Jagannathan S, Punt EL, Gu Y, Arnoult C, Sakkas D, Barratt CL and Publicover SJ. Identification and localization of T-type voltage-operated calcium channel subunits in human male germ cells. Expression of multiple isoforms. *J Biol Chem* 277: 8449–8456, 2002
236 Jay SD, Ellis SB, McCue AF, Williams ME, Vedvick TS, Harpold MM and Campbell KP. Primary structure of the gamma subunit of the DHP-sensitive calcium channel from skeletal muscle. *Science* 248: 490–492, 1990
237 Jay SD, Sharp AH, Kahl SD, Vedvick TS, Harpold MM and Campbell KP. Structural characterization of the dihydropyridine-sensitive calcium channel alpha 2-subunit and the associated delta peptides. *J Biol Chem* 266: 3287–3293, 1991
238 Johnston D, Avery RB and Magee JC. Physiology, pharmacology and function of low voltage-activated Ca^{2+} channels in hippocampal pyramidal neurons. In: *Low-voltage-activated T-type Ca channels*, edited by Tsien RW, Clozel J-P and Nargeot J. Chester, UK: Adis International, 1998, p. 133–142
239 Johnston D, Williams S, Jaffe D and Gray R. NMDA-receptor-independent long-term potentiation. *Annu Rev Physiol* 54: 489–505, 1992
240 Johri AM and Janssen LJ. N-Type Ca^{2+} channels trigger release of excitatory and inhibitory neurotransmitter from nerve endings in canine bronchi. *J Pharmacol Exp Ther* 290: 847–853, 1999
241 Jun K, Piedras-Renteria ES, Smith SM, Wheeler DB, Lee SB, Lee TG, Chin H, Adams ME, Scheller RH, Tsien RW and Shin HS. Ablation of P/Q-type Ca^{2+} channel currents, altered synaptic transmission, and progressive ataxia in mice lacking the alpha(1A)-subunit. *Proc Natl Acad Sci USA* 96: 15245–15250, 1999
242 Jung S, Strotmann R, Schultz G and Plant TD. TRPC6 is a candidate channel involved in recep-

tor-stimulated cation currents in A7r5 smooth muscle cells. *Am J Physiol Cell Physiol* 282: C347–359, 2002
243 Kaneko S, Cooper CB, Nishioka N, Yamasaki H, Suzuki A, Jarvis SE, Akaike A, Satoh M and Zamponi GW. Identification and characterization of novel human Ca(v)2.2 (alpha 1B) calcium channel variants lacking the synaptic protein interaction site. *J Neurosci* 22: 82–92, 2002
244 Karlin A. Emerging structure of the nicotinic acetylcholine receptors. *Nat Rev Neurosci* 3: 102–114, 2002
245 Kasuya H, Onda H, Takeshita M, Okada Y and Hori T. Efficacy and safety of nicardipine prolonged-release implants for preventing vasospasm in humans. *Stroke* 33: 1011–1015, 2002
246 Katz B and Miledi R. Tetrodotoxin-resistant electric activity in presynaptic terminals. *J Physiol* 203: 459–487, 1969
247 Kavalali ET and Plummer MR. Selective potentiation of a novel calcium channel in rat hippocampal neurones. *J Physiol* 480 (Pt 3): 475–484, 1994
248 Kawashima K and Fujii T. The lymphocytic cholinergic system and its biological function. *Life Sci* 72: 2101–2109, 2003
249 Kenakin TP, Bond RA and Bonner TI. Definition of pharmacological receptors. *Pharmacol Rev* 44: 351–362, 1992
250 Kerschbaum HH and Cahalan MD. Single-channel recording of a store-operated Ca^{2+} channel in Jurkat T lymphocytes. *Science* 283: 836–839, 1999
251 Khakh BS. Molecular physiology of P2X receptors and ATP signaling at synapses. *Nat Rev Neurosci* 2: 165–174, 2001
252 Kim D, Song I, Keum S, Lee T, Jeong MJ, Kim SS, McEnery MW and Shin HS. Lack of the burst firing of thalamocortical relay neurons and resistance to absence seizures in mice lacking alpha(1G) T-type Ca^{2+} channels. *Neuron* 31: 35–45, 2001
253 Kiselyov K, Mignery GA, Zhu MX and Muallem S. The N-terminal domain of the IP3 receptor gates store-operated hTrp3 channels. *Mol Cell* 4: 423–429, 1999
254 Kiselyov K, Xu X, Mozhayeva G, Kuo T, Pessah I, Mignery G, Zhu X, Birnbaumer L and Muallem S. Functional interaction between InsP3 receptors and store-operated Htrp3 channels. *Nature* 396: 478–482, 1998
255 Kishimoto T, Sunakawa K, Aoki K, Okamiya Y and Takeshita T. Differences in responses to TC-81 among various arteries in dogs. *J Cardiovasc Pharmacol* 20: 923–931, 1992
256 Kitchens SA, Burch J and Creazzo TL. T-type Ca^{2+} current contribution to Ca^{2+}-induced Ca^{2+} release in developing myocardium. *J Mol Cell Cardiol* 35: 515–523, 2003
257 Klugbauer N, Dai S, Specht V, Lacinova L, Marais E, Bohn G and Hofmann F. A family of gamma-like calcium channel subunits. *FEBS Lett* 470: 189–197, 2000
258 Klugbauer N, Lacinova L, Marais E, Hobom M and Hofmann F. Molecular diversity of the calcium channel alpha2delta subunit. *J Neurosci* 19: 684–691, 1999
259 Klugbauer N, Marais E, Lacinova L and Hofmann F. A T-type calcium channel from mouse brain. *Pflugers Arch* 437: 710–715, 1999
260 Koch WJ, Hui A, Shull GE, Ellinor P and Schwartz A. Characterization of cDNA clones encoding two putative isoforms of the alpha 1 subunit of the dihydropyridine-sensitive voltage-dependent calcium channel isolated from rat brain and rat aorta. *FEBS Lett* 250: 386–388, 1989
261 Kohl BK and Dannhardt G. The NMDA receptor complex: a promising target for novel antiepileptic strategies. *Curr Med Chem* 8: 1275–1289, 2001
262 Koles L, Wirkner K and Illes P. Modulation of ionotropic glutamate receptor channels. *Neurochem Res* 26: 925–932, 2001
263 Komuro H and Rakic P. Selective role of N-type calcium channels in neuronal migration. *Science* 257: 806–809, 1992
264 Koschak A, Reimer D, Huber I, Grabner M, Glossmann H, Engel J and Striessnig J. alpha 1D ($Ca_V1.3$) subunits can form l-type Ca^{2+} channels activating at negative voltages. *J Biol Chem* 276: 22100–22106, 2001
265 Krasowski MD and Harrison NL. General anaesthetic actions on ligand-gated ion channels. *Cell Mol Life Sci* 55: 1278–1303, 1999
266 Kraus R, Reichl B, Kimball SD, Grabner M, Murphy BJ, Catterall WA and Striessnig J. Identification of benz(othi)azepine-binding regions within L-type calcium channel alpha1 subunits. *J Biol Chem* 271: 20113–20118, 1996
267 Kraus RL, Hering S, Grabner M, Ostler D and Striessnig J. Molecular mechanism of diltiazem interaction with L-type Ca^{2+} channels. *J Biol Chem* 273: 27205–27212, 1998

268 Krovetz HS, Helton TD, Crews AL and Horne WA. C-Terminal alternative splicing changes the gating properties of a human spinal cord calcium channel alpha 1A subunit. *J Neurosci* 20: 7564–7570, 2000
269 Kuga T, Kobayashi S, Hirakawa Y, Kanaide H and Takeshita A. Cell cycle—dependent expression of L- and T-type Ca^{2+} currents in rat aortic smooth muscle cells in primary culture. *Circ Res* 79: 14–19, 1996
270 Kullmann DM, Asztely F and Walker MC. The role of mammalian ionotropic receptors in synaptic plasticity: LTP, LTD and epilepsy. *Cell Mol Life Sci* 57: 1551–1561, 2000
271 Kumar PP, Stotz SC, Paramashivappa R, Beedle AM, Zamponi GW and Rao AS. Synthesis and evaluation of a new class of nifedipine analogs with T-type calcium channel blocking activity. *Mol Pharmacol* 61: 649–658, 2002
272 Kunapuli SP and Daniel JL. P2 receptor subtypes in the cardiovascular system. *Biochem J* 336 (Pt 3): 513–523, 1998
273 Kuramoto K, Ichikawa S, Hirai A, Kanada S, Nakachi T and Ogihara T. Azelnidipine and amlodipine: a comparison of their pharmacokinetics and effects on ambulatory blood pressure. *Hypertens Res* 26: 201–208, 2003
274 Kwon YW, Zhong Q, Wei XY, Zheng W and Triggle DJ. The interactions of 1,4-dihydropyridines bearing a 2-(2-aminoethylthio)methyl substituent at voltage-dependent Ca^{2+} channels of smooth muscle, cardiac muscle and neuronal tissues. *Naunyn Schmiedebergs Arch Pharmacol* 341: 128–136, 1990
275 Lacinova L, Klugbauer N and Hofmann F. State- and isoform-dependent interaction of isradipine with the alpha1C L-type calcium channel. *Pflugers Arch* 440: 50–60, 2000
276 Lacinova L, Klugbauer N, Hu M and Hofmann F. Reconstruction of the dihydropyridine site in a non-L-type calcium channel: the role of the IS6 segment. *FEBS Lett* 451: 152–156, 1999
277 Lambert RC, Maulet Y, Mouton J, Beattie R, Volsen S, De Waard M and Feltz A. T-type Ca^{2+} current properties are not modified by Ca^{2+} channel beta subunit depletion in nodosus ganglion neurons. *J Neurosci* 17: 6621–6628, 1997
278 Latour I, Hamid J, Beedle AM, Zamponi GW and Macvicar BA. Expression of voltage-gated Ca^{2+} channel subtypes in cultured astrocytes. *Glia* 41: 347–353, 2003
279 Lee JH, Daud AN, Cribbs LL, Lacerda AE, Pereverzev A, Klockner U, Schneider T and Perez-Reyes E. Cloning and expression of a novel member of the low voltage-activated T-type calcium channel family. *J Neurosci* 19: 1912–1921, 1999
280 Lee KS and Tsien RW. Mechanism of calcium channel blockade by verapamil, D600, diltiazem and nitrendipine in single dialysed heart cells. *Nature* 302: 790–794, 1983
281 Leitold M and Fleissig W. Comparative investigation of different classes of compounds in experimental myocardial infarction in the rat. *Arch Pharmacol* 335: R65, 1987
282 Lenglet S, Louiset E, Delarue C, Vaudry H and Contesse V. Activation of 5-HT(7) receptor in rat glomerulosa cells is associated with an increase in adenylyl cyclase activity and calcium influx through T-type calcium channels. *Endocrinology* 143: 1748–1760, 2002
283 Letts VA, Felix R, Biddlecome GH, Arikkath J, Mahaffey CL, Valenzuela A, Bartlett FS, 2nd, Mori Y, Campbell KP and Frankel WN. The mouse stargazer gene encodes a neuronal Ca^{2+}-channel gamma subunit. *Nat Genet* 19: 340–347, 1998
284 Leuranguer V, Bourinet E, Lory P and Nargeot J. Antisense depletion of beta-subunits fails to affect T-type calcium channels properties in a neuroblastoma cell line. *Neuropharmacology* 37: 701–708, 1998
285 Leuranguer V, Monteil A, Bourinet E, Dayanithi G and Nargeot J. T-type calcium currents in rat cardiomyocytes during postnatal development: contribution to hormone secretion. *Am J Physiol Heart Circ Physiol* 279: H2540–2548, 2000
286 Lewis RS. Calcium signaling mechanisms in T lymphocytes. *Annu Rev Immunol* 19: 497–521, 2001
287 Liu H, Felix R, Gurnett CA, De Waard M, Witcher DR and Campbell KP. Expression and subunit interaction of voltage-dependent Ca^{2+} channels in PC12 cells. *J Neurosci* 16: 7557–7565, 1996
288 Liu X, Wang W, Singh BB, Lockwich T, Jadlowiec J, O'Connell B, Wellner R, Zhu MX and Ambudkar IS. Trp1, a candidate protein for the store-operated Ca^{2+} influx mechanism in salivary gland cells. *J Biol Chem* 275: 3403–3411, 2000
289 Llinas RR, Sugimori M and Cherksey B. Voltage-dependent calcium conductances in mammalian neurons. The P channel. *Ann NY Acad Sci* 560: 103–111, 1989

290 Lloyd GK and Williams M. Neuronal nicotinic acetylcholine receptors as novel drug targets. *J Pharmacol Exp Ther* 292: 461–467, 2000
291 Lohn M, Muzzulini U, Essin K, Tsang SY, Kirsch T, Litteral J, Waldron P, Conrad H, Klugbauer N, Hofmann F et al. Cilnidipine is a novel slow-acting blocker of vascular L-type calcium channels that does not target protein kinase C. *J Hypertens* 20: 885–893, 2002
292 Lory P, Varadi G and Schwartz A. The beta subunit controls the gating and dihydropyridine sensitivity of the skeletal muscle Ca^{2+} channel. *Biophys J* 63: 1421–1424, 1992
293 Lotshaw DP. Role of membrane depolarization and T-type Ca^{2+} channels in angiotensin II and K^+ stimulated aldosterone secretion. *Mol Cell Endocrinol* 175: 157–171, 2001
294 Ludwig A, Flockerzi V and Hofmann F. Regional expression and cellular localization of the alpha1 and beta subunit of high voltage-activated calcium channels in rat brain. *J Neurosci* 17: 1339–1349, 1997
295 Lukas RJ, Changeux JP, Le Novere N, Albuquerque EX, Balfour DJ, Berg DK, Bertrand D, Chiappinelli VA, Clarke PB, Collins AC et al. International Union of Pharmacology. XX. Current status of the nomenclature for nicotinic acetylcholine receptors and their subunits. *Pharmacol Rev* 51: 397–401, 1999
296 MacKenzie AB, Surprenant A and North RA. Functional and molecular diversity of purinergic ion channel receptors. *Ann NY Acad Sci* 868: 716–729, 1999
297 Macrez-Lepretre N, Kalkbrenner F, Schultz G and Mironneau J. Distinct functions of Gq and G11 proteins in coupling alpha1-adrenoreceptors to Ca^{2+} release and Ca^{2+} entry in rat portal vein myocytes. *J Biol Chem* 272: 5261–5268, 1997
298 Madden DR. The structure and function of glutamate receptor ion channels. *Nat Rev Neurosci* 3: 91–101, 2002
299 Malhotra HS and Plosker GL. Barnidipine. *Drugs* 61: 989–996; discussion 997–988, 2001
300 Mangoni M, Leuranguer V, Bourinet E, Nargeot J and Richard S. Block of cardiac Ca^{2+} channels by the new Ca^{2+} antagonist Ro 40-5967: consequences on heart rate and cardiac output. *Biophysical Journal* 72: A256, 1997
301 Mannhold R, Jablonka B, Voigt W, Schonafinger K and Schraven E. Calcium- and calmodulin-antagonism of elnadipine derivatives: Comparative SAR. *Eur J Med Chem* 27: 229–235, 1992
302 Mariot P, Vanoverberghe K, Lalevee N, Rossier MF and Prevarskaya N. Overexpression of an alpha 1H ($Ca_V3.2$) T-type calcium channel during neuroendocrine differentiation of human prostate cancer cells. *J Biol Chem* 277: 10824–10833, 2002
303 Marksteiner R, Schurr P, Berjukow S, Margreiter E, Perez-Reyes E and Hering S. Inactivation determinants in segment IIIS6 of Ca(v)3.1. *J Physiol* 537: 27–34, 2001
304 Martin-Caraballo M and Greer JJ. Voltage-sensitive calcium currents and their role in regulating phrenic motoneuron electrical excitability during the perinatal period. *J Neurobiol* 46: 231–248, 2001
305 Masumiya H, Tanaka Y, Tanaka H and Shigenobu K. Inhibition of T-type and L-type Ca^{2+} currents by aranidipine, a novel dihydropyridine Ca^{2+} antagonist. *Pharmacology* 61: 57–61, 2000
306 Mayhan WG and Heistad DD. Effect of flordipine on cerebral blood flow. *J Pharmacol Exp Ther* 235: 92–97, 1985
307 McDonald T, Pelzer D and Trautwein W. Dual action (stimulation, inhibition) of D600 on contractility and calcium channels in guinea-pig and cat heart cells. *J Physiol* 414: 569–586, 1989
308 McDonough SI and Bean BP. Mibefradil inhibition of T-type calcium channels in cerebellar purkinje neurons. *Mol Pharmacol* 54: 1080–1087, 1998
309 McDonough SI, Boland LM, Mintz IM and Bean BP. Interactions among toxins that inhibit N-type and P-type calcium channels. *J Gen Physiol* 119: 313–328, 2002
310 McEnery MW, Snowman AM, Sharp AH, Adams ME and Snyder SH. Purified omega-conotoxin GVIA receptor of rat brain resembles a dihydropyridine-sensitive L-type calcium channel. *Proc Natl Acad Sci USA* 88: 11095–11099, 1991
311 McNaughton NC, Hainsworth AH, Green PJ and Randall AD. Inhibition of recombinant low-voltage-activated Ca^{2+} channels by the neuroprotective agent BW619C89 (Sipatrigine). *Neuropharmacology* 39: 1247–1253, 2000
312 McNaughton NC, Warre R, Cooper DG, Nasir S, Ranson JL and Randall A. Potent inhibition of a recombinant low voltage-activated Ca^{2+} channel by SB-209712. *Eur J Pharmacol* 407: 53–60, 2000
313 McRory JE, Santi CM, Hamming KS, Mezeyova J, Sutton KG, Baillie DL, Stea A and Snutch TP. Molecular and functional characterization of a family of rat brain T-type calcium channels. *J Biol Chem* 276: 3999–4011, 2001

314 Meldrum BS. Glutamate as a neurotransmitter in the brain: review of physiology and pathology. *J Nutr* 130: 1007S–1015S, 2000
315 Micheli D, Ratti E, Toson G, Trist D and Gaviraghi G. Pharmacological profile of Taludipine GR-53992B, a new long-acting calcium entry blocker. *Br J Pharmacol* 100: 332p, 1990
316 Mignen O and Shuttleworth TJ. I(ARC), a novel arachidonate-regulated, noncapacitative Ca^{2+} entry channel. *J Biol Chem* 275: 9114–9119, 2000
317 Mignen O, Thompson JL and Shuttleworth TJ. Reciprocal regulation of capacitative and arachidonate-regulated noncapacitative Ca^{2+} entry pathways. *J Biol Chem* 276: 35676–35683, 2001
318 Mikami A, Imoto K, Tanabe T, Niidome T, Mori Y, Takeshima H, Narumiya S and Numa S. Primary structure and functional expression of the cardiac dihydropyridine-sensitive calcium channel. *Nature* 340: 230–233, 1989
319 Miljanich GP and Ramachandran J. Antagonists of neuronal calcium channels: structure, function, and therapeutic implications. *Annu Rev Pharmacol Toxicol* 35: 707–734, 1995
320 Minami J, Kawano Y, Makino Y, Matsuoka H and Takishita S. Effects of cilnidipine, a novel dihydropyridine calcium antagonist, on autonomic function, ambulatory blood pressure and heart rate in patients with essential hypertension. *Br J Clin Pharmacol* 50: 615–620, 2000
321 Mintz IM, Adams ME and Bean BP. P-type calcium channels in rat central and peripheral neurons. *Neuron* 9: 85–95, 1992
322 Mintz IM, Venema VJ, Swiderek KM, Lee TD, Bean BP and Adams ME. P-type calcium channels blocked by the spider toxin omega-Aga-IVA. *Nature* 355: 827–829, 1992
323 Mirkhani H, Omrani GR, Ghiaee S and Mahmoudian M. Effects of mebudipine and dibudipine, two new calcium-channel blockers, on rat left atrium, rat blood pressure and human internal mammary artery. *J Pharm Pharmacol* 51: 617–622, 1999
324 Mishra SK and Hermsmeyer K. Selective inhibition of T-type Ca^{2+} channels by Ro 40-5967. *Circ Res* 75: 144–148, 1994
325 Mitchell JW, Larsen JK and Best PM. Identification of the calcium channel alpha 1E (Ca(v)2.3) isoform expressed in atrial myocytes. *Biochim Biophys Acta* 1577: 17–26, 2002
326 Mitterdorfer J, Grabner M, Kraus RL, Hering S, Prinz H, Glossmann H and Striessnig J. Molecular basis of drug interaction with L-type Ca^{2+} channels. *J Bioenerg Biomembr* 30: 319–334, 1998
327 Mitterdorfer J, Sinnegger MJ, Grabner M, Striessnig J and Glossmann H. Coordination of Ca^{2+} by the pore region glutamates is essential for high-affinity dihydropyridine binding to the cardiac Ca^{2+} channel alpha 1 subunit. *Biochemistry* 34: 9350–9355, 1995
328 Mitterdorfer J, Wang Z, Sinnegger MJ, Hering S, Striessnig J, Grabner M and Glossmann H. Two amino acid residues in the IIIS5 segment of L-type calcium channels differentially contribute to 1,4-dihydropyridine sensitivity. *J Biol Chem* 271: 30330–30335, 1996
329 Mittman S, Guo J and Agnew WS. Structure and alternative splicing of the gene encoding alpha1G, a human brain T calcium channel alpha1 subunit. *Neurosci Lett* 274: 143–146, 1999
330 Mittman S, Guo J, Emerick MC and Agnew WS. Structure and alternative splicing of the gene encoding alpha1I, a human brain T calcium channel alpha1 subunit. *Neurosci Lett* 269: 121–124, 1999
331 Mochida S, Westenbroek RE, Yokoyama CT, Zhong H, Myers SJ, Scheuer T, Itoh K and Catterall WA. Requirement for the synaptic protein interaction site for reconstitution of synaptic transmission by P/Q-type calcium channels. *Proc Natl Acad Sci USA* 100: 2819–2824, 2003
332 Mochida S, Yokoyama CT, Kim DK, Itoh K and Catterall WA. Evidence for a voltage-dependent enhancement of neurotransmitter release mediated via the synaptic protein interaction site of N-type Ca^{2+} channels. *Proc Natl Acad Sci USA* 95: 14523–14528, 1998
333 Molderings GJ, Likungu J and Gothert M. N-Type calcium channels control sympathetic neurotransmission in human heart atrium. *Circulation* 101: 403–407, 2000
334 Molyvdas PA and Sperelakis N. Effects of calcium antagonistic drugs on the electrical activity of rabbit sino-atrial node. *Br J Pharmacol* 88: 249–258, 1986
335 Moneer Z and Taylor CW. Reciprocal regulation of capacitative and non-capacitative Ca^{2+} entry in A7r5 vascular smooth muscle cells: only the latter operates during receptor activation. *Biochem J* 362: 13–21, 2002
336 Monteil A, Chemin J, Bourinet E, Mennessier G, Lory P and Nargeot J. Molecular and functional properties of the human alpha(1G) subunit that forms T-type calcium channels. *J Biol Chem* 275: 6090–6100, 2000
337 Monteil A, Chemin J, Leuranguer V, Altier C, Mennessier G, Bourinet E, Lory P and Nargeot J. Specific properties of T-type calcium channels generated by the human alpha 1I subunit. *J Biol*

Chem 275: 16530–16535, 2000
338 Montell C, Birnbaumer L and Flockerzi V. The TRP channels, a remarkably functional family. *Cell* 108: 595–598, 2002
339 Montell C, Birnbaumer L, Flockerzi V, Bindels RJ, Bruford EA, Caterina MJ, Clapham DE, Harteneck C, Heller S, Julius D et al. A unified nomenclature for the superfamily of TRP cation channels. *Mol Cell* 9: 229–231, 2002
340 Morgans CW, Gaughwin P and Maleszka R. Expression of the alpha1F calcium channel subunit by photoreceptors in the rat retina. *Mol Vis* 7: 202–209, 2001
341 Mori Y, Friedrich T, Kim MS, Mikami A, Nakai J, Ruth P, Bosse E, Hofmann F, Flockerzi V, Furuichi T et al. Primary structure and functional expression from complementary DNA of a brain calcium channel. *Nature* 350: 398–402, 1991
342 Mori Y, Nishida M, Shimizu S, Ishii M, Yoshinaga T, Ino M, Sawada K and Niidome T. Ca^{2+} channel alpha(1B) subunit (Ca(V) 2.2) knockout mouse reveals a predominant role of N-type channels in the sympathetic regulation of the circulatory system. *Trends Cardiovasc Med* 12: 270–275, 2002
343 Morita H, Cousins H, Onoue H, Ito Y and Inoue R. Predominant distribution of nifedipine-insensitive, high voltage-activated Ca^{2+} channels in the terminal mesenteric artery of guinea pig. *Circ Res* 85: 596–605, 1999
344 Moulard B, Picard F, le Hellard S, Agulhon C, Weiland S, Favre I, Bertrand S, Malafosse A and Bertrand D. Ion channel variation causes epilepsies. *Brain Res Brain Res Rev* 36: 275–284, 2001
345 Mulryan K, Gitterman DP, Lewis CJ, Vial C, Leckie BJ, Cobb AL, Brown JE, Conley EC, Buell G, Pritchard CA and Evans RJ. Reduced vas deferens contraction and male infertility in mice lacking P2X1 receptors. *Nature* 403: 86–89, 2000
346 Murakami M, Nakagawasai O, Fujii S, Hosono M, Hozumi S, Esashi A, Taniguchi R, Okamura T, Suzuki T, Sasano H et al. Antinociceptive effect of cilnidipine, a novel N-type calcium channel antagonist. *Brain Res* 868: 123–127, 2000
347 Murbartian J, Arias JM, Lee JH, Gomora JC and Perez-Reyes E. Alternative splicing of the rat Ca(v)3.3 T-type calcium channel gene produces variants with distinct functional properties(1). *FEBS Lett* 528: 272–278, 2002
348 Murphy TH, Worley PF and Baraban JM. L-type voltage-sensitive calcium channels mediate synaptic activation of immediate early genes. *Neuron* 7: 625–635, 1991
349 Nakai J, Adams BA, Imoto K and Beam KG. Critical roles of the S3 segment and S3–S4 linker of repeat I in activation of L-type calcium channels. *Proc Natl Acad Sci USA* 91: 1014–1018, 1994
350 Nakajima O, Akioka H and Miyazaki M. Effect of the calcium antagonist benidipine hydrochloride on 24-h ambulatory blood pressure in patients with mild to moderate hypertension in a double-blind study against placebo. *Arzneimittelforschung* 50: 620–625, 2000
351 Nastainczyk W, Ludwig A and Hofmann F. The dihydropyridine-sensitive calcium channel of the skeletal muscle: biochemistry and structure. *Gen Physiol Biophys* 9: 321–329, 1990
352 Naylor MJ, Rancourt DE and Bech-Hansen NT. Isolation and characterization of a calcium channel gene, Cacna1f, the murine orthologue of the gene for incomplete X-linked congenital stationary night blindness. *Genomics* 66: 324–327, 2000
353 Neely A, Olcese R, Baldelli P, Wei X, Birnbaumer L and Stefani E. Dual activation of the cardiac Ca^{2+} channel alpha 1C-subunit and its modulation by the beta-subunit. *Am J Physiol* 268: C732–740, 1995
354 Neely A, Olcese R, Wei X, Birnbaumer L and Stefani E. Ca^{2+}-dependent inactivation of a cloned cardiac Ca^{2+} channel alpha 1 subunit (alpha 1C) expressed in *Xenopus* oocytes. *Biophys J* 66: 1895–1903, 1994
355 Neely A, Wei X, Olcese R, Birnbaumer L and Stefani E. Potentiation by the beta subunit of the ratio of the ionic current to the charge movement in the cardiac calcium channel. *Science* 262: 575–578, 1993
356 Newcomer JW and Krystal JH. NMDA receptor regulation of memory and behavior in humans. *Hippocampus* 11: 529–542, 2001
357 Nielsen KJ, Schroeder T and Lewis R. Structure-activity relationships of omega-conotoxins at N-type voltage-sensitive calcium channels. *J Mol Recognit* 13: 55–70, 2000
358 Niidome T, Kim MS, Friedrich T and Mori Y. Molecular cloning and characterization of a novel calcium channel from rabbit brain. *FEBS Lett* 308: 7–13, 1992
359 Nilius B, Hess P, Lansman JB and Tsien RW. A novel type of cardiac calcium channel in ventricular cells. *Nature* 316: 443–446, 1985

360 Nishikawa M, Gohda M, Shinyama H, Matzno S, Yamanaga K, Kido H and Nakamura N. Calcium channel blocking and vasodilating actions of the novel dihydropyridine derivative AE0047. *Clin Exp Pharmacol Physiol* 25: 347–354, 1998
361 Nishimura S, Takeshima H, Hofmann F, Flockerzi V and Imoto K. Requirement of the calcium channel beta subunit for functional conformation. *FEBS Lett* 324: 283–286, 1993
362 Nordberg A. Nicotinic receptor abnormalities of Alzheimer's disease: therapeutic implications. *Biol Psychiatry* 49: 200–210, 2001
363 Norenberg W and Illes P. Neuronal P2X receptors: localisation and functional properties. *Naunyn Schmiedebergs Arch Pharmacol* 362: 324–339, 2000
364 Normann C, Peckys D, Schulze CH, Walden J, Jonas P and Bischofberger J. Associative long-term depression in the hippocampus is dependent on postsynaptic N-type Ca^{2+} channels. *J Neurosci* 20: 8290–8297, 2000
365 North RA. Molecular physiology of P2X receptors. *Physiol Rev* 82: 1013–1067, 2002
366 Nowycky MC, Fox AP and Tsien RW. Three types of neuronal calcium channel with different calcium agonist sensitivity. *Nature* 316: 440–443, 1985
367 Ogasawara K, Noda A, Yasuda S, Kobayashi M, Yukawa H and Ogawa A. Effect of calcium antagonist on cerebral blood flow and oxygen metabolism in patients with hypertension and chronic major cerebral artery occlusion: a positron emission tomography study. *Nucl Med Commun* 24: 71–76, 2003
368 Olivera BM, McIntosh JM, Cruz LJ, Luque FA and Gray WR. Purification and sequence of a presynaptic peptide toxin from *Conus geographus* venom. *Biochemistry* 23: 5087–5090, 1984
369 Olivier B, van Wijngaarden I and Soudijn W. 5-HT(3) receptor antagonists and anxiety; a preclinical and clinical review. *Eur Neuropsychopharmacol* 10: 77–95, 2000
370 Ostergren J, Isaksson H, Brodin U, Schwan A and Ohman KP. Effect of amlodipine *versus* felodipine extended release on 24-hour ambulatory blood pressure in hypertension. *Am J Hypertens* 11: 690–696, 1998
371 Oury C, Toth-Zsamboki E, Van Geet C, Thys C, Wei L, Nilius B, Vermylen J and Hoylaerts MF. A natural dominant negative P2X1 receptor due to deletion of a single amino acid residue. *J Biol Chem* 275: 22611–22614, 2000
372 Pan JQ and Lipscombe D. Alternative splicing in the cytoplasmic II-III loop of the N-type Ca channel alpha 1B subunit: functional differences are beta subunit-specific. *J Neurosci* 20: 4769–4775, 2000
373 Pan ZH, Hu HJ, Perring P and Andrade R. T-type Ca^{2+} channels mediate neurotransmitter release in retinal bipolar cells. *Neuron* 32: 89–98, 2001
374 Parekh AB, Terlau H and Stuhmer W. Depletion of InsP3 stores activates a Ca^{2+} and K^+ current by means of a phosphatase and a diffusible messenger. *Nature* 364: 814–818, 1993
375 Parsons CG. NMDA receptors as targets for drug action in neuropathic pain. *Eur J Pharmacol* 429: 71–78, 2001
376 Paterson D and Nordberg A. Neuronal nicotinic receptors in the human brain. *Prog Neurobiol* 61: 75–111, 2000
377 Patterson RL, van Rossum DB and Gill DL. Store-operated Ca^{2+} entry: evidence for a secretion-like coupling model. *Cell* 98: 487–499, 1999
378 Pelzer S, Barhanin J, Pauron D, Trautwein W, Lazdunski M and Pelzer D. Diversity and novel pharmacological properties of Ca^{2+} channels in *Drosophila* brain membranes. *Embo J* 8: 2365–2371, 1989
379 Pemberton KE, Hill-Eubanks LJ and Jones SV. Modulation of low-threshold T-type calcium channels by the five muscarinic receptor subtypes in NIH 3 T3 cells. *Pflugers Arch* 440: 452–461, 2000
380 Pepine CJ, Cooper-DeHoff RM, Weiss RJ, Koren M, Bittar N, Thadani U, Minkwitz MC, Michelson EL and Hutchinson HG. Comparison of effects of nisoldipine-extended release and amlodipine in patients with systemic hypertension and chronic stable angina pectoris. *Am J Cardiol* 91: 274–279, 2003
381 Perchenet L, Bénardeau A and Ertel EA. Pharmacological properties of Ca(V)3.2, a low voltage-activated Ca^{2+} channel cloned from human heart. *Naunyn Schmiedebergs Arch Pharmacol* 361: 590–599, 2000
382 Pereverzev A, Mikhna M, Vajna R, Gissel C, Henry M, Weiergraber M, Hescheler J, Smyth N and Schneider T. Disturbances in glucose-tolerance, insulin-release, and stress-induced hyperglycemia upon disruption of the Ca(v)2.3 (alpha1E) subunit of voltage-gated Ca^{2+} channels. *Mol Endocrinol* 16: 884–895, 2002

383 Pereverzev A, Vajna R, Pfitzer G, Hescheler J, Klockner U and Schneider T. Reduction of insulin secretion in the insulinoma cell line INS-1 by over-expression of a $Ca_V2.3$ (alpha1E) calcium channel antisense cassette. *Eur J Endocrinol* 146: 881–889, 2002
384 Perez-Reyes E. Three for T: molecular analysis of the low voltage-activated calcium channel family. *Cell Mol Life Sci* 56: 660–669, 1999
385 Perez-Reyes E, Castellano A, Kim HS, Bertrand P, Baggstrom E, Lacerda AE, Wei XY and Birnbaumer L. Cloning and expression of a cardiac/brain beta subunit of the L-type calcium channel. *J Biol Chem* 267: 1792–1797, 1992
386 Perez-Reyes E, Cribbs LL, Daud A, Lacerda AE, Barclay J, Williamson MP, Fox M, Rees M and Lee JH. Molecular characterization of a neuronal low-voltage-activated T-type calcium channel. *Nature* 391: 896–900, 1998
387 Perez-Reyes E, Wei XY, Castellano A and Birnbaumer L. Molecular diversity of L-type calcium channels. Evidence for alternative splicing of the transcripts of three non-allelic genes. *J Biol Chem* 265: 20430–20436, 1990
388 Perry EK, Martin-Ruiz CM and Court JA. Nicotinic receptor subtypes in human brain related to aging and dementia. *Alcohol* 24: 63–68, 2001
389 Petersen CC, Berridge MJ, Borgese MF and Bennett DL. Putative capacitative calcium entry channels: expression of *Drosophila* trp and evidence for the existence of vertebrate homologues. *Biochem J* 311 (Pt 1): 41–44, 1995
390 Peterson BZ, DeMaria CD, Adelman JP and Yue DT. Calmodulin is the Ca^{2+} sensor for Ca^{2+}-dependent inactivation of L-type calcium channels. *Neuron* 22: 549–558, 1999
391 Petit-Jacques J and Hartzell HC. Effect of arachidonic acid on the L-type calcium current in frog cardiac myocytes. *J Physiol* 493 (Pt 1): 67–81, 1996
392 Philipp S, Trost C, Warnat J, Rautmann J, Himmerkus N, Schroth G, Kretz O, Nastainczyk W, Cavalie A, Hoth M and Flockerzi V. TRP4 (CCE1) protein is part of native calcium release-activated Ca^{2+}-like channels in adrenal cells. *J Biol Chem* 275: 23965–23972, 2000
393 Phillips AM, Bull A and Kelly LE. Identification of a *Drosophila* gene encoding a calmodulin-binding protein with homology to the trp phototransduction gene. *Neuron* 8: 631–642, 1992
394 Picciotto MR, Caldarone BJ, Brunzell DH, Zachariou V, Stevens TR and King SL. Neuronal nicotinic acetylcholine receptor subunit knockout mice: physiological and behavioral phenotypes and possible clinical implications. *Pharmacol Ther* 92: 89–108, 2001
395 Pichler M, Cassidy TN, Reimer D, Haase H, Kraus R, Ostler D and Striessnig J. Beta subunit heterogeneity in neuronal L-type Ca^{2+} channels. *J Biol Chem* 272: 13877–13882, 1997
396 Piedras-Renteria ES, Chen CC and Best PM. Antisense oligonucleotides against rat brain alpha1E DNA and its atrial homologue decrease T-type calcium current in atrial myocytes. *Proc Natl Acad Sci USA* 94: 14936–14941, 1997
397 Placantonakis D and Welsh J. Two distinct oscillatory states determined by the NMDA receptor in rat inferior olive. *J Physiol* 534: 123–140, 2001
398 Plomp JJ, van den Maagdenberg AM, Molenaar PC, Frants RR and Ferrari MD. Mutant P/Q-type calcium channel electrophysiology and migraine. *Curr Opin Investig Drugs* 2: 1250–1260, 2001
399 Plummer MR, Logothetis DE and Hess P. Elementary properties and pharmacological sensitivities of calcium channels in mammalian peripheral neurons. *Neuron* 2: 1453–1463, 1989
400 Porcello DM, Smith SD and Huguenard JR. Actions of U-92032, a T-type Ca^{2+} channel antagonist, support a functional linkage between I(T) and slow intrathalamic rhythms. *J Neurophysiol* 89: 177–185, 2003
401 Pragnell M, De Waard M, Mori Y, Tanabe T, Snutch TP and Campbell KP. Calcium channel beta-subunit binds to a conserved motif in the I-II cytoplasmic linker of the alpha 1-subunit. *Nature* 368: 67–70, 1994
402 Protas L and Robinson RB. Mibefradil, an I(Ca,T) blocker, effectively blocks I(Ca,L) in rabbit sinus node cells. *Eur J Pharmacol* 401: 27–30, 2000
403 Pruneau D, Roy F and Brown NL. Cardiovascular properties of LF 2.0254, a new potent vasoselective calcium channel blocker with a slow onset of action. *Fundam Clin Pharmacol* 4: 223–243, 1990
404 Putney JW, Jr, A model for receptor-regulated calcium entry. *Cell Calcium* 7: 1–12, 1986
405 Putney JW, Jr, Broad LM, Braun FJ, Lievremont JP and Bird GS. Mechanisms of capacitative calcium entry. *J Cell Sci* 114: 2223–2229, 2001
406 Qin N, Olcese R, Bransby M, Lin T and Birnbaumer L. Ca^{2+}-induced inhibition of the cardiac Ca^{2+} channel depends on calmodulin. *Proc Natl Acad Sci USA* 96: 2435–2438, 1999

407 Qin N, Yagel S, Momplaisir ML, Codd EE and D'Andrea MR. Molecular cloning and characterization of the human voltage-gated calcium channel alpha(2)delta-4 subunit. *Mol Pharmacol* 62: 485–496, 2002
408 Ralevic V. The involvement of smooth muscle P2X receptors in the prolonged vasorelaxation response to purine nucleotides in the rat mesenteric arterial bed. *Br J Pharmacol* 135: 1988–1994, 2002
409 Raman IM and Bean BP. Ionic currents underlying spontaneous action potentials in isolated cerebellar Purkinje neurons. *J Neurosci* 19: 1663–1674, 1999
410 Rampe D and Triggle DJ. New synthetic ligands for L-type voltage-gated calcium channels. *Prog Drug Res* 40: 191–238, 1993
411 Randall A and Tsien RW. Pharmacological dissection of multiple types of Ca^{2+} channel currents in rat cerebellar granule neurons. *J Neurosci* 15: 2995–3012, 1995
412 Randall AD and Tsien RW. Contrasting biophysical and pharmacological properties of T-type and R-type calcium channels. *Neuropharmacology* 36: 879–893, 1997
413 Randle JC, Peglion JL and Renaud JF. Inhibition of L-type but not T-type calcium channel current by a new dihydropyridine derivative, S11568. *J Cardiovasc Pharmacol* 17: 348–350, 1991
414 Randriamampita C and Tsien RY. Emptying of intracellular Ca^{2+} stores releases a novel small messenger that stimulates Ca^{2+} influx. *Nature* 364: 809–814, 1993
415 Regan LJ, Sah DW and Bean BP. Ca^{2+} channels in rat central and peripheral neurons: high-threshold current resistant to dihydropyridine blockers and omega-conotoxin. *Neuron* 6: 269–280, 1991
416 Ren D and Hall LM. Functional expression and characterization of skeletal muscle dihydropyridine receptors in *Xenopus* oocytes. *J Biol Chem* 272: 22393–22396, 1997
417 Rettig J, Heinemann C, Ashery U, Sheng ZH, Yokoyama CT, Catterall WA and Neher E. Alteration of Ca^{2+} dependence of neurotransmitter release by disruption of Ca^{2+} channel/syntaxin interaction. *J Neurosci* 17: 6647–6656, 1997
418 Rettig J, Sheng ZH, Kim DK, Hodson CD, Snutch TP and Catterall WA. Isoform-specific interaction of the alpha1A subunits of brain Ca^{2+} channels with the presynaptic proteins syntaxin and SNAP-25. *Proc Natl Acad Sci USA* 93: 7363–7368, 1996
419 Reuter H. The dependence of slow inward current in Purkinje fibres on the extracellular calcium-concentration. *J Physiol* 192: 479–492, 1967
420 Reuter H. Divalent cations as charge carriers in excitable membranes. *Prog Biophys Mol Biol* 26: 1–43, 1973
421 Ringer S. A further contribution regarding the influence of different constituents of the blood on the contraction of the heart. *J Physiol (London)*: 29–43, 1883
422 Rizzuto R, Bernardi P and Pozzan T. Mitochondria as all-round players of the calcium game. *J Physiol* 529 Pt 1: 37–47, 2000
423 Rorsman P, Ashcroft FM and Trube G. Single Ca channel currents in mouse pancreatic B-cells. *Pflugers Arch* 412: 597–603, 1988
424 Rosenthal J, Hittel N and Stumpe KO. Pranidipine, a novel calcium antagonist, once daily, for the treatment of hypertension: a multicenter, double-blind, placebo-controlled dose-finding study. *Cardiovasc Drugs Ther* 10: 59–66, 1996
425 Rossier MF, Burnay MM and Capponi AM. Distinct functions of T- and L-type calcium channels during activation of aldosterone production in adrenal glomerulosa cells. In: *Low-voltage-activated T-type Ca channels*, edited by Tsien RW, Clozel J-P and Nargeot J. Chester, UK: Adis International, 1998, p. 176–185
426 Rossier MF, Burnay MM, Maturana A and Capponi AM. Duality of the voltage-dependent calcium influx in adrenal glomerulosa cells. *Endocr Res* 24: 443–447, 1998
427 Rougier O, Vassort G, Garnier D, Gargouil YM and Coraboeuf E. Existence and role of a slow inward current during the frog atrial action potential. *Pflugers Arch* 308: 91–110, 1969
428 Ruscheweyh R and Sandkuhler J. Role of kainate receptors in nociception. *Brain Res Brain Res Rev* 40: 215–222, 2002
429 Ruth P, Rohrkasten A, Biel M, Bosse E, Regulla S, Meyer HE, Flockerzi V and Hofmann F. Primary structure of the beta subunit of the DHP-sensitive calcium channel from skeletal muscle. *Science* 245: 1115–1118, 1989
430 Saegusa H, Kurihara T, Zong S, Kazuno A, Matsuda Y, Nonaka T, Han W, Toriyama H and Tanabe T. Suppression of inflammatory and neuropathic pain symptoms in mice lacking the N-type Ca^{2+} channel. *Embo J* 20: 2349–2356, 2001

431 Salami M and Fathollahi Y. Do Ca^{2+} channels share NMDA receptors in plasticity of synaptic transmission in the rat visual cortex? *Neuroreport* 11: 3887–3891, 2000
432 Sandmann S, Claas R, Cleutjens JP, Daemen MJ and Unger T. Calcium channel blockade limits cardiac remodeling and improves cardiac function in myocardial infarction-induced heart failure in rats. *J Cardiovasc Pharmacol* 37: 64–77, 2001
433 Sanguinetti MC and Kass RS. Voltage-dependent block of calcium channel current in the calf cardiac Purkinje fiber by dihydropyridine calcium channel antagonists. *Circ Res* 55: 336–348, 1984
434 Sasaki J, Kajiyama G, Kusukawa R, Shichiri M, Sunaga T, Mashiba H, Tanaka N, Nonaka K and Arakawa K. Effects of a new calcium channel blocker, MPC-1304, on blood pressure, serum lipoproteins and serum carbohydrate metabolism in patients with essential hypertension. *Int J Clin Pharmacol Ther* 33: 366–370, 1995
435 Sather WA, Tanabe T, Zhang JF, Mori Y, Adams ME and Tsien RW. Distinctive biophysical and pharmacological properties of class A (BI) calcium channel alpha 1 subunits. *Neuron* 11: 291–303, 1993
436 Schneider T, Wei X, Olcese R, Costantin JL, Neely A, Palade P, Perez-Reyes E, Qin N, Zhou J, Crawford GD et al. Molecular analysis and functional expression of the human type E neuronal Ca^{2+} channel alpha 1 subunit. *Receptors Channels* 2: 255–270, 1994
437 Schramm M, Vajna R, Pereverzev A, Tottene A, Klockner U, Pietrobon D, Hescheler J and Schneider T. Isoforms of alpha1E voltage-gated calcium channels in rat cerebellar granule cells —detection of major calcium channel alpha1-transcripts by reverse transcription-polymerase chain reaction. *Neuroscience* 92: 565–575, 1999
438 Scognamiglio R, Nosadini R, Marin M, Nisti S, Fasoli G, Palisi M, Frigato F, Virgili F, Carraro A and Crepaldi G. Evaluation of the efficacy and tolerability of nitrendipine in reducing both pressure and left ventricular mass in hypertensive type 2 diabetic patients. *Diabetes Care* 20: 1290–1292, 1997
439 Scott VE, De Waard M, Liu H, Gurnett CA, Venzke DP, Lennon VA and Campbell KP. Beta subunit heterogeneity in N-type Ca^{2+} channels. *J Biol Chem* 271: 3207–3212, 1996
440 Seagar MJ, Takahashi M and Catterall WA. Molecular properties of dihydropyridine-sensitive calcium channels. *Ann NY Acad Sci* 522: 162–175, 1988
441 Seino S, Chen L, Seino M, Blondel O, Takeda J, Johnson JH and Bell GI. Cloning of the alpha 1 subunit of a voltage-dependent calcium channel expressed in pancreatic beta cells. *Proc Natl Acad Sci USA* 89: 584–588, 1992
442 Serysheva, II, Ludtke SJ, Baker MR, Chiu W and Hamilton SL. Structure of the voltage-gated L-type Ca^{2+} channel by electron cryomicroscopy. *Proc Natl Acad Sci USA* 99: 10370–10375, 2002
443 Shannon JR, Jordan J, Black BK, Costa F and Robertson D. Uncoupling of the baroreflex by N(N)-cholinergic blockade in dissecting the components of cardiovascular regulation. *Hypertension* 32: 101–107, 1998
444 Sheng ZH, Rettig J, Takahashi M and Catterall WA. Identification of a syntaxin-binding site on N-type calcium channels. *Neuron* 13: 1303–1313, 1994
445 Sheng ZH, Yokoyama CT and Catterall WA. Interaction of the synprint site of N-type Ca^{2+} channels with the C2B domain of synaptotagmin I. *Proc Natl Acad Sci USA* 94: 5405–5410, 1997
446 Shuttleworth TJ. Arachidonic acid activates the non-capacitative entry of Ca^{2+} during $[Ca^{2+}]_i$ oscillations. *J Biol Chem* 271: 21720–21725, 1996
447 Shuttleworth TJ. What drives calcium entry during $[Ca^{2+}]_i$ oscillations?—challenging the capacitative model. *Cell Calcium* 25: 237–246, 1999
448 Shuttleworth TJ and Thompson JL. Discriminating between capacitative and arachidonate-activated Ca^{2+} entry pathways in HEK293 cells. *J Biol Chem* 274: 31174–31178, 1999
449 Shuttleworth TJ and Thompson JL. Muscarinic receptor activation of arachidonate-mediated Ca^{2+} entry in HEK293 cells is independent of phospholipase C. *J Biol Chem* 273: 32636–32643, 1998
450 Sidach SS and Mintz IM. Kurtoxin, a gating modifier of neuronal high- and low-threshold ca channels. *J Neurosci* 22: 2023–2034, 2002
451 Silke B, de la Motte S, Spiers P, Herity NA, Drake M, Kelly J and Harrison FJ. Hemodynamic effects of intravenous elgodipine in coronary artery disease during rest and exercise, and basic pharmacokinetic parameters. *Cardiovasc Drugs Ther* 10: 573–580, 1996
452 Sinnegger MJ, Wang Z, Grabner M, Hering S, Striessnig J, Glossmann H and Mitterdorfer J. Nine L-type amino acid residues confer full 1,4-dihydropyridine sensitivity to the neuronal calcium channel alpha1A subunit. Role of L-type Met1188. *J Biol Chem* 272: 27686–27693, 1997
453 Slish DF, Engle DB, Varadi G, Lotan I, Singer D, Dascal N and Schwartz A. Evidence for the

existence of a cardiac specific isoform of the alpha 1 subunit of the voltage dependent calcium channel. *FEBS Lett* 250: 509–514, 1989
454 Smith MT, Cabot PJ, Ross FB, Robertson AD and Lewis RJ. The novel N-type calcium channel blocker, AM336, produces potent dose-dependent antinociception after intrathecal dosing in rats and inhibits substance P release in rat spinal cord slices. *Pain* 96: 119–127, 2002
455 Sneddon P. Electrophysiology of autonomic neuromuscular transmission involving ATP. *J Auton Nerv Syst* 81: 218–224, 2000
456 Snutch TP and Reiner PB. Ca^{2+} channels: diversity of form and function. *Curr Opin Neurobiol* 2: 247–253, 1992
457 Sohal VS and Huguenard JR. It takes T to tango. *Neuron* 31: 3–4, 2001
458 Soldatov NM, Zuhlke RD, Bouron A and Reuter H. Molecular structures involved in L-type calcium channel inactivation. Role of the carboxyl-terminal region encoded by exons 40–42 in alpha1C subunit in the kinetics and Ca^{2+} dependence of inactivation. *J Biol Chem* 272: 3560–3566, 1997
459 Solle M, Labasi J, Perregaux DG, Stam E, Petrushova N, Koller BH, Griffiths RJ and Gabel CA. Altered cytokine production in mice lacking P2X(7) receptors. *J Biol Chem* 276: 125–132, 2001
460 Son WY, Han CT, Lee JH, Jung KY, Lee HM and Choo YK. Developmental expression patterns of alpha1H T-type Ca^{2+} channels during spermatogenesis and organogenesis in mice. *Dev Growth Differ* 44: 181–190, 2002
461 Soong TW, DeMaria CD, Alvania RS, Zweifel LS, Liang MC, Mittman S, Agnew WS and Yue DT. Systematic identification of splice variants in human P/Q-type channel alpha1(2.1) subunits: implications for current density and Ca^{2+}-dependent inactivation. *J Neurosci* 22: 10142–10152, 2002
462 Soong TW, Stea A, Hodson CD, Dubel SJ, Vincent SR and Snutch TP. Structure and functional expression of a member of the low voltage-activated calcium channel family. *Science* 260: 1133–1136, 1993
463 Sorrentino V and Rizzuto R. Molecular genetics of Ca^{2+} stores and intracellular Ca^{2+} signaling. *Trends Pharmacol Sci* 22: 459–464, 2001
464 Spath M. Current experience with 5-HT3 receptor antagonists in fibromyalgia. *Rheum Dis Clin North Am* 28: 319–328, 2002
465 Spedding M and Paoletti R. Classification of calcium channels and calcium antagonists: progress report. *Cardiovasc Drugs Ther* 6: 35–39, 1992
466 Spedding M and Paoletti R. Classification of calcium channels and the sites of action of drugs modifying channel function. *Pharmacol Rev* 44: 363–376, 1992
467 Spedding M and Vanhoutte PM. Nomenclature of calcium channels and channel modulators: IUPHAR classification. *J Cardiovasc Pharmacol* 22: 906, 1993
468 Sperelakis N. Properties of calcium channels in cardiac muscle and vascular smooth muscle. *Mol Cell Biochem* 99: 97–109, 1990
469 Stahl JS. Calcium channelopathy mutants and their role in ocular motor research. *Ann NY Acad Sci* 956: 64–74, 2002
470 Starmer CF and Grant AO. Phasic ion channel blockade. A kinetic model and parameter estimation procedure. *Mol Pharmacol* 28: 348–356, 1985
471 Starr TV, Prystay W and Snutch TP. Primary structure of a calcium channel that is highly expressed in the rat cerebellum. *Proc Natl Acad Sci USA* 88: 5621–5625, 1991
472 Stea A, Tomlinson WJ, Soong TW, Bourinet E, Dubel SJ, Vincent SR and Snutch TP. Localization and functional properties of a rat brain alpha 1A calcium channel reflect similarities to neuronal Q- and P-type channels. *Proc Natl Acad Sci USA* 91: 10576–10580, 1994
473 Stengel W, Jainz M and Andreas K. Different potencies of dihydropyridine derivatives in blocking T-type but not L-type Ca^{2+} channels in neuroblastoma-glioma hybrid cells. *Eur J Pharmacol* 342: 339–345, 1998
474 Stephens GJ, Page KM, Burley JR, Berrow NS and Dolphin AC. Functional expression of rat brain cloned alpha1E calcium channels in COS-7 cells. *Pflugers Arch* 433: 523–532, 1997
475 Striessnig J. Pharmacology, structure and function of cardiac L-type Ca^{2+} channels. *Cell Physiol Biochem* 9: 242–269, 1999
476 Striessnig J, Grabner M, Mitterdorfer J, Hering S, Sinnegger MJ and Glossmann H. Structural basis of drug binding to L Ca^{2+} channels. *Trends Pharmacol Sci* 19: 108–115, 1998
477 Strom TM, Nyakatura G, Apfelstedt-Sylla E, Hellebrand H, Lorenz B, Weber BH, Wutz K, Gutwillinger N, Ruther K, Drescher B et al. An L-type calcium-channel gene mutated in incomplete X-linked congenital stationary night blindness. *Nat Genet* 19: 260–263, 1998

478 Strong M, Chandy KG and Gutman GA. Molecular evolution of voltage-sensitive ion channel genes: on the origins of electrical excitability. *Mol Biol Evol* 10: 221–242, 1993
479 Strong M and Gutman GA. Missing link in ion channels. *Nature* 362: 26, 1993
480 Stutzin A, Stojilkovic SS, Catt KJ and Rojas E. Characteristics of two types of calcium channels in rat pituitary gonadotrophs. *Am J Physiol* 257: C865–874, 1989
481 Su H, Sochivko D, Becker A, Chen J, Jiang Y, Yaari Y and Beck H. Upregulation of a T-type Ca^{2+} channel causes a long-lasting modification of neuronal firing mode after status epilepticus. *J Neurosci* 22: 3645–3655, 2002
482 Sugawara H, Kurosaki M, Takata M and Kurosaki T. Genetic evidence for involvement of type 1, type 2 and type 3 inositol 1,4,5-trisphosphate receptors in signal transduction through the B-cell antigen receptor. *Embo J* 16: 3078–3088, 1997
483 Sutor B and Zolles G. Neuronal nicotinic acetylcholine receptors and autosomal dominant nocturnal frontal lobe epilepsy: a critical review. *Pflugers Arch* 442: 642–651, 2001
484 Sutton KG, McRory JE, Guthrie H, Murphy TH and Snutch TP. P/Q-type calcium channels mediate the activity-dependent feedback of syntaxin-1A. *Nature* 401: 800–804, 1999
485 Takahashi M, Seagar MJ, Jones JF, Reber BF and Catterall WA. Subunit structure of dihydropyridine-sensitive calcium channels from skeletal muscle. *Proc Natl Acad Sci USA* 84: 5478–5482, 1987
486 Takahashi SX, Mittman S and Colecraft HM. Distinctive modulatory effects of five human auxiliary beta(2) subunit splice variants on L-type calcium channel gating. *Biophys J* 84: 3007–3021, 2003
487 Takamori M, Maruta T and Komai K. Lambert-Eaton myasthenic syndrome as an autoimmune calcium-channelopathy. *Neurosci Res* 36: 183–191, 2000
488 Tanabe T, Beam KG, Adams BA, Niidome T and Numa S. Regions of the skeletal muscle dihydropyridine receptor critical for excitation-contraction coupling. *Nature* 346: 567–569, 1990
489 Tanabe T, Beam KG, Powell JA and Numa S. Restoration of excitation-contraction coupling and slow calcium current in dysgenic muscle by dihydropyridine receptor complementary DNA. *Nature* 336: 134–139, 1988
490 Tanabe T, Mikami A, Numa S and Beam KG. Cardiac-type excitation-contraction coupling in dysgenic skeletal muscle injected with cardiac dihydropyridine receptor cDNA. *Nature* 344: 451–453, 1990
491 Tanabe T, Takeshima H, Mikami A, Flockerzi V, Takahashi H, Kangawa K, Kojima M, Matsuo H, Hirose T and Numa S. Primary structure of the receptor for calcium channel blockers from skeletal muscle. *Nature* 328: 313–318, 1987
492 Tanaka H and Shigenobu K. Efonidipine hydrochloride: a dual blocker of L- and T-type Ca^{2+} channels. *Cardiovasc Drug Rev* 20: 81–92, 2002
493 Tang S, Yatani A, Bahinski A, Mori Y and Schwartz A. Molecular localization of regions in the L-type calcium channel critical for dihydropyridine action. *Neuron* 11: 1013–1021, 1993
494 Taraskevich PS and Douglas WW. Action potentials occur in cells of the normal anterior pituitary gland and are stimulated by the hypophysiotropic peptide thyrotropin-releasing hormone. *Proc Natl Acad Sci USA* 74: 4064–4067, 1977
495 Tareilus E, Roux M, Qin N, Olcese R, Zhou J, Stefani E and Birnbaumer L. A *Xenopus* oocyte beta subunit: evidence for a role in the assembly/expression of voltage-gated calcium channels that is separate from its role as a regulatory subunit. *Proc Natl Acad Sci USA* 94: 1703–1708, 1997
496 Tassonyi E, Charpantier E, Muller D, Dumont L and Bertrand D. The role of nicotinic acetylcholine receptors in the mechanisms of anesthesia. *Brain Res Bull* 57: 133–150, 2002
497 Teramoto T, Niidome T, Miyagawa T, Nishizawa Y, Katayama K and Sawada K. Two types of calcium channels sensitive to omega-agatoxin- TK in cultured rat hippocampal neurones. *Neuroreport* 6: 1684–1688, 1995
498 Thastrup O, Cullen PJ, Drobak BK, Hanley MR and Dawson AP. Thapsigargin, a tumor promoter, discharges intracellular Ca^{2+} stores by specific inhibition of the endoplasmic reticulum Ca^{2+}-ATPase. *Proc Natl Acad Sci USA* 87: 2466–2470, 1990
499 Tobi D, Wiser O, Trus M and Atlas D. N-type voltage-sensitive calcium channel interacts with syntaxin, synaptotagmin and SNAP-25 in a multiprotein complex. *Receptors Channels* 6: 89–98, 1998
500 Todorovic SM, Jevtovic-Todorovic V, Mennerick S, Perez-Reyes E and Zorumski CF. Ca(v)3.2 channel is a molecular substrate for inhibition of T-type calcium currents in rat sensory neurons by nitrous oxide. *Mol Pharmacol* 60: 603–610, 2001

501 Tottene A, Moretti A and Pietrobon D. Functional diversity of P-type and R-type calcium channels in rat cerebellar neurons. *J Neurosci* 16: 6353–6363, 1996
502 Tottene A, Volsen S and Pietrobon D. alpha(1E) subunits form the pore of three cerebellar R-type calcium channels with different pharmacological and permeation properties. *J Neurosci* 20: 171–178, 2000
503 Trepakova ES, Csutora P, Hunton DL, Marchase RB, Cohen RA and Bolotina VM. Calcium influx factor directly activates store-operated cation channels in vascular smooth muscle cells. *J Biol Chem* 275: 26158–26163, 2000
504 Triggle DJ. Calcium, calcium channels, and calcium channel antagonists. *Can J Physiol Pharmacol* 68: 1474–1481, 1990
505 Tsien RW, Ellinor PT and Horne WA. Molecular diversity of voltage-dependent Ca^{2+} channels. *Trends Pharmacol Sci* 12: 349–354, 1991
506 Tsien RW, Fox AP, Hess P, McCleskey EW, Nilius B, Nowycky MC and Rosenberg RL. Multiple types of calcium channel in excitable cells. *Soc Gen Physiol Ser* 41: 167–187, 1987
507 Tuana BS and Murphy BJ. Biochemical analysis of L-type calcium channels from skeletal and cardiac muscle. *Can J Physiol Pharmacol* 68: 1482–1488, 1990
508 Uchitel OD, Protti DA, Sanchez V, Cherksey BD, Sugimori M and Llinas R. P-type voltage-dependent calcium channel mediates presynaptic calcium influx and transmitter release in mammalian synapses. *Proc Natl Acad Sci USA* 89: 3330–3333, 1992
509 Uehara A and Hume JR. Interactions of organic calcium channel antagonists with calcium channels in single frog atrial cells. *J Gen Physiol* 85: 621–647, 1985
510 Ukena D, Boewer C, Oldenkott B, Rathgeb F, Wurst W, Zech K and Sybrecht GW. Tolerance, safety, and kinetics of the new antineoplastic compound dexniguldipine-HCl after oral administration: a phase I dose-escalation trial. *Cancer Chemother Pharmacol* 36: 160–164, 1995
511 Vaca L, Sinkins WG, Hu Y, Kunze DL and Schilling WP. Activation of recombinant trp by thapsigargin in Sf9 insect cells. *Am J Physiol* 267: C1501–1505, 1994
512 van der Lee R, Pfaffendorf M and van Zwieten PA. The differential time courses of the vasodilator effects of various 1,4-dihydropyridines in isolated human small arteries are correlated to their lipophilicity. *J Hypertens* 18: 1677–1682, 2000
513 van Hooft JA and Vijverberg HP. 5-HT(3) receptors and neurotransmitter release in the CNS: a nerve ending story? *Trends Neurosci* 23: 605–610, 2000
514 Vance CL, Begg CM, Lee WL, Haase H, Copeland TD and McEnery MW. Differential expression and association of calcium channel alpha1B and beta subunits during rat brain ontogeny. *J Biol Chem* 273: 14495–14502, 1998
515 Vanegas H and Schaible H. Effects of antagonists to high-threshold calcium channels upon spinal mechanisms of pain, hyperalgesia and allodynia. *Pain* 85: 9–18, 2000
516 Vanhoutte PM, Barnard EA, Cosmides GJ, Humphrey PP, Spedding M and Godfraind T. International Union of Pharmacology Committee on Receptor Nomenclature and Drug Classification. *Pharmacol Rev* 46: 111–116, 1994
517 Vassort G. Adenosine 5'-triphosphate: a P2-purinergic agonist in the myocardium. *Physiol Rev* 81: 767–806, 2001
518 Velena AH, Dubur GJ, Vitolina RO, Kimenis AA, Selga MJ, Zarinsh GV, Narusevicius EV, Macianskiene RA, Gendviliene VI and Simkhovich BZ. Effect of ryodipine on electromechanical parameters of heart and vessels, cAMP phosphodiesterase activity and swelling-contraction cycle of mitochondria. *Arzneimittelforschung* 35: 907–914, 1985
519 Vennekens R, Hoenderop JG, Prenen J, Stuiver M, Willems PH, Droogmans G, Nilius B and Bindels RJ. Permeation and gating properties of the novel epithelial Ca^{2+} channel. *J Biol Chem* 275: 3963–3969, 2000
520 Vennekens R, Voets T, Bindels RJ, Droogmans G and Nilius B. Current understanding of mammalian TRP homologues. *Cell Calcium* 31: 253–264, 2002
521 Viana F, Van den Bosch L, Missiaen L, Vandenberghe W, Droogmans G, Nilius B and Robberecht W. Mibefradil (Ro 40-5967) blocks multiple types of voltage-gated calcium channels in cultured rat spinal motoneurones. *Cell Calcium* 22: 299–311, 1997
522 Voets T, Prenen J, Fleig A, Vennekens R, Watanabe H, Hoenderop JG, Bindels RJ, Droogmans G, Penner R and Nilius B. CaT1 and the calcium release-activated calcium channel manifest distinct pore properties. *J Biol Chem* 276: 47767–47770, 2001
523 Volsen SG, Day NC, McCormack AL, Smith W, Craig PJ, Beattie RE, Smith D, Ince PG, Shaw PJ, Ellis SB et al. The expression of voltage-dependent calcium channel beta subunits in human cerebellum. *Neuroscience* 80: 161–174, 1997

524 Wakamori M, Niidome T, Furutama D, Furuichi T, Mikoshiba K, Fujita Y, Tanaka I, Katayama K, Yatani A, Schwartz A et al. Distinctive functional properties of the neuronal BII (class E) calcium channel. *Receptors Channels* 2: 303–314, 1994
525 Waki M, Sugiyama T, Watanabe N, Ogawa T, Shirahase H and Azuma I. Effect of topically applied iganidipine dihydrochloride, a novel calcium antagonist, on optic nerve head circulation in rabbits. *Jpn J Ophthalmol* 45: 76–83, 2001
526 Walker D and De Waard M. Subunit interaction sites in voltage-dependent Ca^{2+} channels: role in channel function. *Trends Neurosci* 21: 148–154, 1998
527 Wang G, Dayanithi G, Newcomb R and Lemos JR. An R-type Ca^{2+} current in neurohypophysial terminals preferentially regulates oxytocin secretion. *J Neurosci* 19: 9235–9241, 1999
528 Wasling P, Hanse E and Gustafsson B. Long-term depression in the developing hippocampus: low induction threshold and synapse nonspecificity. *J Neurosci* 22: 1823–1830, 2002
529 Watanabe H, Nishio M, Miura M and Iijima T. L-type Ca channel block by highly hydrophilic dihydropyridines in single ventricular cells of guinea-pig hearts. *J Mol Cell Cardiol* 27: 1271–1279, 1995
530 Watanabe T, Kalasz H, Yabana H, Kuniyasu A, Mershon J, Itagaki K, Vaghy PL, Naito K, Nakayama H and Schwartz A. Azidobutyryl clentiazem, a new photoactivatable diltiazem analog, labels benzothiazepine binding sites in the alpha 1 subunit of the skeletal muscle calcium channel. *FEBS Lett* 334: 261–264, 1993
531 Wegener JW, Meyrer H, Rupp J and Nawrath H. Barnidipine block of L-type Ca^{2+} channel currents in rat ventricular cardiomyocytes. *Br J Pharmacol* 130: 2015–2023, 2000
532 Weiss JH and Sensi SL. Ca^{2+}-Zn^{2+} permeable AMPA or kainate receptors: possible key factors in selective neurodegeneration. *Trends Neurosci* 23: 365–371, 2000
533 Welling A, Kwan YW, Bosse E, Flockerzi V, Hofmann F and Kass RS. Subunit-dependent modulation of recombinant L-type calcium channels. Molecular basis for dihydropyridine tissue selectivity. *Circ Res* 73: 974–980, 1993
534 Wen JF, Cui X, Ahn JS, Kim SH, Seul KH, Kim SZ, Park YK, Lee HS and Cho KW. Distinct roles for L- and T-type Ca^{2+} channels in regulation of atrial ANP release. *Am J Physiol Heart Circ Physiol* 279: H2879–2888, 2000
535 Wennemuth G, Westenbroek RE, Xu T, Hille B and Babcock DF. $Ca_V2.2$ and $Ca_V2.3$ (N- and R-type) Ca^{2+} channels in depolarization-evoked entry of Ca^{2+} into mouse sperm. *J Biol Chem* 275: 21210–21217, 2000
536 Wheeler DB, Randall A and Tsien RW. Roles of N-type and Q-type Ca^{2+} channels in supporting hippocampal synaptic transmission. *Science* 264: 107–111, 1994
537 Williams ME, Brust PF, Feldman DH, Patthi S, Simerson S, Maroufi A, McCue AF, Velicelebi G, Ellis SB and Harpold MM. Structure and functional expression of an omega-conotoxin-sensitive human N-type calcium channel. *Science* 257: 389–395, 1992
538 Williams ME, Feldman DH, McCue AF, Brenner R, Velicelebi G, Ellis SB and Harpold MM. Structure and functional expression of alpha 1, alpha 2, and beta subunits of a novel human neuronal calcium channel subtype. *Neuron* 8: 71–84, 1992
539 Williams ME, Marubio LM, Deal CR, Hans M, Brust PF, Philipson LH, Miller RJ, Johnson EC, Harpold MM and Ellis SB. Structure and functional characterization of neuronal alpha 1E calcium channel subtypes. *J Biol Chem* 269: 22347–22357, 1994
540 Williams ME, Washburn MS, Hans M, Urrutia A, Brust PF, Prodanovich P, Harpold MM and Stauderman KA. Structure and functional characterization of a novel human low-voltage activated calcium channel. *J Neurochem* 72: 791–799, 1999
541 Wilson SM, Toth PT, Oh SB, Gillard SE, Volsen S, Ren D, Philipson LH, Lee EC, Fletcher CF, Tessarollo L et al. The status of voltage-dependent calcium channels in alpha 1E knock-out mice. *J Neurosci* 20: 8566–8571, 2000
542 Winterfield JR and Swartz KJ. A hot spot for the interaction of gating modifier toxins with voltage-dependent ion channels. *J Gen Physiol* 116: 637–644, 2000
543 Witcher DR, De Waard M, Liu H, Pragnell M and Campbell KP. Association of native Ca^{2+} channel beta subunits with the alpha 1 subunit interaction domain. *J Biol Chem* 270: 18088–18093, 1995
544 Witcher DR, De Waard M, Sakamoto J, Franzini-Armstrong C, Pragnell M, Kahl SD and Campbell KP. Subunit identification and reconstitution of the N-type Ca^{2+} channel complex purified from brain. *Science* 261: 486–489, 1993
545 Wolf H. Preclinical and clinical pharmacology of the 5-HT3 receptor antagonists. *Scand J Rheumatol Suppl* 113: 37–45, 2000

546 Wolfart J and Roeper J. Selective coupling of T-type calcium channels to SK potassium channels prevents intrinsic bursting in dopaminergic midbrain neurons. *J Neurosci* 22: 3404–3413, 2002
547 Wolfe JT, Wang H, Perez-Reyes E and Barrett PQ. Stimulation of recombinant Ca(v)3.2, T-type, Ca^{2+} channel currents by CaMKIIgamma(C). *J Physiol* 538: 343–355, 2002
548 Woodward JJ. Ethanol and NMDA receptor signaling. *Crit Rev Neurobiol* 14: 69–89, 2000
549 Wu LG, Borst JG and Sakmann B. R-type Ca^{2+} currents evoke transmitter release at a rat central synapse. *Proc Natl Acad Sci USA* 95: 4720–4725, 1998
550 Wu LG and Saggau P. GABAB receptor-mediated presynaptic inhibition in guinea-pig hippocampus is caused by reduction of presynaptic Ca^{2+} influx. *J Physiol* 485 (Pt 3): 649–657, 1995
551 Yaari Y, Hamon B and Lux HD. Development of two types of calcium channels in cultured mammalian hippocampal neurons. *Science* 235: 680–682, 1987
552 Yagil Y, Miyamoto M, Frasier L, Oizumi K and Koike H. Effects of CS-905, a novel dihydropyridine calcium channel blocker, on arterial pressure, renal excretory function, and inner medullary blood flow in the rat. *Am J Hypertens* 7: 637–646, 1994
553 Yamakage M, Chen X, Tsujiguchi N, Kamada Y and Namiki A. Different inhibitory effects of volatile anesthetics on T- and L-type voltage-dependent Ca^{2+} channels in porcine tracheal and bronchial smooth muscles. *Anesthesiology* 94: 683–693, 2001
554 Yamamoto K, Korenaga R, Kamiya A and Ando J. Fluid shear stress activates Ca^{2+} influx into human endothelial cells via P2X4 purinoceptors. *Circ Res* 87: 385–391, 2000
555 Yamamoto K, Korenaga R, Kamiya A, Qi Z, Sokabe M and Ando J. P2X(4) receptors mediate ATP-induced calcium influx in human vascular endothelial cells. *Am J Physiol Heart Circ Physiol* 279: H285–292, 2000
556 Yamasaki T, Ohmagari M, Tamai I, Hayashi K and Matsumura Y. Inhibitory effects of AE0047, a new dihydropyridine Ca^{2+} channel blocker, on renal nerve stimulation-induced renal actions in anesthetized dogs. *J Pharmacol Exp Ther* 293: 1040–1047, 2000
557 Yang Y, Chen X, Margulies K, Jeevanandam V, Pollack P, Bailey BA and Houser SR. L-type Ca^{2+} channel alpha 1c subunit isoform switching in failing human ventricular myocardium. *J Mol Cell Cardiol* 32: 973–984, 2000
558 Yao Y, Ferrer-Montiel AV, Montal M and Tsien RY. Activation of store-operated Ca^{2+} current in *Xenopus* oocytes requires SNAP-25 but not a diffusible messenger. *Cell* 98: 475–485, 1999
559 Yasuda H, Tomita T, Fujita K, Shibata J, Tateda K, Yokota H, Igarashi T, Ogasawara S, Yamazaki M and Oyama Y. Clinical efficacy of niludipine in the treatment of angina pectoris. *Arzneimittelforschung* 34: 614–619, 1984
560 Yi X, Vivien B and Lynch C, 3rd. Clevidipine blockade of L-type Ca^{2+} currents: steady-state and kinetic electrophysiological studies in guinea pig ventricular myocytes. *J Cardiovasc Pharmacol* 36: 592–600, 2000
561 Yokoyama CT, Sheng ZH and Catterall WA. Phosphorylation of the synaptic protein interaction site on N-type calcium channels inhibits interactions with SNARE proteins. *J Neurosci* 17: 6929–6938, 1997
562 Yue L, Peng JB, Hediger MA and Clapham DE. CaT1 manifests the pore properties of the calcium-release-activated calcium channel. *Nature* 410: 705–709, 2001
563 Yunker AM, Sharp AH, Sundarraj S, Ranganathan V, Copeland TD and McEnery MW. Immunological characterization of T-type voltage-dependent calcium channel $Ca_V3.1$ (alpha 1G) and $Ca_V3.3$ (alpha 1I) isoforms reveal differences in their localization, expression, and neural development. *Neuroscience* 117: 321–335, 2003
564 Zanchetti A. Emerging data on calcium-channel blockers: the COHORT study. *Clin Cardiol* 26: II17–20, 2003
565 Zhang H. Clevidipine (the Medicines Company). *Curr Opin Investig Drugs* 3: 1474–1478, 2002
566 Zhang JF, Ellinor PT, Aldrich RW and Tsien RW. Molecular determinants of voltage-dependent inactivation in calcium channels. *Nature* 372: 97–100, 1994
567 Zhang JF, Ellinor PT, Aldrich RW and Tsien RW. Multiple structural elements in voltage-dependent Ca^{2+} channels support their inhibition by G proteins. *Neuron* 17: 991–1003, 1996
568 Zhang JF, Randall AD, Ellinor PT, Horne WA, Sather WA, Tanabe T, Schwarz TL and Tsien RW. Distinctive pharmacology and kinetics of cloned neuronal Ca^{2+} channels and their possible counterparts in mammalian CNS neurons. *Neuropharmacology* 32: 1075–1088, 1993
569 Zhou J, Olcese R, Qin N, Noceti F, Birnbaumer L and Stefani E. Feedback inhibition of Ca^{2+} channels by Ca^{2+} depends on a short sequence of the C terminus that does not include the Ca^{2+}-binding function of a motif with similarity to Ca^{2+}-binding domains. *Proc Natl Acad Sci USA* 94: 2301–2305, 1997

570 Zhuang H, Bhattacharjee A, Hu F, Zhang M, Goswami T, Wang L, Wu S, Berggren PO and Li M. Cloning of a T-type Ca^{2+} channel isoform in insulin-secreting cells. *Diabetes* 49: 59–64, 2000
571 Zitt C, Halaszovich CR and Luckhoff A. The TRP family of cation channels: probing and advancing the concepts on receptor-activated calcium entry. *Prog Neurobiol* 66: 243–264, 2002
572 Zubov AI, Kaznacheeva EV, Nikolaev AV, Alexeenko VA, Kiselyov K, Muallem S and Mozhayeva GN. Regulation of the miniature plasma membrane Ca^{2+} channel I(min) by inositol 1,4,5-trisphosphate receptors. *J Biol Chem* 274: 25983–25985, 1999
573 Zuhlke RD and Reuter H. Ca^{2+}-sensitive inactivation of L-type Ca^{2+} channels depends on multiple cytoplasmic amino acid sequences of the alpha1C subunit. *Proc Natl Acad Sci USA* 95: 3287–3294, 1998
574 Zweifach A and Lewis RS. Mitogen-regulated Ca^{2+} current of T lymphocytes is activated by depletion of intracellular Ca^{2+} stores. *Proc Natl Acad Sci USA* 90: 6295–6299, 1993

The action of calcium antagonists on Ca^{2+} movements in isolated vessels

Experimental pharmacology studies consider short- and long-term effects of CCBs. The most obvious short-term action is the reduction of blood pressure that has prompted the use of calcium antagonists in cardiovascular medicine. This action is the result of a decrease of peripheral resistance due to vasodilatation within the arterial beds. Therefore, a large body of experimental work has been concerned with studies of the mechanism of action of CCBs in arteries. Analytical pharmacology studies of various CCBs have supported the concept of tissue and action selectivity, which has some interest for pharmacotherapy. Studies of the long-term effects have enlightened their action in the prevention of the complications of hypertension including the development of atherosclerosis. Earlier studies have addressed the mechanism of action of calcium antagonists in the vasculature by considering their interaction with Ca^{2+} activator of the contractile machinery. Such approach has required the characterization of calcium movements in the absence and in the presence of calcium antagonists.

Measurements of calcium fluxes and of intracellular calcium in vascular smooth muscles

The observation by Godfraind and Kaba [32, 33] that only contractions directly related to the extracellular concentration of calcium were sensitive to calcium antagonists, provided support to the hypothesis that blockade of calcium entry is an important mechanism of drug action. A further confirmation for this hypothesis has been given by the measurement of unidirectional Ca^{2+} fluxes and by the characterization of the specific binding sites of calcium antagonists in relation to their action. Within the past decade, considerable progress has been made in the understanding of Ca^{2+} movements and distribution in smooth muscle cells. Simultaneous measurements of $[Ca^{2+}]_i$ and contraction in intact smooth muscle, using various intracellular Ca^{2+} indicators have allowed an analysis of the Ca^{2+} sensitivity of contractile elements (for references see [47–49]). Permeabilisation of the cell membrane enabled the measurement of contraction in the presence of steady concentrations of Ca^{2+}, of ATP and of other substances in the cell. Calcium-imaging techniques have revealed an uneven distribution of Ca^{2+} within the cell and have localized spots of concentration increase in the form of Ca^{2+} sparks and of propagating $Ca^{2+}{}_i$ waves.

Before the estimate of $[Ca^{2+}]_i$ using intracellular Ca^{2+} indicators, contraction was considered as an accurate indicator of $[Ca^{2+}]_i$, because, at that time, the complexity of regulation of smooth muscle contraction was not perceived. Simultaneous measurements of $[Ca^{2+}]_i$ and of contraction have shown that factors other than $[Ca^{2+}]_i$ increase are involved in the excitation-contraction process.

Measurements by radioactive calcium

Analysis with $^{45}Ca^{2+}$ of the calcium distribution in an artery showed that the amount of Ca^{2+} bound outside the cell membrane is much greater than the amount of free Ca^{2+} in the cytoplasm and/or the amount of Ca^{2+} entering the cell during a contractile stimulation. It was not possible to discriminate between Ca^{2+} bound to the membrane surface and Ca^{2+} in the cytoplasm by just immersing vessels in physiological solution containing $^{45}Ca^{2+}$, because changes in transmembrane Ca^{2+} fluxes occurring after a stimulus were not perceivable under such experimental conditions (see [40, 41, 101]). Several approaches have been developed to estimate the importance of calcium changes in a slowly-exchanging tissue fraction supposed to be intracellular. In 1962, Briggs [8, 9] incubated rabbit aortic strips with solutions containing $^{45}Ca^{2+}$ for 30 to 60 min followed by a 10 to 15 min washout period with identical non-radioactive solutions in order to remove $^{45}Ca^{2+}$ from the extracellular space. With this procedure, it was possible to remove a rapidly exchanging Ca^{2+} fraction and to estimate the capacity of a slowly-exchanging Ca^{2+} fraction. It was found that high KC1, epinephrine and norepinephrine increased the level of $^{45}Ca^{2+}$ remaining after the washout in non-radioactive solution. Thus, the quantity of Ca^{2+} in a slowly-exchanging fraction appeared to vary with the contraction. However, the time course of this increase in $^{45}Ca^{2+}$ was slower than that of contraction and the decrease in $^{45}Ca^{2+}$ following removal of the stimulant was much slower than the decrease in muscle tension, suggesting that this method could just measure $^{45}Ca^{2+}$ in a cellular fraction in which Ca^{2+} gradually accumulated during a contraction. Neither the cellular location nor the physiological role of this Ca^{2+} fraction has ever been defined.

Measurement of the lanthanum-inaccessible calcium fraction of smooth muscles has provided a valuable approach to Ca^{2+}-fluxes measurements. Due to their higher charge density, La^{3+} ions were expected to have a greater affinity than Ca^{2+} for any anionic groups that binds Ca^{2+}. Based upon anatomical evidence indicating that La^{3+} is restricted to the extracellular compartment, it was found in smooth muscle preparations that La^{3+} replaced $^{45}Ca^{2+}$ at superficial membrane sites and prevented $^{45}Ca^{2+}$ uptake by intracellular Ca^{2+} stores [40, 41, 101]. Van Breemen et al. [98] attempted to remove the extracellular $^{45}Ca^{2+}$ by washing the tissue in a physiological salt solution (PSS) containing 2×10 mM $LaCl^{3+}$ after completion of $^{45}Ca^{2+}$ uptake and before measurement of tissue $^{45}Ca^{2+}$. In rabbit aorta depolarized with a high KC1 solution they observed that during the contraction, Ca^{2+} uptake was increased from a resting level of about 50 mmol/kg of wet tissue to 150 mmol/kg of wet tissue. However, with their procedure, they did not discover change in $^{45}Ca^{2+}$ uptake when contractions were produced by norepinephrine. However increased $^{45}Ca^{2+}$ uptake was noticed when muscle strips were preincubated with Ca^{2+}-free PSS before the norepinephrine-induced contraction [19]. These results suggested that $^{45}Ca^{2+}$ uptake increased only under non-physiological conditions and supported the hypothesis that norepinephrine-stimulated contraction of rabbit aorta was due mainly to Ca^{2+} release from intracellular stores. In 1976, Godfraind [28] improved the lanthanum method by making use of a high concentration (50 mM) of LaCl3, thereby minimizing the loss of $^{45}Ca^{2+}$ during the washout with La^{3+} solution. He found that, at physiological concentration, norepinephrine increases the rate but not the total amount of $^{45}Ca^{2+}$ uptake in the rat aorta (see Fig. 1). Karaki and Weiss [51] and Van Breemen et al. [99] finally found that high KC1 and norepinephrine increased the rate of $^{45}Ca^{2+}$ uptake in the rabbit aorta. Norepinephrine also transiently increases the rate of $^{45}Ca^{2+}$ efflux [18, 28] by decreasing Ca^{2+} amount on high affinity Ca^{2+} binding sites but not on low affinity Ca^{2+} sites [51–53, 56]. These results provided support for the model that in addition to the activation of membrane calcium channels occurring in some vessels, in all vessels norepinephrine and various vasoconstrictors may release Ca^{2+} from intracellular stores that have been identified with sarcoplasmic reticulum. With the lanthanum method, increases in total $^{45}Ca^{2+}$ uptake could be detected under non-physiological conditions. In rabbit aorta, Karaki and Weiss [54, 55] found that inhibition of mitochondrial function with antimycin A, oligomycin, potassium cyanide (KCN) and hypoxia reduced KC1-induced increase in $^{45}Ca^{2+}$ uptake indicating that a portion of $^{45}Ca^{2+}$ uptake was not associated with contraction and represented an incremental uptake of Ca^{2+} into mitochondria.

Such experiments pointed to the fact that the response to norepinephrine is different in various vessels. In the rabbit aorta norepinephrine increased Ca uptake in the La^{3+} resistant compartment only in the presence of high KCl, resulting in increased mitochondrial Ca^{2+} uptake [51, 54]. On the other hand, in the rat aorta, norepinephrine-evoked ^{45}Ca entry in the La^{3+}-resistant compartment did not require depolarization by KCl and was observed in physiological conditions [28]. A similar action was later found in various vessels including rat mesenteric arteries and human coronary arteries bathed in physiological solution.

Measurements by fluorescent indicators

Measurements of intracellular Ca^{2+} changes by fluorescent indicators have provided additional information on the relation between $[Ca^{2+}]_i$ and smooth muscle contraction.

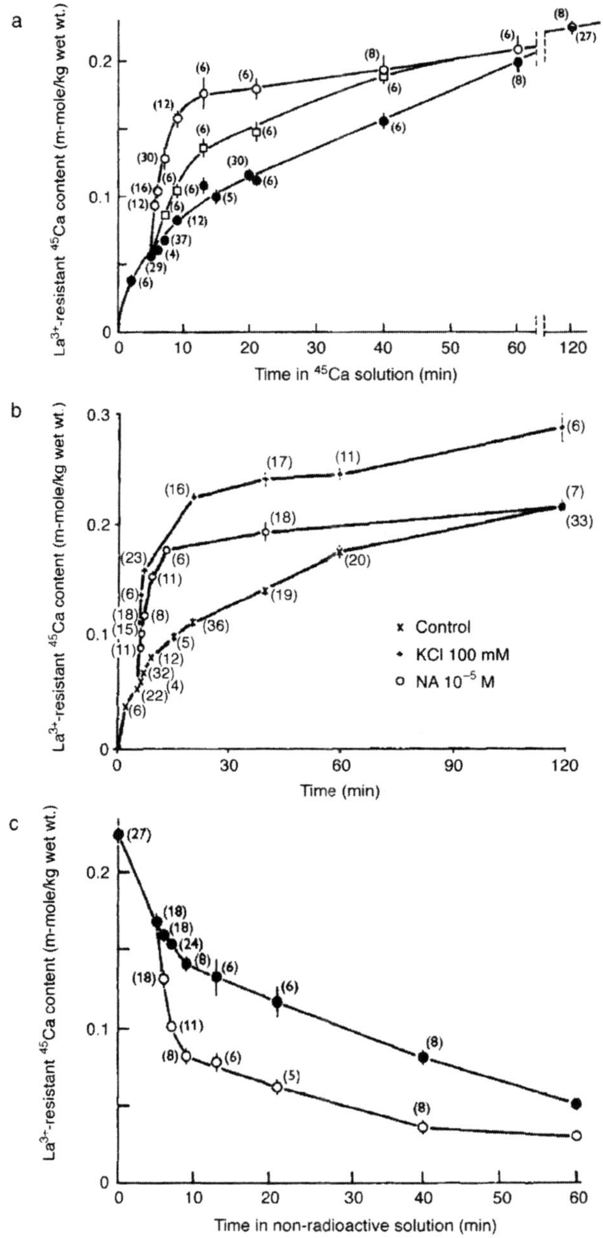

Figure 1. (a) ^{45}Ca influx and efflux evoked by noradrenaline and KCl-depolarisation in vascular smooth muscle cells (VSMCs) of isolated rat aorta. (●) Ca influx in resting tissue; (□) Ca influx in the presence of noradrenaline 10^{-8} M; (○) Ca influx in the presence of noradrenaline 10^{-5} M. Note the dose-related response of Ca influx that is related to activation of α_1-adrenoceptors [28]. (b) Comparison of Ca influx evoked by noradrenaline and KCl-depolarisation. Note a net Ca increase with KCl [36]. (c) Ca efflux evoked by noradrenaline 10^{-5} M [28].

Aequorin

Aequorin is a Ca^{2+} binding protein extracted from the jelly fish, *Aequorea aequorea*. This protein emits light at 465 nm in the presence of Ca^{2+}. Ridgway and Ashley [82] injected this photoprotein into barnacle single muscle fibers and measured $[Ca^{2+}]_i$ by monitoring changes in aequorin light. Their method was applied to a single smooth muscle cell by Fay et al. [22]. Morgan and Morgan [73, 74] loaded the 21 kDa photoprotein into smooth muscle cells of ferret portal vein by transiently increasing the membrane permeability using a high concentration of EGTA, and measured $[Ca^{2+}]_i$ and contraction in isolated smooth muscle strips. They found that high KC1 induced a sustained increase in $[Ca^{2+}]_i$ during sustained contraction; both were related to the extracellular Ca^{2+} concentration. This supported the general view that the high KCl-induced contraction is due to an increase in $[Ca^{2+}]_i$ resulting from activation of Ca^{2+} influx. In contrast, stimulation of the α-adrenoceptors of ferret portal vein by phenylephrine induced a rapid rise of $[Ca^{2+}]_i$ to a maximum from which it decreased rapidly to a lower level and then declined more slowly, staying only slightly above basal $[Ca^{2+}]_i$. At the same time, the muscle tension rapidly increased to reach maximum level and remained elevated as long as the stimulation was maintained. During the phenylephrine-induced sustained contraction, removal of external Ca^{2+} decreased $[Ca^{2+}]_i$ to a level lower than the basal one, but the contraction was only partially inhibited. From these results, the authors concluded that the contractions induced by phenylephrine and high KC1 were due to elevation of $[Ca^{2+}]_i$ above baseline, but that in addition, phenylephrine increased the effectiveness of Ca^{2+} on the contractile apparatus. This observation that at a given $[Ca^{2+}]_i$, receptor agonists produce a larger force than high KC1 during the period of force maintenance has been extended to various vessels from different species including ferret aorta, rabbit aorta, guinea pig aorta, swine carotid artery and canine and bovine trachea (for ref see Karaki et al. [49]).

Other fluorescent indicators

The fluorescent Ca^{2+} indicator, quin2, was synthesized by Tsien [97]. This was soon followed by the second generation of indicators including fura-2 and indo-1 [43]. These indicators are not membrane-permeable, an acetoxymethyl radical is attached to these molecules in order to allow them to enter the cells. After loading smooth muscle cells with the acetoxymethyl esters of these indicators, the acetoxymethyl moiety is cleaved by endogenous esterases and the indicator is trapped in the cell.

Measurements of $[Ca^{2+}]_i$ by the fluorescent indicators in smooth muscle tissues are much more difficult than in single cells. Abe and Karaki (1989) have elegantly solved most of the difficulties. They showed that fura-2/AM is insoluble in physiological solutions: only a small amount disperses as particles of various sizes, but most of the particles are so large they are not able to diffuse in the extracellular space of the smooth muscle tissues. To solubilize fura-2/AM, they added small amounts of detergent and applied strong ultrasonic waves. Using this procedure, smooth muscle tissues can be loaded with fura-2/AM, allowing simultaneous measurements of $[Ca^{2+}]_i$ and contraction. $[Ca^{2+}]_i$ measured with fura-2 showed better correlation with contraction than did $[Ca^{2+}]_i$ measured with aequorin. Therefore, most authors have used newly-synthesized fluorescent indicators instead of aequorin. An example of simultaneous recording of Ca signal and contraction is given in Figure 2 (unpublished experiment).

Furthermore, the use of confocal microscopy has shown the complexity of the calcium waves within the cell and has illustrated the interplay between various calcium stores. To make the story short, as was shown by various investigators (for further information, see [49]), the main contributors to increases in $[Ca^{2+}]_i$ and tension are an entry of Ca^{2+} through voltage-dependent channels opened by KCl-evoked sustained depolarization or during a transitory depolarization related to action potentials (AP) evoked by various agonists and a Ca^{2+} release from store sites in the cell by the action of IP3 or by Ca^{2+} itself according to the mechanism known as Ca-induced Ca-release (CICR). The entry of Ca^{2+} during an AP triggers CICR from up to 20 or more subplasmalemmal store sites (seen as hot spots, using fluorescent indicators). Ca^{2+} waves then spread from these hot spots, which results in a rise in $[Ca^{2+}]_i$ throughout the cell. Spontaneous transient releases of stored Ca^{2+}, previously detected as spontaneous transient outward currents (STOCs), are seen as sparks when fluorescent indicators are used. Sparks occur at certain preferred locations named frequent discharge sites (FDSs) and these and hot spots may represent aggregations of sarcoplasmic reticulum scattered throughout the cytoplasm. Activation of receptors for excitatory signal molecules generally

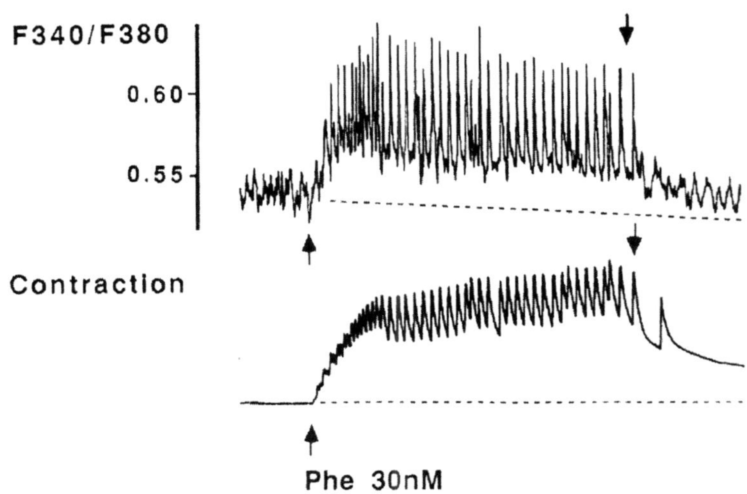

Figure 2. Contraction and Fura-2 Ca signal evoked by phenylephrine in isolated rat aorta (unpublished experiment).

depolarizes the cell while it increases the production of IP3 (causing calcium store release) and diacylglycerols (which activate protein kinases). Activation of receptors for inhibitory signal molecules increases the activity of protein kinases through increases in cAMP or cGMP and often hyperpolarizes the cell. Other receptors are linked to tyrosine kinases, which trigger signal cascades interacting with trimeric G-protein systems. Multiple cellular mechanisms have been implicated in receptor-mediated smooth muscle contraction but all of them ultimately converge on increased phosphorylation of myosin light chain [91]. Classically this has been attributed to activation of a phospholipase (PL) C leading to mobilization of Ca^{2+} from intracellular stores and/or to activation of voltage-operated Ca^{2+} channels. In recent years a variety of additional signalling pathways has been implicated in receptor-mediated contraction of vascular and other smooth muscle, including activation of a PLD [1], of store-operated Ca^{2+} channels [64], of protein kinase C [16, 17], of various types of tyrosine kinases including the src family, of phosphatidylinositol-3-kinases (PI-3-kinases), of extracellular signal-regulated kinase (ERK) forms of the mitogen-activated protein kinases (MAPK) and of Rho-associated protein kinases (for ref, see [49]).

Calcium antagonists act at the level of one of these processes in smooth muscles: the voltage-dependent calcium entry. In intact arteries, the L-arginine-NO pathway has been identified as another target as this will be addressed below.

Actions of CCBs in isolated arteries

There is a general agreement to recognize that the increase in $[Ca^{2+}]_i$ in smooth is the result of different Ca^{2+} influx pathways including receptor-linked and voltage-dependent Ca^{2+} channels (Cav). High KC1 induces membrane depolarization, which, in turn, opens the voltage-dependent Ca^{2+} channels. Inorganic agents such as La^{3+} and organic molecules including verapamil, nifedipine (and many other organic agents) block those channels. Norepinephrine releases Ca^{2+} from storage sites to induce initial transient contractions and may evoke membrane depolarization that subsequently opens VOCs; other channels (SOCs) are also open when the internal calcium stores are empty. The situation might become more complex with vasoconstrictors such as endothelin-1 that opens various calcium entry channels and non-selective cationic channels, depending on the concentration of the peptide [106–108]. The complexity increases when considering vessels isolated with an intact endothelium that has been shown to influence intracellular processes involved in vasoconstriction. Recent insight on the physiology of vascular contraction supports the early choice of K-depolarized arteries in order to gain information on the interaction of calcium antagonists with VOCs and vessel contractility.

Role of endothelium

Since Furchgott and Zawadzki [24] first described the endothelium-dependent relaxations to acetylcholine in the aorta of the rabbit, it has been established that the endothelium can mediate, wholly or partly, the relaxing effect of a large number of agents. This effect of endothelium is due to the release of factors termed EDRF(s) [23, 45]. Endothelium also modulates the contractile action displayed by a wide variety of vasoconstrictor agonists [21, 61, 62]. Furchgott's discovery has prompted an extensive work dealing with the nature and the tissular distribution of EDRFs responsible for vasorelaxation [68]. It is now recognized that endothelial cells synthesize and release vasoactive mediators in response to various neurohumoural substances including bradykinin and acetylcholine and to physical stimuli (e.g., cyclic stretch or fluid shear stress). The best-characterized endothelium-derived relaxing factors are nitric oxide and prostacyclin. In some blood vessels endothelium releases continuously nitric oxide, this release being largely increased by the stimuli quoted above. Three NO-synthase isoforms function in animals and each gene is located on a different chromosome (for ref. [93]). Two enzymes are constitutively expressed in cells, eNOS (NOSII) in endothelium and nNOS (NOSI) in nervous tissue, they synthesize NO in response to increased Ca^{2+}. An inducible NOS (iNOS also NOSIII) is synthesized in response to inflammatory or pro-inflammatory mediators, it usually produces large amount of NO. NO is formed from L-arginine and it diffuses to the target site. The initial step by which NO mediates vascular relaxation is likely to be activation of soluble guanylate cyclase, leading to an elevation of the content of cGMP in vascular smooth muscle [20, 79].

In the early 1980s, it was known that the endothelium markedly modifies the response to vasoconstrictor agonists in various arteries as was initially shown in canine and porcine coronary arteries and in the aorta of rat and rabbit [13, 21]. Endothelium removal in the isolated aorta of the rat enhanced the contractile response to different α-adrenergic agonists, especially partial agonists, which only cause weak contractions in intact preparations [31]. When comparing concentration-response curves from different α-adrenergic agonists in the presence and the absence of endothelium, it appeared that the removal of the endothelium shifted the concentration-response curves to the different agonists to the left, with an enhancement of the maximal developed tension. This observation was most pronounced for oxymetazoline, clonidine, and UK14,304; these compounds had only a negligible effect in the presence of endothelium. Treatment of the aortas without endothelium with a permeable analog of cGMP (8-bromo-cGMP) reduced the contractile response to norepinephrine. Measurement of calcium fluxes showed that the removal of the endothelium evoked a small, but significant, increase of ^{45}Ca entry in unstimulated preparations. The norepinephrine-dependent ^{45}Ca entry was two-fold higher in preparations without endothelium than in those with endothelium (Fig. 3). In the preparations with endothelium, blockade of guanylate cyclase (with methylene

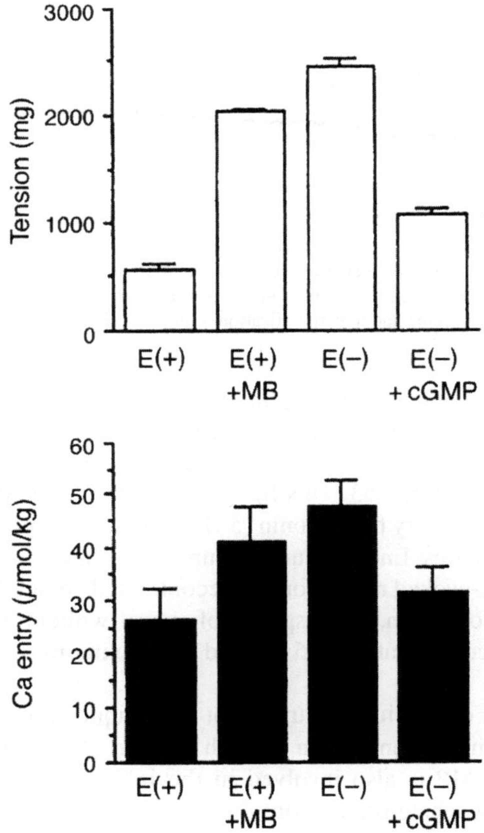

Figure 3. Influence of endothelium and of cGMP on contraction and ^{45}Ca entry evoked by noradrenaline. Upper panel: Tonic contractile force (expressed in milligrams) developed by rings of rat aorta stimulated with noradrenaline (10^{-8} M). Each value is mean of six determinations, and S.E. is indicated on the graph. E(+), preparations with endothelium intact treated with methylene blue for 10 min before noradrenaline; E(–), preparations where endothelium was removed; E(–) + cGMP. preparations where endothelium was removed and treated with 8-bromo-cGMP (0.1 mM for 30 min before noradrenaline). Lower panel: ^{45}Ca influx (expressed in nmol/kg wet weight) in preparations treated with noradrenaline (10^{-8} M for 2 min). Each value is the mean of 12 determinations, and the S.E. is indicated on the graph. The symbols in the lower panel are the same as those in the upper panel. From [29], modified.

blue), enhanced the norepinephrine-dependent ^{45}Ca entry to levels similar to those found in preparations without endothelium. These observations showed the involvement of the l-arginine-NO pathway in both ^{45}Ca entry and contraction evoked by adrenergic agonists. It appeared to be related to the efficacy of the given adrenergic agonist indicating that the efficacy of vasoconstrictor could be related to the gating of calcium channels controlled by EDRF through production of cGMP [29]. This gating action is likely indirect due to an effect

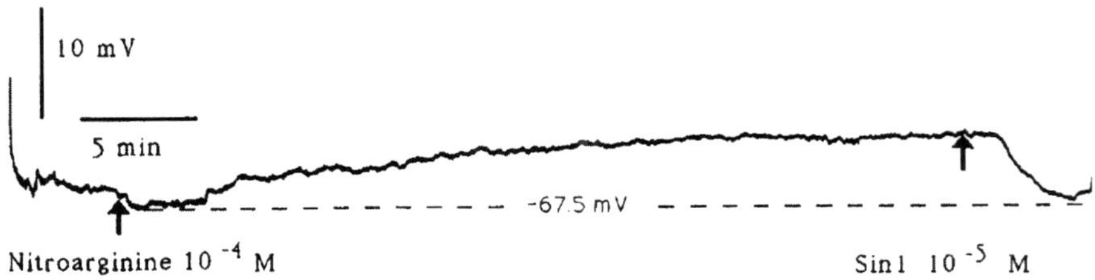

Figure 4. Effect of nitroarginine, a blocker of NO-synthase, and of the subsequent addition of Sin-1, which spontaneously released NO, on the membrane potential of rat aorta smooth muscle cell. Note depolarization with nitroarginine and hyperpolarisation with Sin-1. From [60], modified.

of NO on membrane potential [6, 60]. In rat aorta and other vessels, NO hyperpolarizes the cells by a direct action on K channels (Fig. 4). Another example of the role of endothelium on the responsiveness of arteries to vasoconstrictors is given by Figure 1, page 153. This figure illustrates the contractile response of isolated rat basilar artery to serotonin (5 HT), known as a physiological stimulant of cerebral arteries. Endothelium dysfunction is indicated by reduction of acetycholine (Ach)-evoked relaxation of precontracted vessel. When compared to vessel with endothelium, the response of vessel without endothelium was observed at lower concentration of 5 HT and the maximum response was about 40% higher [86a].

However, effect on calcium influx is not the unique action of NO on agonist-evoked calcium movements in smooth muscle. As shown by Lang and Lewis [61, 62] cGMP is also involved in the inhibition of agonist-induced inositol 1,4,5-triphosphate production; this leads to inhibition of the intracellular calcium release also implicated in regulation of vascular tone. NO has many other effects on cell function. The action of the increase of cellular cGMP on both $[Ca^{2+}]_i$ and contraction has been examined by Salomone et al. [87], as Figure 5 illustrates, for a given cytosolic concentration of Ca, the contractile force was lower in preparations exposed to BrcGMP than in controls, indicating that cGMP could decrease the affinity of contractile machinery for Ca. Much evidence suggests that the initial phase of agonist-induced force generation is related to increase in intracellular Ca^{2+}. However, the maintained portion of contraction is also regulated by a Ca^{2+}-sensitization mechanism mediated by the activity of RhoA/Rho-kinase. NO is known to stimulate an increase in cGMP levels, leading to the activation of cGMP-dependent protein kinase (cGK). Studies have reported recombinant cGK to phosphorylate RhoA, destabilizing the membrane binding of RhoA, thus providing a mechanism by which NO may inhibit RhoA/Rho-kinase activity and thereby decrease the contractile force evoked by an agonist inducing the translocation of RhoA [12].

Some endothelium-dependent relaxations and hyperpolarizations can be partially or totally resistant to inhibitors of cyclooxygenases and nitric oxide (NO) synthases and can occur without an increase in intracellular levels of

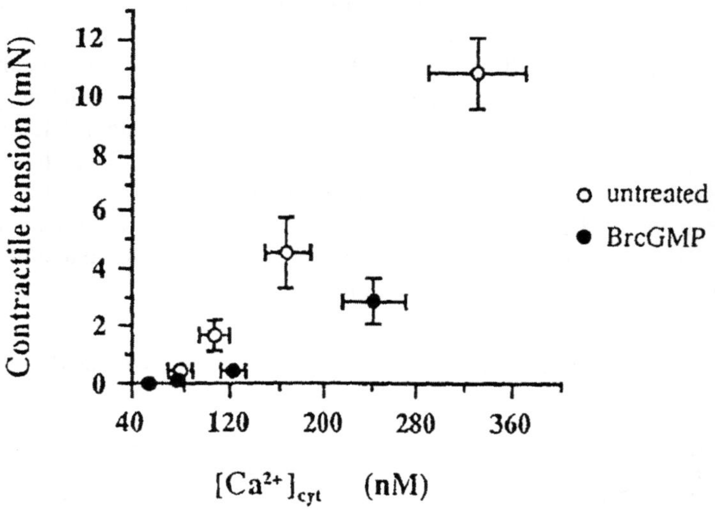

Figure 5. Contractile force of isolated rat aorta as a function of cytosolic Ca^{2+} concentration before (untreated) and after exposure to 0.1 mM Br-cGMP. Modified from [87].

cyclic nucleotides in the smooth muscle cells, indicating the existence of an additional pathway that involved smooth muscle hyperpolarization attributed to the putative endothelial factor called endothelium-derived hyperpolarizing factor (EDHF). The hyperpolarization originally attributed to the release of the endothelium-derived hyperpolarizing factor (EDHF) was assumed to diffuse to and activate smooth muscle K^+ channels. More recent evidence suggests that endothelial cell receptor activation by acetylcholine and other neurohumoural substances opens endothelial cell K^+ channels. Several mechanisms have been proposed to link this pivotal step to the subsequent smooth muscle hyperpolarization. The endothelial hyperpolarization could spread to the adjacent smooth muscle cells through myo-endothelial gap junctions or the efflux of K^+ through the endothelial potassium channels could elicit the hyperpolarization of the surrounding myocytes by activating K_{IR} channels and/or the Na^+–K^+-ATPase. These mechanisms are not necessarily mutually exclusive [10]. Hyperpolarization of smooth muscle produces relaxation by reducing both the open probability of voltage-dependent Ca^{2+} channels and the turnover of intracellular phosphatidylinositides, thus decreasing the intracellular Ca^{2+} concentration $[Ca^{2+}]_i$. The contribution of EDHF-mediated responses as a mechanism for endothelium-dependent relaxation increases as the vessel size decreases. In some tissues, the activation of cytochrome P450 and the resulting generation of EETs might regulate the hyperpolarization of the endothelial cells. The relative proportion of each EDHF mechanism almost certainly depends on numerous parameters including the state of activation of the vascular smooth muscle, the density of myo-endothelial gap junctions and the level of the expression of cytochrome P450 and the appropriate isoforms of Na^+–K^+-ATPase and/or K_{IR} channels. There are species differences that are the subject of experimental studies. In mice, EDHF-mediated responses in resistance vessels are at least as important as endothelium-derived NO in mediating agonist-induced, endothelium-dependent vasodilatation because neither deletion of the gene encoding endothelial NO synthase nor inhibition of NO-synthase attenuates agonist-induced vasodilator responses *in vivo* and *in vitro* [7]. A role for EDHF in endothelium-dependent vasorelaxation is assumed in the presence of a cyclo-oxygenase inhibitor when the relaxation is not sensitive to a blocker of NO-synthase, the enzyme responsible for the formation of NO (Fig. 6).

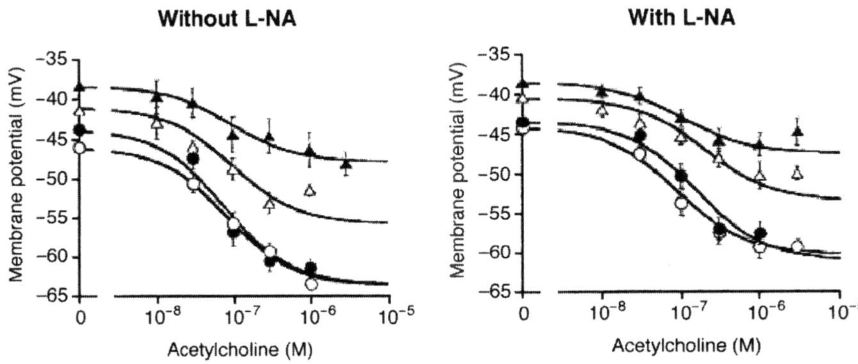

Figure 6. Relaxation to acetylcholine of pre-contracted rat mesenteric arteries isolated from various strains, all showing a residual hyperpolarisation that is attributed to EDHF after exposure to LNNA, a blocker of NO-synthase. Modified from [25].

Inhibition of K-depolarization evoked contraction

Because, depolarization-induced contraction is primarily maintained by a sustained increased in intracellular Ca^{2+}, this mode of activation seems particularly suitable for the study of the interaction of CCBs with calcium channels in various controlled conditions.

In resting conditions, when an isolated rat aorta is bathed in physiological solution containing ^{45}Ca, the specific activity of intracellular calcium increases slowly with the duration of incubation and reaches a plateau after 1 or 2 hr, when inward and outward movements of ^{45}Ca become equal. The initial rate of uptake of ^{45}Ca may be taken as reflecting an inward influx. When the intracellular fraction is completely loaded with ^{45}Ca, the initial rate of ^{45}Ca loss after transfer to a non-radioactive solution depends mainly on outward movements. The calcium influx rate under resting conditions is about 0.014 and 0.03 $pmol \cdot cm^{-2} \cdot s^{-1}$, respectively, in the rat aorta and in the rabbit aorta. This calcium influx has been termed "passive Ca^{2+} leak", because it is thought to occur through pathways that differ from those involved in calcium influx evoked by stimulating agents. This calcium influx through leak channels is resistant to Ca antagonists. As shown by our group some years ago [36], noradrenaline and KCl stimulations evoke a 20-fold increase in the rate of calcium influx through channels sensitive to calcium antagonists. This stimulated influx is blocked by calcium antagonists at concentrations reducing the contractile response, and inhibition of contraction may be related to blockade of voltage-operated Ca^{2+} channels, since dose-effect curves relating the degree of inhibition of Ca influx and of contraction to the concentration of the Ca antagonist are superimposed as this is shown on Figure 7 for nifedipine. In isolated smooth muscle cells voltage-clamped with a single-patch electrode technique

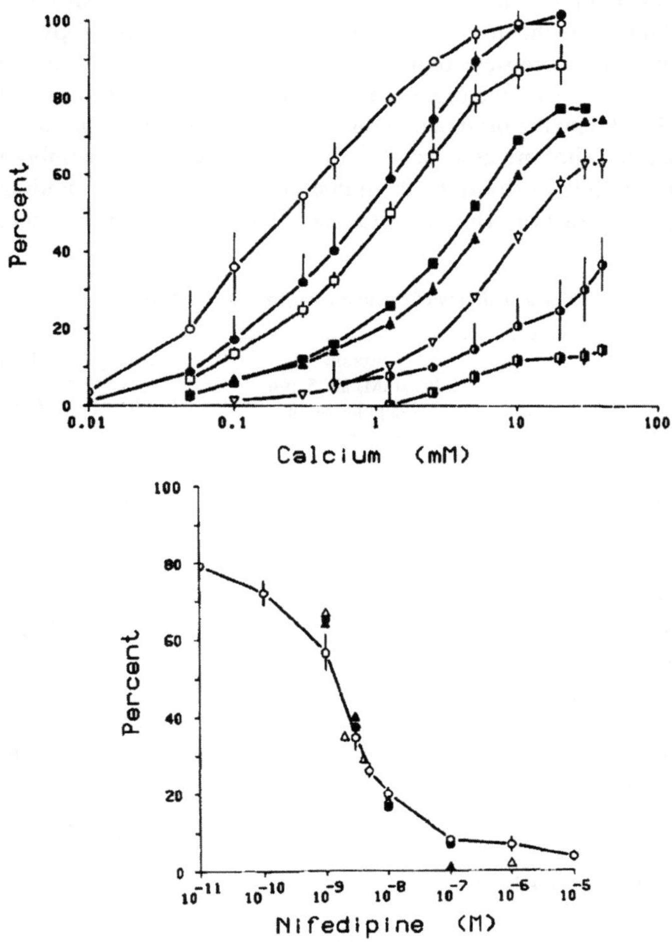

Figure 7. Action of various concentrations of nifedipine on Ca evoked contraction and Ca influx. Upper panel: contraction in isolated rat aorta with various concentration of nifedipine, from 3×10^{-10} up to 10^{-6} M. Lower panel: Reduction by nifedipine of rat aorta K-contraction (○), Ca influx in depolarized aorta (△), K-contraction in rat mesenteric artery (●) and Ca influx in depolarized mesenteric artery (▲), modified from [26].

(whole cell recording), Klockner and Isenberg [57] have observed that the dihydropyridine niguldipine reduced Ca^{2+} currents at pharmacologically active concentrations. A similar observation had been made by Terada et al. [96] with the calcium antagonist flunarizine. Mironneau [67] showed that when measured in similar conditions, the IC50 value of isradipine on Ca^{2+} currents was similar to the IC50 value on contraction. Thus, data obtained from electrophysiological studies are consistent with those obtained from radiochemistry.

With various dihydropyridines so far studied, there is a close similarity between IC50 values obtained on intact tissue and Ki values measured in binding studies performed on microsomal preparations. This shows that the pharmacological action of calcium antagonists may be related to specific binding sites. Furthermore, the use of enantiomeric pairs of dihydropyridines has demonstrated the stereoselectivity of the binding confirming its specificity (Tab. 1) [35, 88]. Using the digitonin shift method, allowing to identify activities associated with the plasma membrane, we observed that dihydropyridine-specific binding sites are associated with the plasmalemmal membrane of the smooth muscle cell, as shown by the higher amount of specific binding sites in the microsomal fraction. Binding sites have been identified in mitochondria,

Table 1. Chirality on action and affinity of calcium antagonists (for ref. see [27])

Drug	Action IC_{50} (nM) at 35 min K-depolarization	Affinity K_d or K_i (nM)	
		Intact tissue	Membranes
(+) Isradipine			
rat aorta	0.092	0.068	0.085
rat mesenteric artery	0.033	0.025	0.055
rat cerebral microvessels		0.024	
(–) Isradipine			
rat aorta	12.3		14.9
rat mesenteric artery	5.0		
rat cerebral microvessels			
(–) Nimodipine			
rat aorta	0.234		0.546
rat cerebral microvessels		0.23	0.100
(+) Nimodipine			
rat aorta	1.371		2.89
rat cerebral microvessels		2.0	
S(+) 312			
rat aorta	0.14		
rat cerebral microvessels		0.12	
R(–) 312			
rat aorta	2.98		
rat cerebral microvessels		2.4	

they show low affinity binding that is enhanced by Ca^{2+} at high ionic strength. This is at variance with the binding sites found on plasmalemma membranes. Furthermore, these mitochondrial sites do not exhibit stereoselectivity and are not involved in the regulation of smooth muscle tone [88].

Kinetic studies have pointed out disparities between CCBs for inhibition of contraction. Confirming our previous experiments performed in rat aorta, Figure 8 shows the time course of human coronary artery preparations evoked by KCl before and after treatment with: nifedipine, nisoldipine, diltiazem and verapamil. The pattern of inhibition of the contraction differs according to the calcium-channel blocker used. With nifedipine, diltiazem and verapamil, the inhibition of KCl-evoked contraction increases little with time during a 30 min stimulation period. On the other hand, with nisoldipine the inhibition develops more gradually. This time-dependent pattern of inhibition of KCl-evoked con-

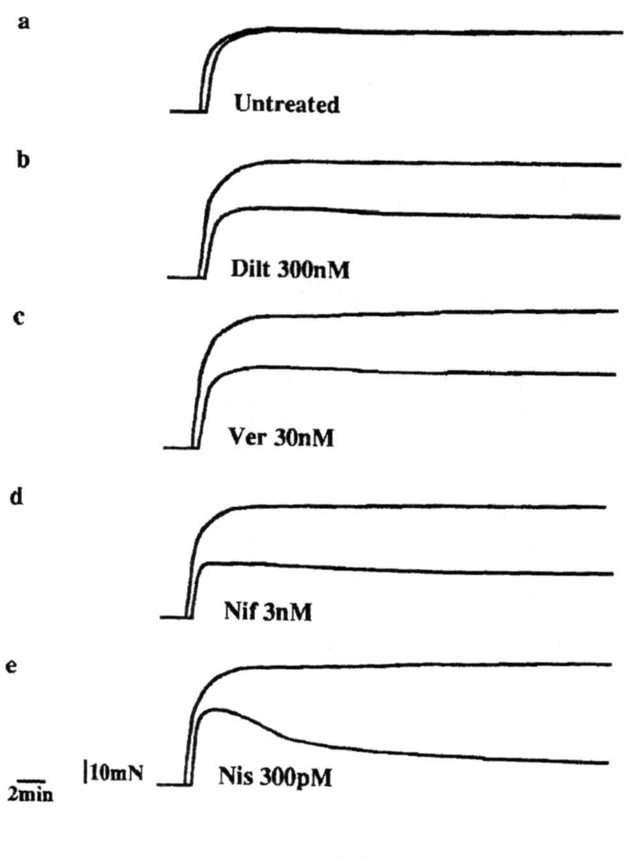

Figure 8. Typical tracings of the contractile response to 100 mM KCl of human coronary artery before and after a 90 min exposure to calcium antagonists: a, control; b, diltiazem; c, verapamil; d, nifedipine; e, nisoldipine. Note that nisoldipine inhibition increases with prolonged depolarization. From [30], modified.

tractions could be reproduced in successive contractions, separated by a resting period of 30 min in physiological solution in the presence of the drug, indicating that the pre-incubation time before stimulation was not the factor responsible for the discrepancies between CCBs. Figure 9 shows with (+)isradipine that the kinetics of inhibition during depolarization is superimposed on the kinetics of binding to calcium channels in membranes isolated from smooth muscle. A similar observation was done with lacidipine [86]. This suggests that depolarization induces a conformational change in the calcium channels, resulting in an increased affinity for dihydropyridines, and that this high-affinity form is similar to that found in isolated membranes. This hypothesis has been confirmed in isolated rat mesenteric arteries by Morel and Godfraind [71, 72] who have studied how the resting membrane potential influences both the pharmacological effect and the specific binding of calcium antagonists in intact arteries. A typical study with (+)isradipine [(+)PN 200-110] has been reported by Morel and Godfraind in rat mesenteric arteries. The time course of the K^+ contraction of the rat mesenteric artery in the presence of (+)PN 200-110 is characterized by a time-dependent decrease in tension until a steady-state inhibition is reached, as already shown for other dihy-

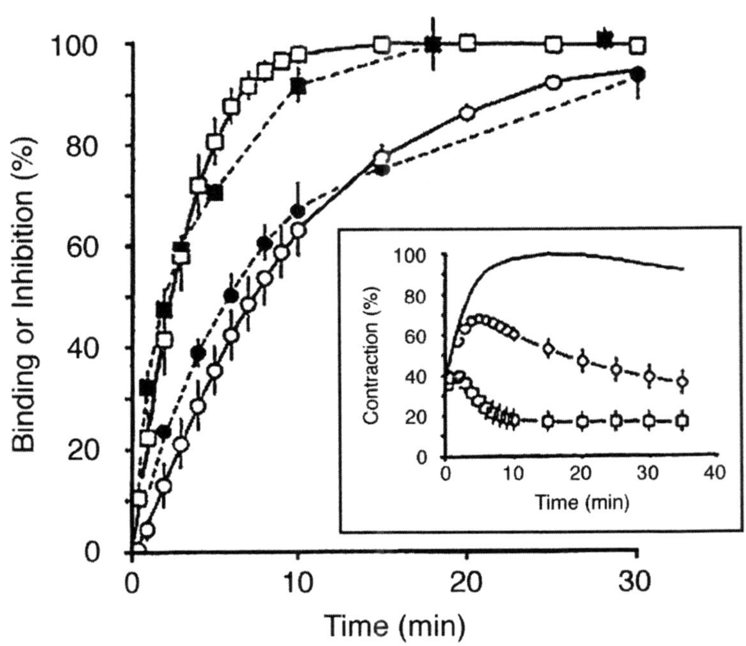

Figure 9. Comparison between kinetics of ^3H-(+)PN 200-110 association with its specific binding site (● = 0.1 nM; ■ = 0.3 nM) and (+)PH 200-10 inhibition of K^+-evoked contraction of rat aorta (○ = 0.1; □ = 0.3 nM (+)PN 200-110). Inset: Mechanical responses to KCl depolarisation of rat aortic rings with control (upper curve), rings treated with 0.1 (○) or 0.3 nM (□) (+)PH 200-110. Reprinted from [102], with the permission of the copyright holder, American Heart Association, Dallas.

dropyridines in the rat aorta. Dose-effect curves for inhibition measured 2 and 30 min after initiation of depolarization are characterized by IC50 values equal to 270 ± 65 and 33 ± 3 pM, respectively. The inhibitory potency of (–)PN 200-110 is also time-dependent, IC50 values measured at 2 and 30 min in K^+ solution being equal to 16 ± 4 and 5 ± 3 nM, respectively. Thus, the effect of PN 200-110 is stereoselective, the (+) enantiomer being markedly more potent than the (–) enantiomer. ^{3}H-(+)PN 200-110 binding has been determined in mesenteric arteries bathed in normal and high K^+ solutions. Non-specific binding is not different in polarized and in depolarized arteries. On the contrary, as shown in Figure 10, the specific binding is markedly enhanced in depolarized arteries. Experimental estimates of the specific binding are well fitted by one hyperbolic curve, indicating a one-to-one binding of (+)PN 200-110 to a single class of sites. Fitting of the data reveals that membrane depolarization sig-

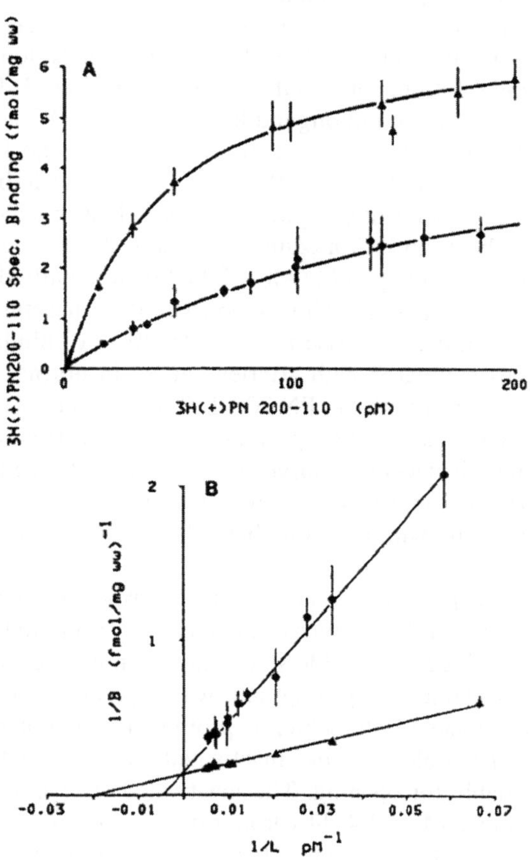

Figure 10. Binding of ^{3}H-(+)PN 200-110 to isolated mesenteric arteries. (A) Saturation study of the specific binding of ^{3}H-(+)PN 200-110 in mesenteric arteries bathed in physiological solution (●) and in KCl depolarising solution (▲). Each point represents the mean ± SE of measurements obtained from 6–18 rings. (B) Double-reciprocal plot of the same data. Modified [71].

nificantly lowers apparent Kd, while maximum binding capacity is not significantly affected. Reciprocal plot of the same data (Fig. 10B) shows that both curves intersect at the same point on the 1/B axis, confirming that the Bmax value is not different in arteries bathed in physiological and in K^+-depolarizing solutions. The Kd value obtained in depolarized arteries (25 pM) is similar to that reported for (+)PN 200-110 in membrane preparations from other tissues and is close to the IC50 measured after 35 min of depolarization. These data indicate that, like its pharmacological effect, the binding of PN 200-110 to intact tissue is stereospecific and voltage-dependent.

Analysis of the interaction of various CCBs with specific binding in isolated arteries at various resting potentials has revealed interesting differences between molecules. For instance, we have compared the effects of nifedipine, (+)PN 200-110 and flunarizine on specific binding of ^{3}H-(+)PN 200-110 in intact mesenteric arteries [72]. Segments of mesenteric arteries were incubated either for 90 min in physiological solution in the presence of 100-pM ^{3}H(+)PN 200-110 or for 60 min in physiological solution followed by 30 min in KCl depolarizing solution, both solutions containing 40 pM ^{3}H-(+)PN 200-110. These concentrations of radioligand labelled about 30% and 50% of the total number of binding sites, respectively, in polarized and in depolarized arteries. Nifedipine and (+)PN 200-110 inhibited the specific binding of ^{3}H-(+)PN 200-110 dose-dependently in polarized, as well as in depolarized arteries. In arteries incubated in KCl medium, the curve describing the displacement of the tritiated ligand by cold (+)PN 200-110 was shifted to the left of that obtained in NaCl medium. This is consistent with saturation studies, which showed a significant increase in ^{3}H(+)PN 200-110 binding affinity in depolarized arteries compared with arteries bathed in normal physiological solution [71]. By contrast with (+) PN 200-110, the effectiveness of nifedipine is not significantly modified by prolonged depolarization, and Ki values calculated from the displacement curves obtained in polarized and in depolarized arteries are not significantly different indicating a similar degree of interaction of nifedipine with calcium channels in both resting and depolarized tissue.

The modulated receptor model may help to describe the interaction of calcium antagonists with $Ca_V1.2$ (L-type) channels. According to this model, the channel can exist in three convertible states: the resting state, when the channel is closed but available for opening, and which predominates in polarized cells; the open or activated state, which is promoted by depolarization pulses beyond a certain threshold; and the inactivated state, when the channel is closed, but unavailable for opening. The inactivated state is favored by prolonged depolarization. Most 1,4-dihydropyridines bind preferentially to the inactivated state of $Ca_V1.2$ channels. Therefore, depolarizing holding potentials that increase the proportion of inactivated channels, but fail to open them, enhance their inhibitory potency. As resting and inactivated channels are in equilibrium, drug binding to inactivated channels decreases the proportion of channels that are available for activation. If K_L and K_H are dissociation constants for low-affinity and high-affinity states, respectively, and L is the fraction of channels in the resting state in the absence of the drug, the model that is schematically illustrated by Figure 11 predicts that at any given holding potential, the concentration dependence of drug binding, and thus of calcium current inhibition, follows a simple adsorption isotherm with an apparent dissociation constant that is given by:

$$Kapp = 1/[(L/K_L) + (1 - L)/K_H].$$

Electrophysiological data are also consistent with this model. In canine ventricle myocytes, K_L and K_H for nitrendipine are equal to 730 and 0.25 nM, respectively [4], in smooth muscle cells from the rat mesenteric artery [4] and dog saphenous vein [104], K_L values were estimated to be 222 and 10 nM and K_H values 0.46 and 0.25 nM, respectively. For nisoldipine, Nelson and Worley [76] estimated, in rabbit mesenteric artery exposed to 1 μM Bay K 8644,

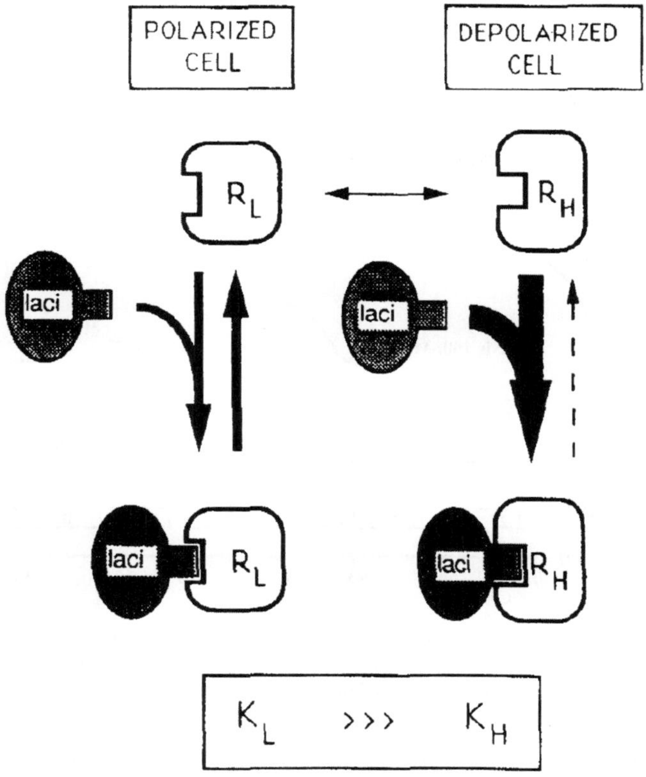

Figure 11. Cartoon representation of binding sites for lacidipine (laci) on calcium channels in polarized and depolarized cells. The high-affinity configuration (low dissociation constant, K_H) is related to the inactivated state of the channels. The low-affinity configuration (high dissociation constant, K_L) is related to the resting state.

apparent dissociation constants of 12.1 and 1.9 nM, respectively, for depolarization of the holding potential from –100 to –55 mV.

The role of the pre-existing membrane potential in the sensitivity of a given tissue to the action of a calcium antagonist in isolated rat aorta is illustrated in Figure 12 for nisoldipine and for lead compounds of the three main classes of

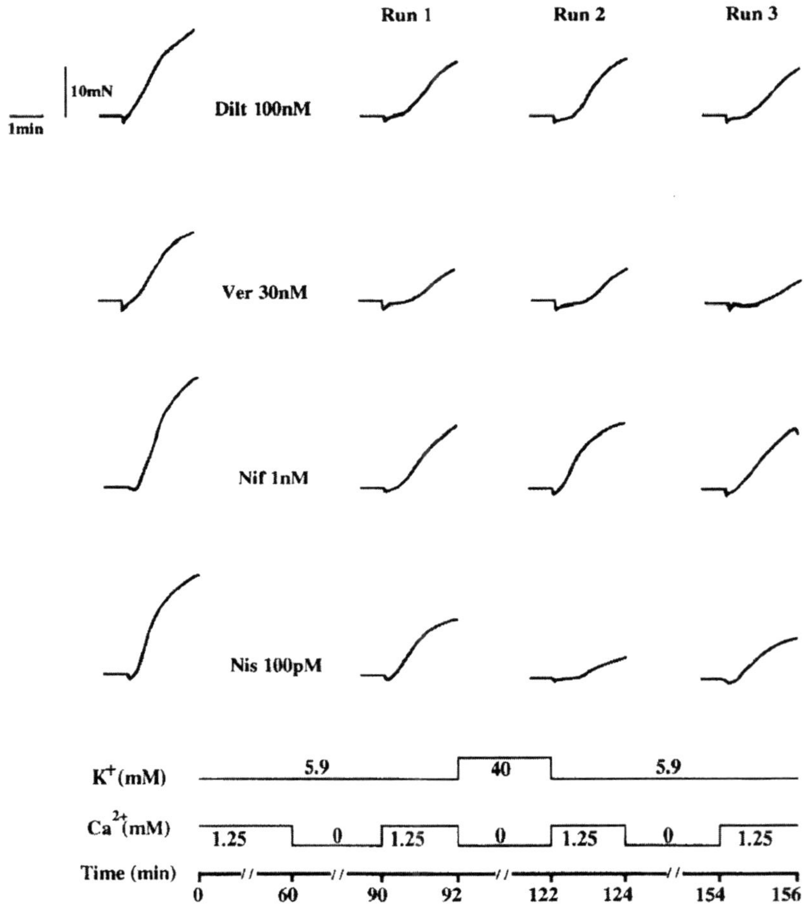

Figure 12. Inhibition produced by calcium antagonists on KCI-induced contraction of rat aorta after preincubation in physiological solution or in 40 mM KCI solution. After recording of control contractions, aortic rings were preincubated for 60 min in the presence of calcium antagonists (at the concentration shown on the figure) in physiological solution. They were then incubated for 30 min in zero Ca^{2+} physiological solution with calcium antagonists before contraction was elicited by exposure to 100 mM KCI solution for 2 min, in the continuous presence of calcium antagonists (run I). Aortic rings were thereafter incubated for 30 min in zero Ca^{2+}, 40 mM KCI-depolarising solution containing the same concentration of calcium antagonists before a second run of contraction was recorded. At the end of this contraction, aortic rings were incubated further in zero Ca^{2+} physiological solution with calcium antagonists and a third run of contraction was recorded. Dilt, diltiazem; Ver, verapamil; Nif, nifedipine; Nis, nisoldipine. Redrawn from [30].

calcium antagonists (nifedipine, verapamil and diltiazem) [30]. The inhibition of the contraction in response to a short test pulse of KCl was tested after an incubation of vascular rings in the presence of a fixed concentration of nisoldipine, nifedipine, verapamil and diltiazem for 60 min in physiological solution followed by 30 min incubation either in physiological solution (KCl = 5.9 mM) or in 40-mM KCl-depolarizing solution. This study showed that the effectiveness of nisoldipine as an inhibitor of the contraction was enhanced after preincubation of the tissue in 40 mM KCl (run 2). With verapamil, diltiazem and nifedipine as inhibitors, incubation in 40 mM KCl did not produce increased inhibition. The increased inhibition of nisoldipine observed after preincubation in high KCl solution was reversed when arteries were further equilibrated in normal physiological solution (run 3); there was no change in the action of the other CCBs. Such experiments allowed the pharmacological identification of CCBs with a higher affinity for inactivated than for closed channels. Those may be termed voltage-dependent CCBs. They belong to the group characterized by a high vasoselectivity.

Because the apparent affinity of the voltage-dependent CCBs for Ca^{2+} channels is related to the resting membrane potential, the degree of initial inhibition of a vasoconstrictor stimulus may differ along the vascular tree, since the resting membrane potential varies between vessels. For instance, cerebral microvessels, which display a resting membrane potential less negative than peripheral vessels, are more sensitive to nimodipine, a voltage-dependent CCB, than conduit arteries. In addition to its tissue distribution, this account for the selectivity of nimodipine for the cerebral circulation [70].

Inhibition by CCBs of agonist-evoked contraction of vascular smooth muscles

As was summarized above, the contraction of vascular smooth muscle, evoked by neurotransmitters and autacoids, is the result of several factors: a) depolarisation, which is responsible for stimulation of calcium entry; b) calcium release from intracellular stores, which activates a further refilling by external calcium; and c) increase in the sensitivity of the contractile proteins to calcium. It is likely that the relative importance of these mechanisms of activation is not identical for different agonists, which are not necessarily present *in vivo* at the concentration required to observe an appreciable response in an organ bath. Several authors have attempted to establish the relation existing between $[Ca^{2+}]_i$ changes and the force of contraction of isolated vessels following the activation by catecholamines, prostanoids, endothelin, angiotensin II, PDGF and other vasoconstrictors. Those studies have revealed differences of this relation among vessels. They have also shown that the origin of activator calcium may vary and that is not always related to depolarization and consequently to the activation of VOCs. As far cathecholamines are concerned, as reviewed by Karaki et al. [49] experimental results indicate that activation of the α_1-adrenoceptor releases Ca^{2+} in rat aorta and portal vein. However, this receptor is not coupled to Ca^{2+} release in ferret aorta and only weakly coupled to Ca^{2+} release in rat tail artery. This receptor may also be directly coupled to the L-type Ca^{2+} channel and to Ca^{2+} sensitizing mechanism in some types of smooth muscle. In contrast, the activation of α_2-adrenoceptor, which increases $[Ca^{2+}]_i$ stimulates neither phosphoinositide turnover nor Ca^{2+} release from intracellular stores. In isolated cell studies, pre-treatment of cells with pertussis toxin abolishes the elevation of $[Ca^{2+}]_i$ suggesting the involvement of a Gi-like GTP-binding protein. By measuring simultaneously $[Ca^{2+}]_i$ and contraction in ferret portal vein, Morgan and Morgan [74] have shown that phenylephrine produces a larger force than high KC1 for a similar augmentation of $[Ca^{2+}]_i$. Similar results were obtained in guinea pig aorta [46], swine carotid artery [80] and rat aorta [50]. In rat and rabbit mesenteric artery permeabilized by α-toxin, Nishimura et al. [77] have shown that norepinephrine augmented the contraction induced by Ca^{2+}. The response to norepinephrine was increased by GTP and inhibited by guanosine-5'-O-β–thiodiphosphate (GDPβS), suggesting that the change in Ca^{2+} sensitivity is mediated by a GTP-binding protein coupled with the α-adrenoceptor. It is therefore not surprising, considering the complexity of the Ca signaling processes including the L-type Ca^{2+} influx, that verapamil reduced the norepinephrine-stimulated Ca entry more than the contraction as was observed in rat aorta [50].

Endothelin

Endothelin-1 (ET-1) is a 21-amino acid peptide produced by the endothelium of the vascular wall [103], it exhibits a very powerful vasoconstrictor action in various animal and human vessels both *in vitro* and *in vivo*. Therefore, endothelin has been proposed to be one of the factors responsible for the pathogenesis of coronary ischaemic syndromes and of hypertension. However, *in vivo* studies have shown that the action of endothelin is surprisingly more complex than that predicted from *in vitro* studies. Indeed, as shown by D'Orleans Juste et al. [14], endothelin can produce a decrease in perfusion pressure in some vascular beds and even a transitory fall in blood pressure. This action of endothelin, which has been attributed to the release of endothelium-derived relaxing factors (EDRF) in the venous side of the circulation, may be reproduced on isolated veins *in vitro* [37]. The ability of endothelin to release EDRF is not limited to the venous endothelium, it has been shown that endothelin triggers NO formation via ET_B receptors on the endothelium of arteries. The resulting activation of soluble guanylate cyclase, stimulates cGMP production is followed by the relaxation of the artery as was shown for the rat thoracic aorta [75]. Other studies have shown that endothelin may also exhibit at sub-threshold concentration an action that is detectable only when the artery is exposed to another vasoactive agent. This action appears to be different from the direct vasoconstrictor action and may be ascribed as a pre-conditioning effect, resulting in the amplification of the response to the other vasoconstrictors. Figure 13 illustrates a pre-conditioning action of endothelin,

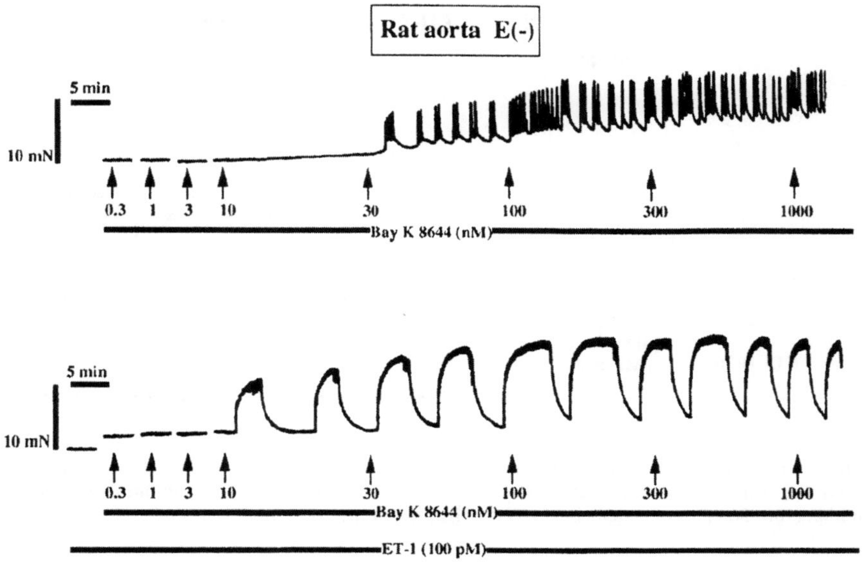

Figure 13. Potentiation by a sub-threshold concentration of endothelin-1 (ET-1) of the contractile response to BayK8644 of isolated rat aorta without endothelium [E(–)]. Modified from [34].

using an activator of $Ca_V1.2$ (L-type) as an agonist. It shows how the vasoconstrictor action of this agent is amplified by a sub-threshold concentration of ET-1. Amplification was also observed with adrenoceptor agonists and was related to increased Ca entry during receptor stimulation [34], an effect amplified by high-salt diet [90]. This amplification is not limited to rat aorta, as it has been observed in many vessel with various agonists including cerebral arteries stimulated by serotonin, the physiological regulator of their tone [85] and human coronary arteries also stimulated by serotonin, a putative pathophysiological transmitter (Fig. 14) [3].

Endothelin-1 by acting on the ET_A receptor, increases IP3 production and releases Ca^{2+} to induce an initial transient increase in $[Ca^{2+}]_i$ in some types of smooth muscle. However, this Ca^{2+} increase is not always coupled to myosin light chain (MLC) phosphorylation or contraction. Endothelin-1 also opens the L-type Ca^{2+} channel to induce a sustained increase in $[Ca^{2+}]_i$ and a sustained contraction. Non-L-type Ca^{2+} entry pathway may also be activated. In some smooth muscles, the Ca^{2+} sensitivity of contractile elements is increased by endothelin-1. Activation of the ET_A receptor elicits sustained contractions with sustained increases in $[Ca^{2+}]_i$ in various vessels *in vitro* including: rat aorta, rat carotid artery [78], swine carotid artery [81], rabbit mesenteric artery [105] and human coronary arteries [3]. The initial portion of the increase in $[Ca^{2+}]_i$ is due to the formation of IP3 [65], which is resulting in Ca^{2+} release. Sustained increases in $[Ca^{2+}]_i$ due to endothelin-1 are inhibited by removal of

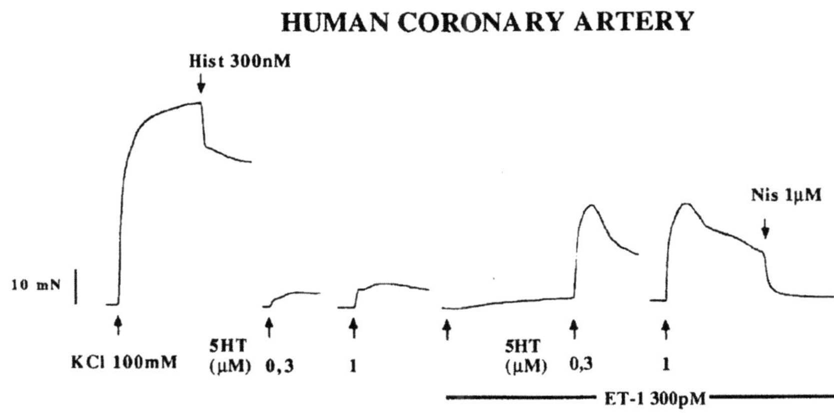

Figure 14. Typical recording of contraction of a human proximal artery segment with two concentrations (0.3–1 μM) of serotonin (Ser), before and after 90 min incubation with a sub-threshold concentration (100–300 pM) of endothelin-1 (ET-1). Hist, histamine. Modified from [3].

external Ca^{2+} and, also, by CCBs in swine coronary artery [42], in rat aorta [84], in rabbit mesenteric artery [105], in rabbit aorta [5] and in human coronary arteries [3]. The sensitivity to CCBs suggests that endothelin-1 opens the L-type Ca^{2+} channel and elicits a sustained increase in $[Ca^{2+}]_i$ although the processes involved appear more numerous. When ET-1 concentration is low, oscillatory contractions are observed that are related to oscillations of the intracellular Ca concentration (Fig. 15). Different non-specific voltage operated channels are also involved in the entry of calcium [106]. The endothelin-1-induced contraction is greater than that induced by high KC1 at a given

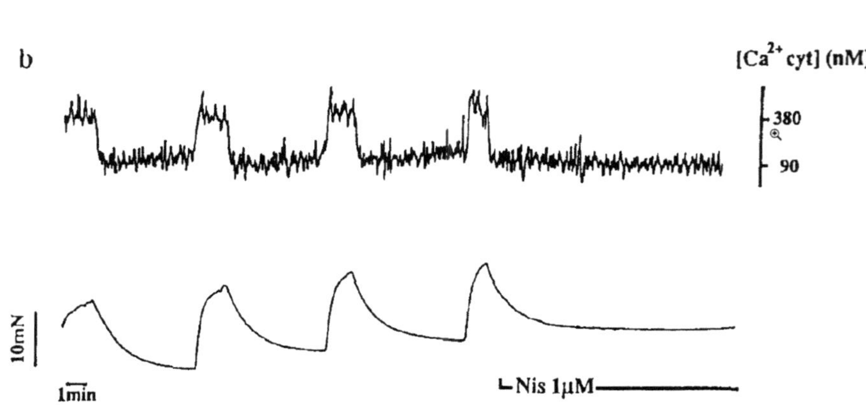

Figure 15. Fura-2 loaded human coronary artery. Typical recording of changes in cytosolic calcium (Ca^{2+} cyt, upper tracing) and in force development (lower tracing) during spontaneous activity, showing the action of nisoldipine Nis, 1 μM). Modified from [38].

$[Ca^{2+}]_i$ in rat aorta [84], and swine coronary artery [58, 59]. Endothelin-1 also augments the Ca^{2+}-induced contraction in permeabilized smooth muscle [94]. Endothelin-1 elicits a greater MLC phosphorylation than high KC1 at a given $[Ca^{2+}]_i$ in swine carotid artery [80], rat aorta [44] and rabbit mesenteric artery [105]. In rabbit mesenteric artery, the increase in MLC phosphorylation is not altered by changes in $[Ca^{2+}]_i$, suggesting that it could result from C kinase activation rather than from MLC kinase activation [95]. Endothelin-1 also acts on the ET_B receptors localized on smooth muscle membrane, which may be coupled to Ca^{2+} influx pathway and Ca^{2+} sensitization but not to phosphatidylinositol turnover. Stimulation of the ET_B receptor, therefore, increases $[Ca^{2+}]_i$ and induced contraction which is greater than that induced by high KC1 at a given $[Ca^{2+}]_i$ without inducing Ca^{2+} release. In swine pulmonary vein, porcine coronary artery endothelin-1 acts on the ET_B receptor and increases both $[Ca^{2+}]_i$ and Ca^{2+} sensitivity although it does not induce Ca^{2+} release, indicating that the ET_B receptor is coupled to Ca^{2+} influx but not to Ca^{2+} release [94].

When considering the action of CCBs on ET-1-evoked vasoconstriction, it appears that, due to the complexity of ET-1 intracellular pathways leading to contraction, the direct vasoconstrictor action is not everywhere sensitive to the presence of calcium antagonists, indicating that L-type Ca currents are not everywhere involved in contraction. Whereas the pre-conditioning action identified by the amplified response to other vasoconstrictors is highly sensitive even in vessels where the direct action is resistant to CCBs [34]. The amplifying action of a given agent does not necessarily involve calcium channels, several other pathways may operate as for instance an increase of the sensitivity of the contractile machinery to the activation by calcium. In addition to the regulation of $[Ca^{2+}]_i$ at the level of calcium channels, IP3CaR and/or CalCaR, an induction of contraction by the stimulation of a receptor may be modulated by activation of MLC kinase (MLCK) and phosphorylation of MLC [49]. A first mechanism is the inhibition of Ca^{2+}-calmodulin-dependent protein kinase II (CaMKII), which phosphorylates MLC kinase inhibiting its activity. A second mechanism is the inhibition of MLC phosphatase (PPase). Arachidonic acid, produced by receptor-mediated activation of phospholipase A2, may directly inhibit phosphatase. C kinase and tyrosine kinase may also inhibit phosphatase by inhibiting the endogenous inhibitor of phosphatase. A third mechanism is the increase of free calmodulin concentration. A fourth mechanism is to activate actin independently of MLC phosphorylation. The complexity of the mechanisms activated by ET-1 indicates that CCBs could not be expected to blunt all the effects of this peptide on vascular tone.

Endothelin immunoreactivity has been detected in human plasma [15], but at very low circulating levels. It is likely that the actual concentration at the site of arterial spasm or in the interstitium surrounding the vascular smooth muscle may be higher than in plasma. However, it is likely that it does not reach the level of concentration required *in vitro* in order to evoke contraction of vascular smooth muscle. Most likely, *in vivo*, the low level of endothelin produced by endothelium may merely amplify the constrictor effect of other circulating hormones or autacoids. In the case of the coronary circulation, clinical studies have emphasized the role of serotonin in acute ischaemic heart diseases [39], and potentiation by low level of endothelin or serotonin locally released from activated platelets may contribute to the pathogenesis of ischaemic heart disease.

Cathecholamines

Stimulation of α1-adrenoceptors by noradrenaline increases cytosolic free calcium and produces a contraction. This contraction may be characterized by an initial fast component followed by a sustained tonic component. It has been known for a long time [32, 33] that the initial fast component of the contraction evoked by high concentration of noradrenaline persisted in the absence of extracellular calcium, implying that noradrenaline releases calcium from intracellular stores. It is now well established that activation of α_1-adrenoceptors causes the hydrolysis of inositol phospholipids through the coupling of the adrenoceptor with phospholipase C. Inositol 1,4,5-triphosphate released into the cytosol then induces the release of calcium from internal stores, which is responsible for the initial phase of the contraction [66]. The tonic-sustained component is partly dependent on the noradrenaline-dependent calcium influx related to the opening of channels allowing calcium to enter the cell according to its electrochemical gradient [28]. Calcium antagonists prevent this increased calcium entry without affecting resting calcium fluxes or intracellular calcium release. It has been observed that they are less potent against calcium entry stimulated by receptors than by high potassium depolarisation [36]. Therefore, some authors [11, 92] have hypothesized the existence of calcium channels gated by receptor activation (ROCs) and calcium channels gated by potential (VDCs) [6a], the former being less sensitive and the latter being more sensitive to the action of calcium antagonists. Morel and Godfraind [69] have investigated whether the apparent existence of two different calcium entry pathways with differing sensitivity to calcium antagonists could be related to different degrees of activation of L-type calcium channels ($Ca_V1.2$) by noradrenaline and K-depolarisation. The analysis of the effect of nisoldipine in rat aorta shows that although agonists and depolarization-induced responses have different sensitivities to this dihydropyridine, this does not necessarily mean that responses are mediated by different calcium channels. While the potency of nisoldipine is higher against the 100 mM KCl-induced contraction than against the noradrenaline-induced contraction when measures of the inhibition are performed after prolonged contraction, there is no significant difference between the IC50 value of nisoldipine on calcium entry and contraction induced by 100 mM KCl solution or by noradrenaline, when the responses are measured after a short duration of stimulation. Furthermore, the inhibitory potency of nisoldipine on the response evoked by brief application of noradrenaline may be increased by pre-incubation of the tissue with the dihydropyridine in depolarizing solution. This suggests that noradrenaline-evoked contractions depend, at least partly, on the same nisoldipine-sensitive calcium entry pathway as depolarization-induced contraction.

Modulation of the voltage-dependent binding sites of the dihydropyridines by noradrenaline has been confirmed in radioligand experiments. Noradrenaline produces an increase in the affinity of both nisoldipine and isradipine, comparable to that of 20 mM KCl, which is likely to be the result of the small depolarization produced by noradrenaline. Thus, nisoldipine inhibition of noradrenaline-induced effects is modulated by the preexisting membrane potential of the tissue, which, in turn, modulates the affinity of the binding sites for nisoldipine. Furthermore, noradrenaline, by its depolarising effect, modulates the interaction of nisoldipine with its binding sites on calcium channels in intact tissue and, in turn, its own inhibition by nisoldipine.

Electrophysiological studies may also help to demonstrate this activation of voltage-operated calcium channels by noradrenaline [63]. In rat aorta, noradrenaline produces a dose-dependent depolarization of the vascular smooth muscle [60]. This depolarization of vascular smooth muscle may be characterized by the existence of two thresholds: a lower one for a sustained tonic depolarization, and the other for the activation of oscillatory potentials. These oscillatory potentials are absent when calcium is removed from the extracellular fluid, indicating that they are the result of the activation of voltage-operated calcium channels that are blocked by calcium antagonists, a finding that is in agreement with the results of calcium removal experiments.

There have been many publications describing the sensitivity to calcium-channel blockers of responses to adrenoceptors stimulation. It has been postulated that responses sensitive to calcium antagonists were related to activation of α_2-adrenoceptors and that resistant responses were due to activation of α_1-adrenoceptors. This hypothesis was derived mainly from *in vivo* studies on pithed rats, in which it was observed that vasoconstriction evoked by α_1-adrenoceptor agonists, such as phenylephrine, was relatively insensitive to calcium-channel blockers, whereas the vasoconstriction evoked by an α_2-agonist, such as B-HT 920, was highly sensitive [100]. However, in pithed rats, calcium-channel blockers inhibited vasoconstriction effects evoked by other α_2-adrenoceptor agonists, such as St 587 and (–)-dobutamine. Such a discrepancy has been explained by a relationship between receptor reserve and adrenoceptor agonist efficacy to inhibition by calcium antagonists [83]. *In vitro* studies on the response of blood vessels to α_2-adrenoceptor agonists have pointed to the complexity of the factors involved [89], and experiments in pithed rats have not allowed discrimination between the sensitivity of subtypes of $\alpha 1$-receptors to calcium antagonists [89].

In contrast, depolarization-induced contraction is primarily maintained by a sustained increased in intracellular Ca^{2+}. *In vitro* studies on endothelium-denuded arteries have shown that the maximum response to the $\alpha 2$-agonist clonidine is reduced more by calcium antagonists than the maximum response to noradrenaline, findings that were in agreement with *in vivo* studies [31]. Calcium antagonists are non-competitive antagonists of vasoconstrictors;

therefore, their inhibitory action should be largely dependent upon receptor reserve in a given tissue and upon the intrinsic activity of the agonist utilized. We have shown that the intrinsic activity of clonidine, a partial agonist, is much lower than that of noradrenaline, which may explain why the former is more sensitive to blockade by calcium antagonists [2].

References

1 Aburto T, Jinsi A, Zhu Q and Deth RC. Involvement of protein kinase C activation in alpha 2-adrenoceptor-mediated contractions of rabbit saphenous vein. *Eur J Pharmacol* 277: 35–44, 1995
2 Alosachie I and Godfraind T. The modulatory role of vascular endothelium in the interaction of agonists and antagonists with alpha-adrenoceptors in the rat aorta. *Br J Pharmacol* 95: 619–629, 1988
3 Balligand JL and Godfraind T. Effect of nisoldipine on contractions evoked by endothelin-1 in human isolated distal and proximal coronary arteries and veins. *J Cardiovasc Pharmacol* 24: 618–625, 1994
4 Bean BP, Sturek M, Puga A and Hermsmeyer K. Calcium channels in muscle cells isolated from rat mesenteric arteries: modulation by dihydropyridine drugs. *Circ Res* 59: 229–235, 1986
5 Benchekroun MT, Gros-Louis N, Bkaily G and D'Orleans-Juste P. R-type calcium channel involved in endothelin-1-induced contraction of rabbit aorta. *J Cardiovasc Pharmacol* 26 Suppl 3: S300–302, 1995
6 Bolotina VM, Najibi S, Palacino JJ, Pagano PJ and Cohen RA. Nitric oxide directly activates calcium-dependent potassium channels in vascular smooth muscle. *Nature* 368: 850–853, 1994
6a Bolton TB. Mechanisms of action of transmitters and other substances on smooth muscle. *Physiol Rev* 59: 606–718, 1979
7 Brandes RP, Schmitz-Winnenthal FH, Feletou M, Godecke A, Huang PL, Vanhoutte PM, Fleming I and Busse R. An endothelium-derived hyperpolarizing factor distinct from NO and prostacyclin is a major endothelium-dependent vasodilator in resistance vessels of wild-type and endothelial NO synthase knockout mice. *Proc Natl Acad Sci USA* 97: 9747–9752, 2000
8 Briggs AH. Calcium movements during potassium contracture in isolated rabbit aortic strips. *Am J Physiol* 203: 849–852, 1962
9 Briggs AH and Shibata S. Ca and ouabain interaction on vascular smooth muscle. *Proc Soc Exp Biol Med* 121: 274–278, 1966
10 Busse R, Edwards G, Feletou M, Fleming I, Vanhoutte PM and Weston AH. EDHF: bringing the concepts together. *Trends Pharmacol Sci* 23: 374–380, 2002
11 Cauvin C and van Breemen C. Different Ca^{2+} channels along the arterial tree. *J Cardiovasc Pharmacol* 7 Suppl 4: S4–10, 1985
12 Chitaley K and Webb RC. Nitric oxide induces dilation of rat aorta via inhibition of rho-kinase signaling. *Hypertension* 39: 438–442, 2002
13 Cocks TM and Angus JA. Endothelium-dependent relaxation of coronary arteries by noradrenaline and serotonin. *Nature* 305: 627–630, 1983
14 D'Orleans-Juste P, Finet M, de Nucci G and Vane JR. Pharmacology of endothelin-1 in isolated vessels: effect of nicardipine, methylene blue, hemoglobin, and gossypol. *J Cardiovasc Pharmacol* 13 Suppl 5: S19–22; discussion S45, 1989
15 Davenport AP, Ashby MJ, Easton P, Ella S, Bedford J, Dickerson C, Nunez DJ, Capper SJ and Brown MJ. A sensitive radioimmunoassay measuring endothelin-like immunoreactivity in human plasma: comparison of levels in patients with essential hypertension and normotensive control subjects. *Clin Sci (Lond)* 78: 261–264, 1990
16 Dessy C, Kim I, Sougnez CL, Laporte R and Morgan KG. A role for MAP kinase in differentiated smooth muscle contraction evoked by alpha-adrenoceptor stimulation. *Am J Physiol* 275: C1081–1086, 1998
17 Dessy C, Matsuda N, Hulvershorn J, Sougnez CL, Sellke FW and Morgan KG. Evidence for

involvement of the PKC-alpha isoform in myogenic contractions of the coronary microcirculation. *Am J Physiol Heart Circ Physiol* 279: H916–923, 2000
18 Deth R and van Breemen C. Agonist induced release of intracellular Ca^{2+} in the rabbit aorta. *J Membr Biol* 30: 363–380, 1977
19 Deth R and van Breemen C. Relative contributions of Ca^{2+} influx and cellular Ca^{2+} release during drug induced activation of the rabbit aorta. *Pflugers Arch* 348: 13–22, 1974
20 Diamond J and Chu EB. Possible role for cyclic GMP in endothelium-dependent relaxation of rabbit aorta by acetylcholine. Comparison with nitroglycerin. *Res Commun Chem Pathol Pharmacol* 41: 369–381, 1983
21 Egleme C, Godfraind T and Miller RC. Enhanced responsiveness of rat isolated aorta to clonidine after removal of the endothelial cells. *Br J Pharmacol* 81: 16–18, 1984
22 Fay FS, Shlevin HH, Granger WC, Jr and Taylor SR. Aequorin luminescence during activation of single isolated smooth muscle cells. *Nature* 280: 506–508, 1979
23 Furchgott RF, Cherry PD, Zawadzki JV and Jothianandan D. Endothelial cells as mediators of vasodilation of arteries. *J Cardiovasc Pharmacol* 6 Suppl 2: S336–343, 1984
24 Furchgott RF and Zawadzki JV. The obligatory role of endothelial cells in the relaxation of arterial smooth muscle by acetylcholine. *Nature* 288: 373–376, 1980
25 Ghisdal P, Godfraind T and Morel N. Effect of nitro-L-arginine on electrical and mechanical responses to acetylcholine in the superior mesenteric artery from stroke-prone hypertensive rat. *Br J Pharmacol* 128: 1513–1523, 1999
26 Godfraind T. Actions of nifedipine on calcium fluxes and contraction in isolated rat arteries. *J Pharmacol Exp Ther* 224: 443–450, 1983
27 Godfraind T. Calcium antagonists and vasodilatation. *Pharmacol Ther* 64: 37–75, 1994
28 Godfraind T. Calcium exchange in vascular smooth muscle, action of noradrenaline and lanthanum. *J Physiol* 260: 21–35, 1976
29 Godfraind T. EDRF and cyclic GMP control gating of receptor-operated calcium channels in vascular smooth muscle. *Eur J Pharmacol* 126: 341–343, 1986
30 Godfraind T, Dessy C and Salomone S. A comparison of the potency of selective L-calcium channel blockers in human coronary and internal mammary arteries exposed to serotonin. *J Pharmacol Exp Ther* 263: 112–122, 1992
31 Godfraind T, Egleme C and Al Osachie I. Role of endothelium in the contractile response of rat aorta to alpha-adrenoceptor agonists. *Clin Sci (Lond)* 68 Suppl 10: 65 s-71 s, 1985
32 Godfraind T and Kaba A. Blockade or reversal of the contraction induced by calcium and adrenaline in depolarized arterial smooth muscle. *Br J Pharmacol* 36: 549–560, 1969
33 Godfraind T and Kaba A. Inhibition by cinnarizine and chlorpromazine of the contraction induced by calcium and adrenaline in vascular smooth muscle. *Br J Pharmacol* 35: P354–355, 1969
34 Godfraind T, Mennig D, Morel N and Wibo M. Effect of endothelin-1 on calcium channel gating by agonists in vascular smooth muscle. *J Cardiovasc Pharmacol* 13 Suppl 5: S112–117; discussion S123, 1989
35 Godfraind T, Miller R and Wibo M. Calcium antagonism and calcium entry blockade. *Pharmacol Rev* 38: 321–416, 1986
36 Godfraind T and Miller RC. Specificity of action of Ca^{2+} entry blockers. A comparison of their actions in rat arteries and in human coronary arteries. *Circ Res* 52: I81–91, 1983
37 Godfraind T and Salomone S. Functional interaction of lacidipine with calcium channels in vascular smooth muscle. *J Cardiovasc Pharmacol* 18 Suppl 11: S1–6, 1991
38 Godfraind T, Salomone S, Dessy C, Verhelst B, Dion R and Schoevaerts JC. Selectivity scale of calcium antagonists in the human cardiovascular system based on *in vitro* studies. *J Cardiovasc Pharmacol* 20 Suppl 5: S34–41, 1992
39 Golino P, Piscione F, Willerson JT, Cappelli-Bigazzi M, Focaccio A, Villari B, Indolfi C, Russolillo E, Condorelli M and Chiariello M. Divergent effects of serotonin on coronary-artery dimensions and blood flow in patients with coronary atherosclerosis and control patients. *N Engl J Med* 324: 641–648, 1991
40 Goodman FR and Weiss GB. Dissociation by lanthanum of smooth muscle responses to potassium and acetylcholine. *Am J Physiol* 220: 759–766, 1971
41 Goodman FR and Weiss GB. Effects of lanthanum on ^{45}Ca movements and on contractions induced by norepinephrine, histamine and potassium in vascular smooth muscle. *J Pharmacol Exp Ther* 177: 415–425, 1971
42 Goto K, Kasuya Y, Matsuki N, Takuwa Y, Kurihara H, Ishikawa T, Kimura S, Yanagisawa M and

Masaki T. Endothelin activates the dihydropyridine-sensitive, voltage-dependent Ca^{2+} channel in vascular smooth muscle. *Proc Natl Acad Sci USA* 86: 3915–3918, 1989
43 Grynkiewicz G, Poenie M and Tsien RY. A new generation of Ca^{2+} indicators with greatly improved fluorescence properties. *J Biol Chem* 260: 3440–3450, 1985
44 Hori M, Sato K, Sakata K, Ozaki H, Takano-Ohmuro H, Tsuchiya T, Sugi H, Kato I and Karaki H. Receptor agonists induce myosin phosphorylation-dependent and phosphorylation-independent contractions in vascular smooth muscle. *J Pharmacol Exp Ther* 261: 506–512, 1992
45 Ignarro LJ and Kadowitz PJ. The pharmacological and physiological role of cyclic GMP in vascular smooth muscle relaxation. *Annu Rev Pharmacol Toxicol* 25: 171–191, 1985
46 Jiang MJ, Chan CF and Chang YL. Intracellular calcium and myosin light chain phosphorylation during U46619-activated vascular contraction. *Life Sci* 54: 2005–2013, 1994
47 Karaki H. Ca^{2+} localization and sensitivity in vascular smooth muscle. *Trends Pharmacol Sci* 10: 320–325, 1989
48 Karaki H. The intracellular calcium-force relationship in vascular smooth muscle. Time- and stimulus-dependent dissociation. *Am J Hypertens* 3: 253S-256S, 1990
49 Karaki H, Ozaki H, Hori M, Mitsui-Saito M, Amano K, Harada K, Miyamoto S, Nakazawa H, Won KJ and Sato K. Calcium movements, distribution, and functions in smooth muscle. *Pharmacol Rev* 49: 157–230, 1997
50 Karaki H, Sato K and Ozaki H. Different effects of verapamil on cytosolic Ca^{2+} and contraction in norepinephrine-stimulated vascular smooth muscle. *Jpn J Pharmacol* 55: 35–42, 1991
51 Karaki H and Weiss GB. Alterations in high and low affinity binding of ^{45}Ca in rabbit aortic smooth muscle by norepinephrine and potassium after exposure to lanthanum and low temperature. *J Pharmacol Exp Ther* 211: 86–92, 1979
52 Karaki H and Weiss GB. Dissociation of varied actions of norepinephrine on ^{45}Ca uptake and release at different sites in rabbit aortic smooth muscle. *J Pharmacol Exp Ther* 215: 363–368, 1980
53 Karaki H and Weiss GB. Effects of stimulatory agents on mobilization of high and low affinity site ^{45}Ca in rabbit aortic smooth muscle. *J Pharmacol Exp Ther* 213: 450–455, 1980
54 Karaki H and Weiss GB. Inhibitors of mitochondrial Ca^{2+} uptake dissociate potassium-induced tension responses from increased ^{45}Ca retention in rabbit aortic smooth muscle. *Blood Vessels* 18: 28–35, 1981
55 Karaki H and Weiss GB. Modification by decreased temperature and hypoxia of ^{45}Ca movements in stimulated smooth muscle of rabbit aorta. *Gen Pharmacol* 18: 363–368, 1987
56 Karaki H and Weiss GB. Qualitative differences in ^{45}Ca efflux from membrane sites in vascular smooth muscle when washout conditions are varied. *Gen Pharmacol* 11: 483–489, 1980
57 Klockner U and Isenberg G. The dihydropyridine niguldipine modulates calcium and potassium currents in vascular smooth muscle cells. *Br J Pharmacol* 97: 957–967, 1989
58 Kodama M, Kanaide H, Abe S, Hirano K, Kai H and Nakamura M. Endothelin-induced Ca-independent contraction of the porcine coronary artery. *Biochem Biophys Res Commun* 160: 1302–1308, 1989
59 Kodama M, Yamamoto H and Kanaide H. Myosin phosphorylation and Ca^{2+} sensitization in porcine coronary arterial smooth muscle stimulated with endothelin-1. *Eur J Pharmacol* 288: 69–77, 1994
60 Krippeit-Drews P, Morel N and Godfraind T. Effect of nitric oxide on membrane potential and contraction of rat aorta. *J Cardiovasc Pharmacol* 20 Suppl 12: S72–75, 1992
61 Lang D and Lewis MJ. Endothelium-derived relaxing factor inhibits the formation of inositol trisphosphate by rabbit aorta. *J Physiol* 411: 45–52, 1989
62 Lang D and Lewis MJ. Inhibition of inositol 1,4,5-trisphosphate formation by cyclic GMP in cultured aortic endothelial cells of the pig. *Br J Pharmacol* 102: 277–281, 1991
63 Large WA. Three membrane-conductance mechanisms activated by noradrenaline in vascular smooth muscle. *Z Kardiol* 80 Suppl 7: 55–57, 1991
64 Low AM, Kwan CY and Daniel EE. Evidence for two types of internal Ca^{2+} stores in canine mesenteric artery with different refilling mechanisms. *Am J Physiol* 262: H31–37, 1992
65 Marsden PA, Danthuluri NR, Brenner BM, Ballermann BJ and Brock TA. Endothelin action on vascular smooth muscle involves inositol trisphosphate and calcium mobilization. *Biochem Biophys Res Commun* 158: 86–93, 1989
66 Minneman KP. Alpha 1-adrenergic receptor subtypes, inositol phosphates, and sources of cell

Ca^{2+}. *Pharmacol Rev* 40: 87–119, 1988
67 Mironneau J. Pharmacology of Ca^{2+} channels in smooth muscle. *Z Kardiol* 80 Suppl 7: 43–46, 1991
68 Moncada S and Higgs A. The L-arginine-nitric oxide pathway. *N Engl J Med* 329: 2002–2012, 1993
69 Morel N and Godfraind T. Characterization in rat aorta of the binding sites responsible for blockade of noradrenaline-evoked calcium entry by nisoldipine. *Br J Pharmacol* 102: 467–477, 1991
70 Morel N and Godfraind T. Pharmacological properties of voltage-dependent calcium channels in functional microvessels isolated from rat brain. *Naunyn Schmiedebergs Arch Pharmacol* 340: 442–451, 1989
71 Morel N and Godfraind T. Prolonged depolarization increases the pharmacological effect of dihydropyridines and their binding affinity for calcium channels of vascular smooth muscle. *J Pharmacol Exp Ther* 243: 711–715, 1987
72 Morel N and Godfraind T. Selective modulation by membrane potential of the interaction of some calcium entry blockers with calcium channels in rat mesenteric artery. *Br J Pharmacol* 95: 252–258, 1988
73 Morgan JP and Morgan KG. Alteration of cytoplasmic ionized calcium levels in smooth muscle by vasodilators in the ferret. *J Physiol* 357: 539–551, 1984
74 Morgan JP and Morgan KG. Stimulus-specific patterns of intracellular calcium levels in smooth muscle of ferret portal vein. *J Physiol* 351: 155–167, 1984
75 Moritoki H, Hisayama T, Takeuchi S, Kondoh W and Imagawa M. Relaxation of rat thoracic aorta induced by the Ca^{2+}-ATPase inhibitor, cyclopiazonic acid, possibly through nitric oxide formation. *Br J Pharmacol* 111: 655–642, 1994
76 Nelson MT and Worley JF. Dihydropyridine inhibition of single calcium channels and contraction in rabbit mesenteric artery depends on voltage. *J Physiol* 412: 65–91, 1989
77 Nishimura J, Khalil RA, Drenth JP and van Breemen C. Evidence for increased myofilament Ca^{2+} sensitivity in norepinephrine-activated vascular smooth muscle. *Am J Physiol* 259: H2–8, 1990
78 Ozaki H, Sato K, Sakata K and Karaki H. Endothelin dissociates muscle tension from cytosolic Ca^{2+} in vascular smooth muscle of rat carotid artery. *Jpn J Pharmacol* 50: 521–524, 1989
79 Rapoport RM, Draznin MB and Murad F. Endothelium-dependent relaxation in rat aorta may be mediated through cyclic GMP-dependent protein phosphorylation. *Nature* 306: 174–176, 1983
80 Rembold CM. Modulation of the $[Ca^{2+}]$ sensitivity of myosin phosphorylation in intact swine arterial smooth muscle. *J Physiol* 429: 77–94, 1990
81 Rembold CM and Weaver BA. $[Ca^{2+}]$, not diacylglycerol, is the primary regulator of sustained swine arterial smooth muscle contraction. *Hypertension* 15: 692–698, 1990
82 Ridgway EB and Ashley CC. Calcium transients in single muscle fibers. *Biochem Biophys Res Commun* 29: 229–234, 1967
83 Ruffolo RR, Jr and Nichols AJ. The relationship of receptor reserve and agonist efficacy to the sensitivity of alpha-adrenoceptor-mediated vasopressor responses to inhibition by calcium channel antagonists. *Ann NY Acad Sci* 522: 361–376, 1988
84 Sakata K, Ozaki H, Kwon SC and Karaki H. Effects of endothelin on the mechanical activity and cytosolic calcium level of various types of smooth muscle. *Br J Pharmacol* 98: 483–492, 1989
85 Salomone S, Dessy C, Morel N and Godfraind T. Inhibition by bosentan, an endothelin antagonist, of the hypersensitivity to Ca^{2+} channel activator evoked by salt-loading in basilar artery of stroke-prone spontaneously hypertensive rats. *Life Sci* 59: PL247–253, 1996
86 Salomone S and Godfraind T. Radioligand and functional estimates of the interaction of the 1,4-dihydropyridines, isradipine and lacidipine, with calcium channels in smooth muscle. *Br J Pharmacol* 109: 100–106, 1993
86a Salomone S, Morel N and Godfraind T. Role of nitric oxide in the contractile response to 5-hydroxy-tryptamine of the basilar artery from Wistar Kyoto and stroke-prone rats. *Br J Pharmacol* 121: 1051–1058, 1997
87 Salomone S, Morel N and Godfraind T. Effects of 8-bromo cyclic GMP and verapamil on depolarization-evoked Ca^{2+} signal and contraction in rat aorta. *Br J Pharmacol* 114: 1731–1737, 1995
88 Salomone S, Wibo M, Morel N and Godfraind T. Binding sites for 1,4-dihydropyridine Ca^{2+}-channel modulators in rat intestinal smooth muscle. *Naunyn Schmiedebergs Arch Pharmacol* 344: 698–705, 1991
89 Schwietert HR, Mathy MJ, Wilhelm D, Wilffert B, Pfaffendorf M and van Zwieten PA. Alpha

1-adrenoceptor-mediated Ca^{2+}-entry from the extracellular fluid and Ca^{2+}-release from intracellular stores: no role for alpha 1A,B-adrenoceptor subtypes in the pithed rat. *J Auton Pharmacol* 12: 125–136, 1992
90 Smith L, Payne JA, Sedeek MH, Granger JP and Khalil RA. Endothelin-induced increases in Ca^{2+} entry mechanisms of vascular contraction are enhanced during high-salt diet. *Hypertension* 41: 787–793, 2003
91 Somlyo AP and Somlyo AV. Signal transduction and regulation in smooth muscle. *Nature* 372: 231–236, 1994
92 Spedding M and Cavero I. 'Calcium antagonists': a class of drugs with a bright future. Part II. Determination of basic pharmacological properties. *Life Sci* 35: 575–587, 1984
93 Stuehr DJ. Mammalian nitric oxide synthases. *Biochim Biophys Acta* 1411: 217–230, 1999
94 Sudjarwo SA, Hori M, Tanaka T, Matsuda Y and Karaki H. Coupling of the endothelin ETA and ETB receptors to Ca^{2+} mobilization and Ca^{2+} sensitization in vascular smooth muscle. *Eur J Pharmacol* 289: 197–204, 1995
95 Sudjarwo SA and Karaki H. Role of protein kinase C in the endothelin-induced contraction in the rabbit saphenous vein. *Eur J Pharmacol* 294: 261–269, 1995
96 Terada K, Ohya Y, Kitamura K and Kuriyama H. Actions of flunarizine, a Ca^{2+} antagonist, on ionic currents in fragmented smooth muscle cells of the rabbit small intestine. *J Pharmacol Exp Ther* 240: 978–983, 1987
97 Tsien RY. New calcium indicators and buffers with high selectivity against magnesium and protons: design, synthesis, and properties of prototype structures. *Biochemistry* 19: 2396–2404, 1980
98 Van Breemen C, Farinas BR, Gerba P and McNaughton ED. Excitation-contraction coupling in rabbit aorta studied by the lanthanum method for measuring cellular calcium influx. *Circ Res* 30: 44–54, 1972
99 van Breemen C, Hwang O and Meisheri KD. The mechanism of inhibitory action of diltiazem on vascular smooth muscle contractility. *J Pharmacol Exp Ther* 218: 459–463, 1981
100 van Zwieten PA and Timmermans PB. Receptor subtypes involved in the action of calcium entry blockers. *Ann NY Acad Sci* 522: 351–360, 1988
101 Weiss GB and Goodman FR. Effects of lanthanum on contraction, calcium distribution and ^{45}Ca movements in intestinal smooth muscle. *J Pharmacol Exp Ther* 169: 46–55, 1969
102 Wibo M, DeRoth L and Godfraind T. Pharmacologic relevance of dihydropyridine binding sites in membranes from rat aorta: kinetic and equilibrium studies. *Circ Res* 62: 91–96, 1988
103 Yanagisawa M, Kurihara H, Kimura S, Tomobe Y, Kobayashi M, Mitsui Y, Yazaki Y, Goto K and Masaki T. A novel potent vasoconstrictor peptide produced by vascular endothelial cells. *Nature* 332: 411–415, 1988
104 Yatani A, Seidel CL, Allen J and Brown AM. Whole-cell and single-channel calcium currents of isolated smooth muscle cells from saphenous vein. *Circ Res* 60: 523–533, 1987
105 Yoshida M, Suzuki A and Itoh T. Mechanisms of vasoconstriction induced by endothelin-1 in smooth muscle of rabbit mesenteric artery. *J Physiol* 477 (Pt 2): 253–265, 1994
106 Zhang XF, Iwamuro Y, Enoki T, Okazawa M, Lee K, Komuro T, Minowa T, Okamoto Y, Hasegawa H, Furutani H, Miwa S and Masaki T. Pharmacological characterization of Ca^{2+} entry channels in endothelin-1-induced contraction of rat aorta using LOE 908 and SKandF 96365. *Br J Pharmacol* 127: 1388–1398, 1999
107 Zhang XF, Iwamuro Y, Okamoto Y, Kawanabe Y, Masaki T and Miwa S. Endothelin-1-induced contraction of rat thoracic aorta depends on calcium entry through three types of calcium channel. *J Cardiovasc Pharmacol* 36: S105–106, 2000
108 Zhang XF, Iwamuro Y, Okamoto Y, Miwa S and Masaki T. [Analysis of Ca^{2+} entry channels in endothelin-1-induced contraction of rat aorta using new blockers]. *Nippon Yakurigaku Zasshi* 114 Suppl 1: 103P–109P, 1999

The tissue selectivity of calcium antagonists

The term "tissue selectivity" is used for an agent showing varying degrees of potency between tissues, with a preferential action in a given one. Tissue selectivity is well-known in the field of α-adrenoceptors, where α_1- and α_2-agonists and antagonists differ by the ratio of activity at the level of a given tissue. Usually, this is related to their respective affinities for α_1- and α_2-adrenoceptors. Selectivity is not equivalent to specificity, which refers to a given agent interacting with only one type of receptor. This interaction has been documented mainly in the field of histaminergic receptors, where H_1-antagonists do not interact with H_2-receptors and *vice versa*. A question that has been raised several times [18, 19] is the existence of tissue selectivity for calcium antagonists. In other words, does any selectivity exist in the pharmacology of calcium channels? Several factors may be involved in tissue selectivity as reported in Table 1. We do not intend to review each of those factors for every compounds, which would be impossible because all have not been submitted to extensive studies. Nevertheless, some examples need to be given.

Characteristics of the drug

The IUPHAR classification of CCBs (see Chapter 2) is based on channel selectivity, a strong indication for a lack of specificity among the various drugs. Figure 1 illustrates a study of various compounds, considering their relative potency on L- and T-type currents. All CCBs tested blocked both T and

Table 1. Factors affecting the tissue selectivity of Ca^{2+} antagonists

1. Characteristics of the drug:

   Ca channel selectivity (L, T, N type). Site of action within the channel. Selectivity window. Voltage and/or frequency dependency. Ratio Ca^{2+} antagonistic/Ca^{2+} agonistic action. Physicochemical properties (pKa, partition coefficient). Susceptibility to tissue metabolism.

2. Properties of the tissue:

   Relative contribution of various Ca^{2+} pools to final response. Density and types of Ca^{2+} channels. Level of resting potential. Gating control of Ca^{2+} channels. Pharmacokinetic determinants.

3. Characteristics of the stimuli:

   Level, duration and frequency of depolarization. Nature of activated kinase(s).

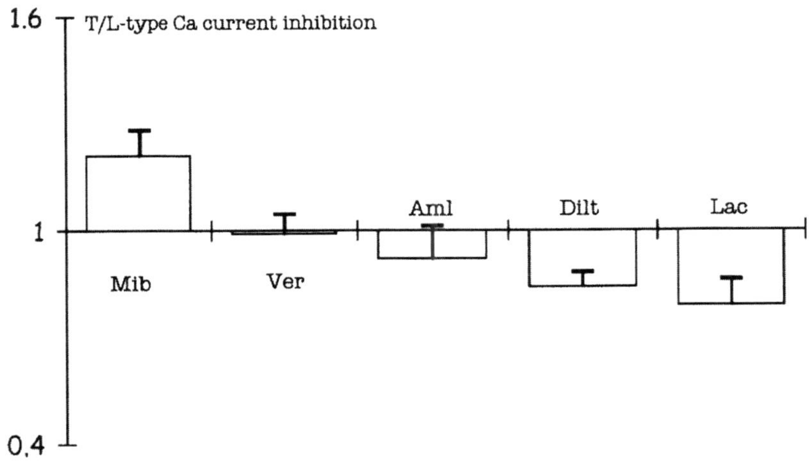

Figure 1. Calcium channel selectivity: T-type *versus* L-type Ca current selectivity of mibefradil (Mib), verapamil (Ver), amlodipine (Aml), dittiazem (Dilt) and lacidipine (Lac); modified from [9].

L channels, but their selectivity was differing, mibefradil being the most selective for T-channels and lacidipine being the most selective for L-channels [9]. As far as what can be considered as a pleiotropic agent, amlodipine appears to be a good example. As shown by Furukawa et al. [12], it has a strong blocking action on both L- and N-type calcium channels expressed in oocytes. The potency of the amlodipine block on the N-type Ca^{2+} channel is comparable to that on the L-type Ca^{2+} channel. The concentration dose-effect curves are nearly superimposed. At –100 mV holding potential, the IC50 values for amlodipine block on the L-type and N-type Ca^{2+} channel are 2.4 and 5.8 μM, respectively. The blocking action of amlodipine on the N-type Ca^{2+} channel is dependent on holding potential and extracellular pH, as has been observed with amlodipine block on L-type Ca^{2+} channel. A depolarized holding potential and high pH enhanced the blocking action of amlodipine. The time course of block development by amlodipine is similar for L-type and N-type Ca^{2+} channels, but it is slower than the time course of block development by nifedipine for L-type Ca^{2+} channel. Amlodipine appears also to be active on T-type currents. Bénardeau and Ertel [4] have reported an IC50 value of 5.6 μM for T-channel block in guinea-pig atria. It is of note that in this concentration range, amlodipine is a powerful ACE inhibitor, which through the preservation of bradykinine stimulates the release of NO from endothelial cells [42]. This latter effect is important in view of the synergism for vascular relaxation existing between NO and calcium antagonists [21, 32]. Those various properties of amlodipine need to be taken into account when examining the therapeutic mode of action of this drug.

Figure 2 [38] illustrates a comparison of the blockade of N-type currents by various DHPs. It shows that cilnidipine is highly potent against N-type current.

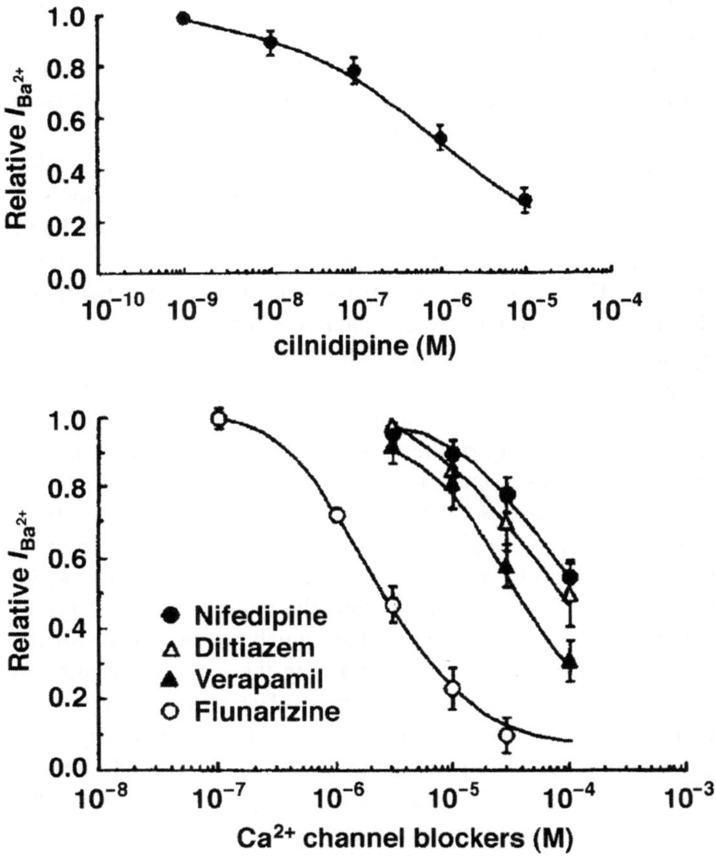

Figure 2. Blockade of N-type current measured as high voltage-activated Ba^{2+} currents ($I_{Ba^{2+}}$) by cilnidipine and other CCBs; modified from [37].

It may be anticipated that those CCBs acting at the level of N-type currents and thereby impairing catecholamines release from nerve endings, should blunt the sympathetic reflex following vasodilatation. This is the basis of another difference of selectivity between drugs. Nifedipine is highly selective for L-type current, being active at concentrations three to four orders of magnitude lower on L- than on T-type current. Therefore, it is appropriate to consider the selectivity window, which can be related not only to the ratio of active concentrations blocking L-type channels and other channels (T- or N-type) but also to the ratio of active concentrations blocking L-type channels and other membrane processes (such as receptors, other channels or transporters). For instance D600 blocks not only L-type channels but also the α-adrenoceptors [22]. Dihydropyridines may also block Na channels, but at higher concentration than calcium channels [43]. Another example is flunarizine, which does not only interfere with various voltage-operated calcium channels, but which is also acting on the release of dopamine by nerve terminals [35]. Great attention has been devoted to the selectivity for other ion channels, in particular K-channels, verapamil has the lowest ratio CaCh/KCh of the drugs tested. It is acting at nearly the same concentration on both channels; the consequences of this property have not been evaluated [23, 24].

As already pointed out in Chapter 2, the α_1-subunit of L-type calcium channels is one among the five subunits constitutive of those channels. Its importance is due to the fact that it has the properties of calcium channels when inserted in lipid bilayer. Furthermore, it contains the receptor binding sites for the various CCBs. The α_1 subunits of the various calcium channels are coded by different genes. L-type calcium channels found in heart and vessels are splicing products of a same gene. The isoforms are distributed differently among various cardiac and smooth muscles. The numerical identifier corresponds to the Ca_V channel α_1 subunit gene subfamily (1 through 3 at present) and the order of discovery of the α_1 subunit within that subfamily (1 through m). According to this nomenclature, the Ca_V1 subfamily ($Ca_V1.1$ through $Ca_V1.4$) includes channels, which mediate L-type Ca^{2+} currents. The Ca_V2 subfamily ($Ca_V2.1$ through $Ca_V2.3$) includes channels, which mediate P/Q-type, N-type, and R-type Ca^{2+} currents, respectively. The Ca_V3 subfamily ($Ca_V3.1$ through $Ca_V3.3$) includes channels, which mediate T-type Ca^{2+} currents. Lowercase letters are used to distinguish alternatively spliced variants; $Ca_V1.2a$ corresponds to channels containing the cardiac variant and $Ca_v1.2b$ corresponds to the smooth muscle variant. The pharmacology of those two variants presents some dissimilarity characterized by small differences in sensitivity to some CCBs. Two transcripts coding for the IS6 segment of the $\alpha_1 1.2a$ subunit and for the IS6 segment of the $\alpha_1 1.2b$ subunit, have been shown to be selectively expressed in cardiac and vascular smooth muscle, respectively [39a]. On Table 2 are reported binding and functional data collected from publications of our laboratory; they show concordant values of various estimates of the equilibrium dissociation constant of nifedipine on intact isolated rat mesenteric artery and on the recombinant $\alpha_1 1.2b$ subunit. Interestingly, as illustrated by Figure 3, the two splice types have different sensitivity for nisoldipine. a dihydropyridine (DHP) Ca^{2+} channel blocker with a high vascular selectivity [22]. Nisoldipine is thus a more potent blocker of inward current in

Table 2. Collected data of binding and functional studies with nifedipine. Values are in nM. Data from Godfraind and colleagues [13, 29]

Isolated rat mesenteric artery	Binding (K_i)	^{45}Ca Influx (I_{50})	Contraction (IC_{50})	Calcium current whole cell K_i patch
100 mM KCl	1.2	1.9	1.9	
Recombinant Ca Channel				
$\alpha_1 1.2b$				1.9

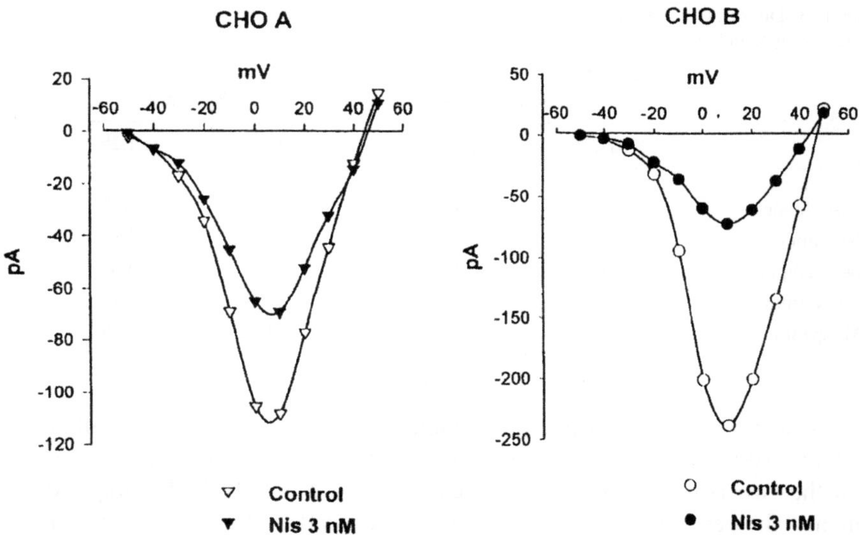

Figure 3. Inhibition of L-type Ca current by nisoldipine. L-type Ca currents were monitored under whole cell patch clamp conditions in CHO cells transfected with $\alpha_1 1.2a$ (CHOA) and $\alpha_1 1.2b$ (CHOB); modified from [29].

cells transfected with $\alpha_1 1.2b$ isoform cDNA than in those transfected with $\alpha_1 1.2a$ isoform cDNA. We have examined if this property is shared by other DHP and non-DHP Ca^{2+} channel blockers [29]. We used Chinese hamster ovary cells (CHO) transfected either with cDNA encoding for the $\alpha_1 1.2a$ or with cDNA encoding for the $\alpha_1 1.2b$ subunit of the L-type Ca^{2+} channel, issuing respectively from rabbit heart and lung smooth muscle [39]. The Ca^{2+} channel blocking activity of three neutral DHP derivatives, (+)-PN 200-110, nifedipine and nisoldipine, which show different degrees of vascular selectivity [15, 22], and one positively-charged derivative SDZ 207-180 [26] was compared to that of the phenylalkylamine verapamil, which is equipotent in cardiac and vascular tissue (see below) and to that of pinaverium bromide, a non-DHP compound with a quaternary ammonium, reported to show intestinal selectivity [8]. The voltage-dependent current mediated by the $\alpha 1$ subunit of the L-type Ca^{2+} channel ($I\alpha_1$) was recorded with the whole-cell configuration of the patch-clamp technique using barium ions as charge carrier. Binding affinity of Ca^{2+} channel blockers was also assessed in displacement studies using the Ca^{2+} channel ligand [^{3}H]-(+)-PN 200-110. Experimental results (Tab. 3) show that neutral dihydropyridines (nifedipine, nisoldipine, (+)-PN 200-110) were more potent inhibitors of $\alpha_1 1.2b$ subunit than of $\alpha_1 1.2a$ subunit. This difference was more marked at a holding potential of –100 mV than at -50 mV. SDZ 207-180 (an ionized dihydropyridine) exhibited the same potency on the two isoforms. Pinaverium (ionized non-dihydropyridine deriv-

Table 3. Dissociation constants (nM) of various CCBs in splice variants at two holding potentials. Data from Morel et al. [29]

	K-100 mV		K-50 mV	
	$\alpha_1$1.2a	$\alpha_1$1.2b	$\alpha_1$1.2a	$\alpha_1$1.2b
Nisoldipine	2.1	0.5	0.33	0.15
Nifedipine	47	10	6.9	3.7
(+)Isradipine	15	2.2	0.82	0.46
Pinaverium	1.8	3.3	0.34	1.3
Verapamil	29	23	0.95	0.96

ative) was two- and four-fold more potent on $\alpha_1$1.2a than on $\alpha_1$1.2b subunit at Vh of −100 mV and -50 mV, respectively. Effects of verapamil were identical on the two isoforms at both voltages. [^{3}H]-(+)-PN 200-110 binding experiments showed that neutral dihydropyridines had a higher affinity for the $\alpha_1$1.2b than for the $\alpha_1$1.2a subunit. SDZ 207-180 had the same affnity for the two isoforms and pinaverium had a higher affinity for the $\alpha_1$1.2a subunit than for the $\alpha_1$1.2b subunit.

All these results show marked differences among Ca^{2+} channel blockers in their selectivity not only for the three subfamilies of calcium channels but also for the $\alpha_1$1.2a and $\alpha_1$1.2b subunits. It is therefore not surprising that the pharmacological profile is not uniform among the various CCBs, even among those belonging to a same chemical family.

Properties of the tissue and characteristics of the stimuli

In order to characterize the factors related to the properties of the tissue and the characteristics of the stimuli, we may focus on some *in vitro* studies describing the selectivity of calcium antagonists in the cardiovascular system. These studies deal not only with a comparison of the sensitivity of arteries and myocardium to the action of calcium antagonists, but also with a comparison among arteries. It is shown just below that the results of such a comparison are differing between species. Therefore, data obtained with human preparations are important for any robust extrapolation from the laboratory to a clinical situation. Indeed, clinically-relevant information deals not only with the vasodepressor potency of a given agent, but also with its cardiodepressor potency.

Table 4 summarizes a comparison of the effects of nifedipine in cardiac and artery preparations from various origins: rat, rabbit, guinea pig and human. It is noteworthy that the potency ratios expressed as a ratio of IC50 of nifedipine for cardiac inotropism over IC50 of nifedipine for depolarized vessel contraction are dissimilar with the highest value for rat and the lowest for guinea pig. In a study performed in the guinea-pig, Spedding et al. [34] showed that

Table 4. Comparison of nifedipine effects on inotropism (isolated cardiac muscles) and vascular contraction (isolated vessels), in different species

Species	IC_{50} (nM) on inotropism (electrically paced hearts)	IC_{50} (nM) on vascular contraction (K^+-stimulated)	Ratio (heart/vessels)
Rat	1000 [1,2]	1.40 [3]	714
Rabbit	300 [4]	8.9 [5]	33.7
Guinea pig	44.06 [6]	14.1 [7]	3.1
Human	67 [8]	4.7 [9]	14.2

(1) Ventricle [7]
(2) Ventricle [11]
(3) Aorta [41]
(4) Atria [27]
(5) Aorta [27]
(6) Papillary muscle [34]
(7) Mesenteric artery [34]
(8) Ventricle [16]
(9) Coronary arteries [16]

the ratio of IC50 values estimated in the isolated heart and in isolated vessels is 0.3 for diltiazem, 1.3 for verapamil and 3.1 for nifedipine. Experiments from Triggle's laboratory are in complete agreement with the results just mentioned [36].

The radioligand ^3H(+)-isradipine, was used in order to estimate the apparent affinity of dihydropyridine-binding sites in plasma membranes prepared from human coronary artery and myocardium. Binding data expressed as Ki or Kd values are reported in Table 5 for nisoldipine, nifedipine and isradipine.

Table 5. Binding parameters of nisoldipine, nifedipine and (+)-isradipine, in membranes of human coronary arteries and myocardium compared with functional parameters

Drug	K_i or K_d (nM)	IC_{50} (nM)
Nisoldipine		
. coronary artery	0.093 ± 0.029	0.062 [1]
. myocardium	0.030 ± 0.005	310 [2]
Nifedipine		
. coronary artery	4.84 ± 1.98	3.7 [1]
. myocardium	2.40 ± 0.89	67 [2]
(+)-Isradipine		
. coronary artery	0.115 ± 0.017	/
. myocardium	0.077 ± 0.010	100 [3]

(+)-Isradipine binding was measured directly by titrated ligand.
Nisoldipine and nifedipine binding was measured in competition experiments. Values were obtained from 3–4 different membrane preparations; each experiment was performed at least three times. IC_{50} = concentration producing 50% reduction of the calcium antagonist-sensitive contraction of coronary artery to serotonin 10^{-5} M and electrically paced ventricular preparations. Mean ± SE.
[1] [15]; [2] [16]; [3] [6].

These values show that the sequence of affinity was nisoldipine > isradipine > nifedipine. They also show that the apparent affinity was about two-fold higher in the myocardium than in coronary artery. The dissociation constant values may be compared to functional values of IC50 obtained in other experiments [22]. Functional estimates of IC50 of calcium antagonists in human coronary arteries exposed to serotonin were close to the radioligand estimates of the apparent dissociation constant in plasma membranes prepared from this tissue. This was not the case for myocardium. Functional IC50 values in human heart were much higher than radiochemical Ki (or Kd) values estimated in plasma membranes prepared from human heart. There was a 10,000-fold difference for nisoldipine, a 1,298-fold difference for isradipine and a 27-fold difference for nifedipine. The different sensitivity of cardiac and vascular preparations to dihydropyrine calcium antagonists is illustrated by Figure 4, which shows dose-inhibition curves of the contraction of human coronary artery stimulated by a 100 mM K^+-depolarising solution and of the electrically-paced human myocardium, both preparations being exposed to nifedipine or to nisoldipine. Nisoldipine is much less active than nifedipine in cardiac preparation and much more active in human coronary artery. Differences between calcium antagonists are also illustrated in Figure 5, which represents a log scale of the reciprocal of the concentration needed to block 50% of the contractile activity (IC50) in human coronary artery, in internal mammary artery and in myocardium. It shows that diltiazem and verapamil have the same potency in both arteries and in myocardium. On the other hand, for nisoldipine, the potency sequence is coronary artery >> mammary artery >> myocardium, whereas for nifedipine, the sequence is coronary artery = mammary artery >> myocardium [22]. More recent experiments [33], using preparations from human atria and aortic vasa vasorum, confirm the vasoselectivity of nisoldipine and the cardioselectivity of verapamil. Sarsero et al. [33] also reported that the sequence of vascular/cardiac (V/C) ratios was mibefradil >> felodipine > nifedipine = amlodipine >> verapamil.

Several factors might be involved in the difference in sensitivity between heart and vessels. There are sarcolemmal Ca channels in cardiac myocytes, which serve to bring Ca into the cell (L- and T-type Ca channels). This Ca influx contributes an inward current tending to make (or keep) the membrane potential more positive, but this Ca also serves as an important second messenger in the excitation-contraction (E-C) coupling, leading to activation of contraction. There are also intracellular Ca-release channels, which are responsible for releasing Ca from the sarcoplasmic reticulum (SR) and endoplasmic reticulum (ER; ryanodine and IP_3 receptors). The Ca released from the SR greatly amplifies the function of Ca that enters via the sarcolemma in the activation of contraction [5]. The sarcolemmal Ca channels are crucial to control of cardiac contractility. The intracellular Ca release channels (or ryanodine receptors) respond to triggering events mediated by sarcolemmal ion currents and are largely responsible for releasing of an amount of Ca^{2+} much larger that the Ca^{2+} entering as a L-type current. This released Ca activates the myofila-

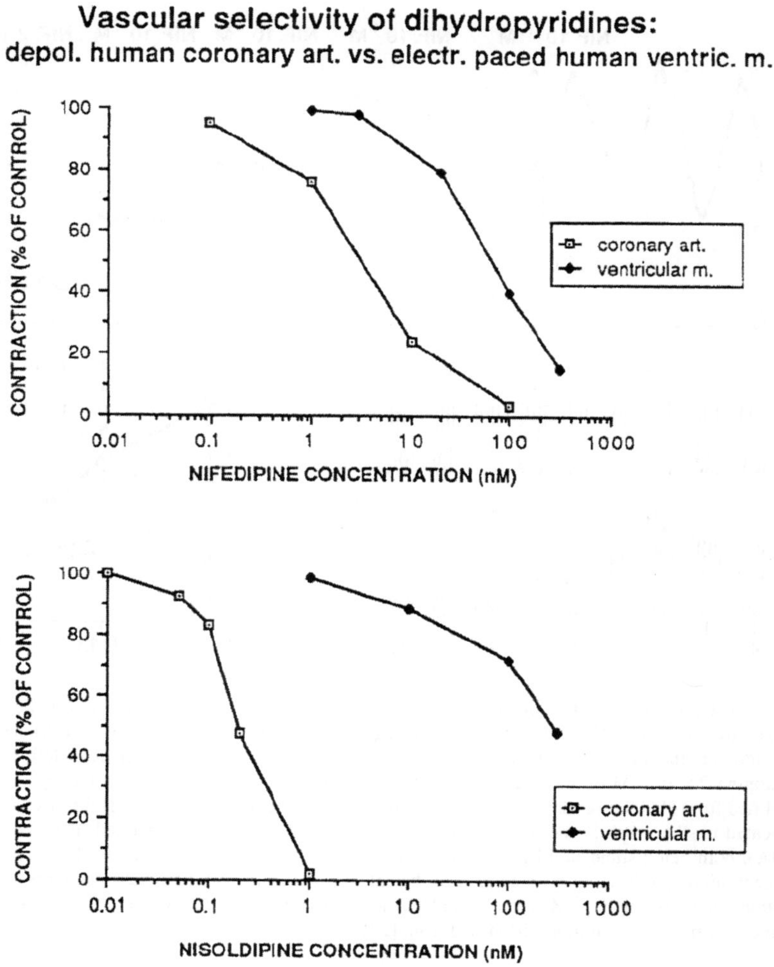

Figure 4. Inhibitory action of nifedipine and nisoldipine on the contraction of human ventricular muscle isolated preparations (electrically paced) and on K-depolarized isolated human coronary artery segments; modified from [16].

ments to produce contraction. The basic mechanism of cardiac excitation-contraction coupling operates as a calcium-induced calcium release. Calcium enters the cell from the extracellular fluid once the voltage-dependent L-type Ca^{2+} channels are open. This results in an increase of $[Ca^{2+}]_i$ in the space between the sarcolemma and sarcoplasmic reticulum (SR) and this leads to the opening of the SR Ca^{2+} release channel or ryanodine receptors (RyR), which are more numerous that the L-type channels. According to Wibo et al. [40], the ratio is 1 over 9. This E-C mechanism is influenced in different circumstances. These include autonomic modulation, L-arginine-NO pathway activation and

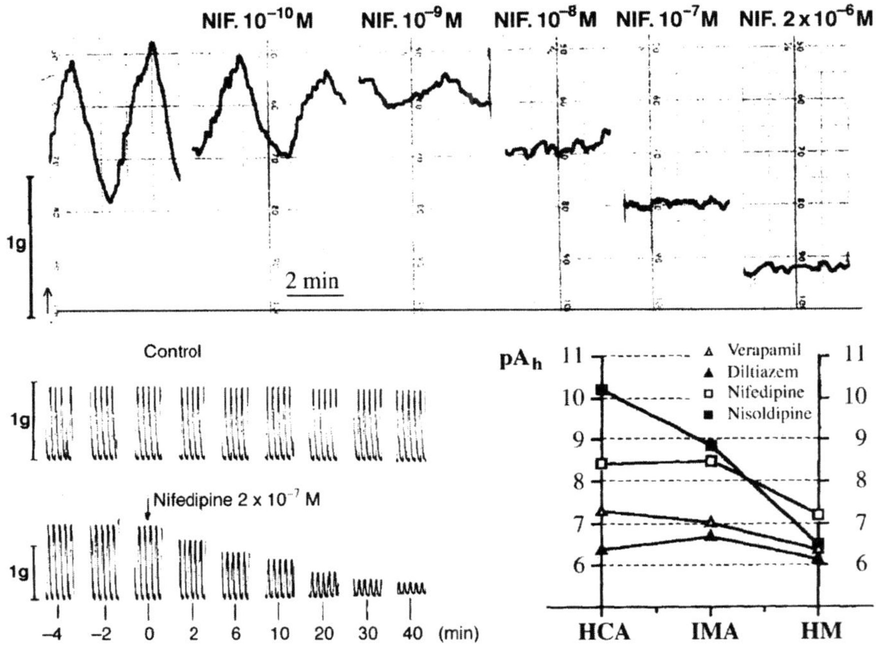

Figure 5. Upper panel: Effect of increasing concentrations of nifedipine on the contractile activity evoked by serotonin (5HT) 10^{-5} M in isolated segment of human coronary artery (HCA), serotonin was added at the arrow and maintained as shown by the continuous line. Lower panel left: Effect of nifedipine 2×10^{-7} M on electrically stimulated human trabecular muscle from the rigt ventricle, modified from [16]. Lower panel right: Logarithmic scale of the reciprocal of the IC50 (pA_h) of CCBs indicated on the graph in the human coronary artery (HCA), the human internal mammary artery (IMA), both being stimulated by serotonin and the human myocardium (HM). IC50 values are the concentrations producing 50% reduction of the calcium-antagonist-sensitive component to the tonic contraction evoked by 10^{-5} M serotonin in HCA and IMA or of the contraction of electrically paced human ventricular preparations. Modified from [22].

pathological conditions related or not to hypertension and atherosclerosis [3, 28]. The opening of calcium channels is the result of cardiac action potentials that may have a variety of different shapes. The classical long plateau, essential for preventing re-excitation and arrhythmias is prominent in physiological conditions.

As already pointed out above, the α_1-subunit of L-type calcium channels is one among the five subunits constitutive of those channels. Its importance is due to the fact that it has the properties of calcium channels when inserted in lipid bilayers. Furthermore, it contains the receptor binding sites for the various CCBs. The $\alpha 1$ subunits of the various calcium channels are coded by different genes. L-type calcium channels found in heart and vessels are splicing products of a same gene. The two splice types have different affinities for dihydropyridines, but the same affinity for verapamil, an observation consistent with the absence of selectivity of this drug as observed in pharmacological studies (see above). The isoforms are distributed differently among various cardiac and smooth muscles. However, the affinity ratio of DHPs existing between isoforms is not high enough in order to take into account the differences between heart and vessels observed in pharmacological experiments and other factors need to be considered [29].

Feron et al. [10] have reported that the splicing process is tissue-dependent and is regulated during development. During development, there is a profound modification of the localization of L-type Ca channels from the peripheral plasma membrane to the junctional structures (Fig. 6) [40]. The functional consequence results in a lower sensitivity to calcium channel blockers of adult over neonatal hearts (Fig. 7) [40].

Time-course experiments reported on pages 95 and 96 may provide additional information on the tissue selectivity. Like in rat aorta, in human coronary artery *in vitro*, the inhibitory action of nisoldipine on contractions evoked by a depolarizing stimulus is characterized by a marked time-dependency, in

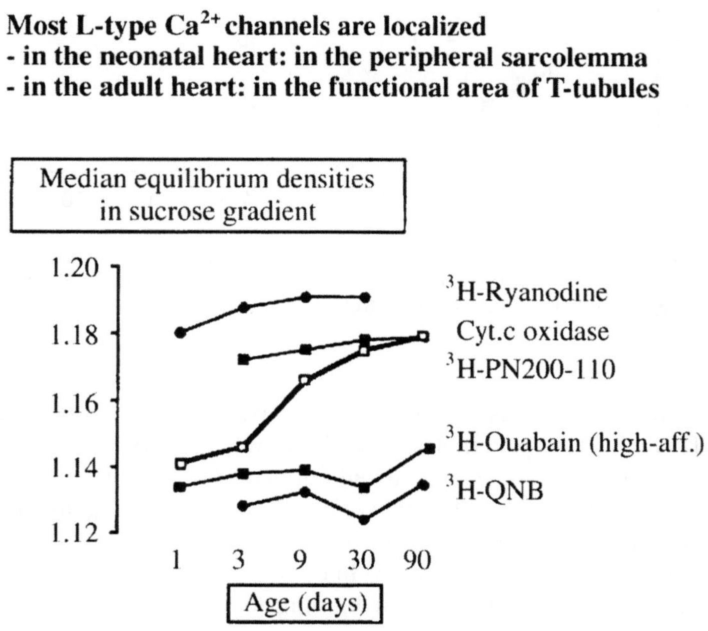

Figure 6. Median equilibrium density in sucrose gradient of markers of plasma membrane and of sarcoplasmic reticulum. After equilibration of microsomal fractions in density gradient, ryanodine receptors are characterized by a heavy distribution pattern that does not change appreciably between days 1 and 30 after birth. In neonatal tissue, 1,4-dihydropyridine receptors are found mainly in low-density subfractions, together with other sarcolemmal constituents, whereas in adult tissue, they are recovered predominantly in high-density subfractions, together with ryanodine receptors. Thus, after birth, and in parallel with the development of T tubules, there is a progressive concentration of $Ca_v1.2$ (L-type Ca^{2+}) channels in junctional structures of high equilibrium density, where they are situated close to the Ca^{2+} release channels of the sarcoplasmic reticulum. In adult ventricle, L-type channels are, on an average, threefold more abundant in T tubules area than in external sarcolemma; modified from [40].

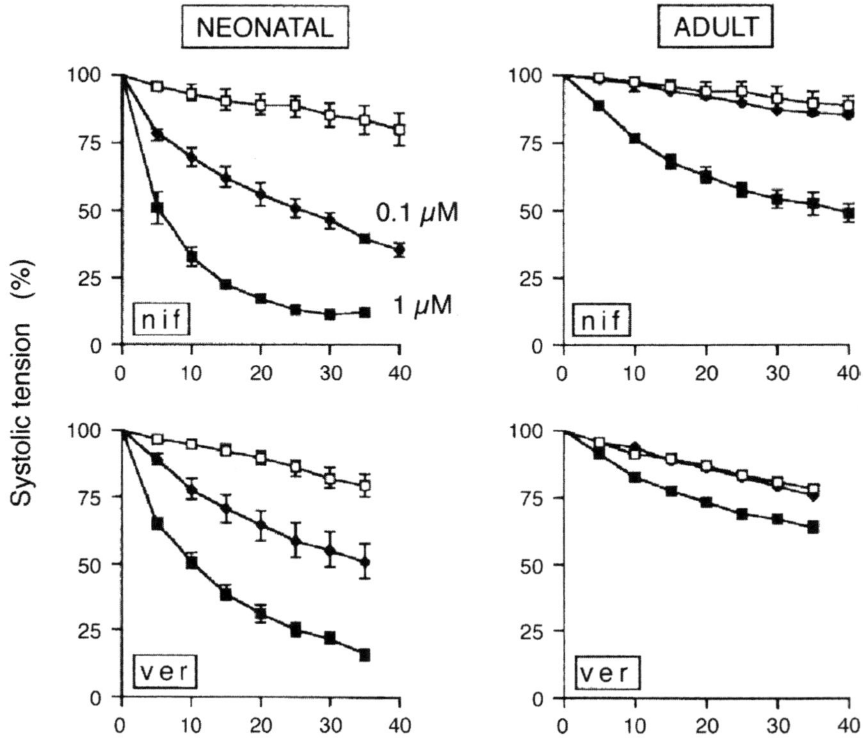

Figure 7. Negative inotropic effect of the CCBs nifedipine (nif) and verapamil in neonatal and adult rat ventricles. Ordinate: contraction in per cent of control. Abcissa: time after addition of the CCBs at the concentration of 0.1 and 1 μM to the organ bath (min). Modified from [40].

which inhibition increases slowly after depolarization to attain a steady-state-value. This inhibitory pattern has been observed with other dihydropyridines, but was not obvious with verapamil and diltiazem (see Fig. 8, p. 95). In depolarized arteries preincubated with verapamil and diltiazem, the inhibitory action is immediate and sustained for the duration of the depolarization. The kinetics of inhibition by dihydropyridines of the contraction of depolarized arteries follows the kinetics of their binding to receptor sites located at the outer mouth of the channels as illustrated above for isradipine. Depolarization induces a conformational change in the dihydropyridine receptor sites resulting in a state of higher affinity. For a drug such as nisoldipine, occupation of this site is made possible at very low concentrations (10–300 pM), but appreciable time is needed to attain a steady state. This combination of voltage- and time-dependency contributes to the tissue selectivity, which may be related to disparities in the modulation of calcium channels due to physiological differences in the duration of the stimuli. The slow time-course of association of nisoldipine with its receptors in depolarized tissues might account for its comparatively low potency in cardiac muscle, as compared with vascular smooth muscle. Binding sites in isolated membranes show the same affinity as binding sites in intact tissues submitted to prolonged exposure to high KCl solution (which completely depolarizes muscle cells). The rate of association in intact depolarized tissues follows a pseudo-first-order kinetics similar to the association rate constant for purified calcium channels [41]. Therefore, the concentration of nisoldipine required to occupy the same proportion of channels may be estimated at any time of exposure to the drug. The time-course of occupation may be calculated for a short systolic depolarisation (±0.4 sec), as well as for a time required to fully activate a smooth muscle (±6 min). Assuming an occupation of 50% of receptor sites at the end of the stimulus, this computation shows that the ratio of concentrations required in cardiac *versus* arterial muscle is equal to 1,500. This theoretical value is similar to that observed when the relative sensitivity to nisoldipine was assessed *in vitro* in human coronary artery and in human myocardium myocardium as illustrated on Figure 4. [16]. The rate model described above may account for differences in sensitivity between arteries and myocardium since the triggering process of the cardiac contraction involves L-type channels. *In vivo* studies are fully consistent with *in vitro* studies as far as concerned the sensitivity difference in contractility between coronary bed and myocardium [31].

The inhibition of the response to a given vasoconstrictor may be different between arteries exposed to the same CCB. Study of the sensitivity to nisoldipine of the contraction of human coronary artery and of internal mammary artery stimulated by serotonin (Fig. 8) shows that the curves relating inhibition by nisoldipine of serotonin-evoked tonic contraction in those two arteries are not superimposed: inhibition of the tonic contraction to serotonin is much more important in human coronary artery than in human internal mammary

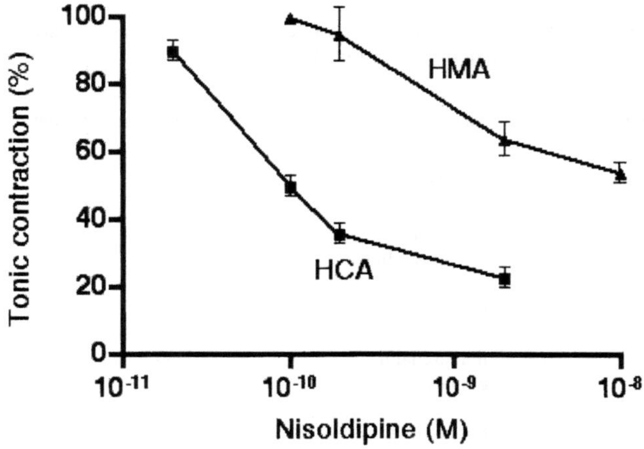

Figure 8. Dose-inhibition curves of serotonin-evoked tonic contraction of human coronary artery (HCA: ■) and human internal mammary artery (HMA: ▲). Modified from [15].

artery. This confirms our earlier reports that inhibition of contractile responses may be related to the type of vessel, resistance arteries being more inhibited than conduit arteries [17, 20]. Another illustration of heterogeneity is related to the mode of activation of the contraction as reported on Table 6, which shows that maximum contractions of rat aorta evoked by noradrenaline or phenylephrine were less inhibited than maximum contractions evoked by α_2 agonists such as clonidine and oxymetazoline. Such observations have been extended to various calcium antagonists and to various vessels. For instance, Figure 9 illustrates the contraction evoked by ET-1 in human isolated distal and proximal coronary arteries exposed or not to nisoldipine (1 μM) [2]. It shows that the maximal contraction of the distal artery was inhibited by 51% whereas the maximal contraction of the proximal segment was inhibited by 35%. They emphasize the hypothesis that vascular heterogeneity may be, at least partly, related to the proportion of contractile responses resistant or not to calcium-channel blockade [14]. It is likely that the interaction of agonists with their receptors activates an intracellular pathway involving protein kinase C and resulting in an increase in the sensitivity of the contractile proteins to calcium [25, 30]. The importance of this mechanism that is independent of Ca entry is likely to vary between different smooth muscles and to play a role in vascular selectivity.

Among factors responsible for heterogeneity among vessels, not only the specificity of the blocker and its voltage-dependency but also its tissue pharmacokinetics needs to be taken into account. For instance, Angelico et al. [1] have observed in isolated rabbit aorta stimulated by high KCl that 50% relaxation was reached at different times according to the CCB tested. At 10 nM concentration 50% relaxation was reached after 210 min with lercanidipine, 278 min with amlodipine, 135 min with lacidipine, 75 min with nitrendipine and 70 min with felodipine. On the other hand, when studying the heart ven-

Table 6. Maximal inhibition (in per cent) of the contraction evoked by various agonists in isolated rat aorta exposed to calcium antagonists. Data from [14]

Calcium antagonist	Vasoconstrictor	% inhibition of contraction
Cinnarizine	noradrenaline	60
	phenylephrine	64
	clonidine	92
	oxymetazoline	93
D600	noradrenaline	100
Nifedipine	noradrenaline	50
	clonidine	84
Flunarizine	noradrenaline	50
	clonidine	84
Nisoldipine	Noradrenaline (E+)	40
	Noradrenaline (E-)	30

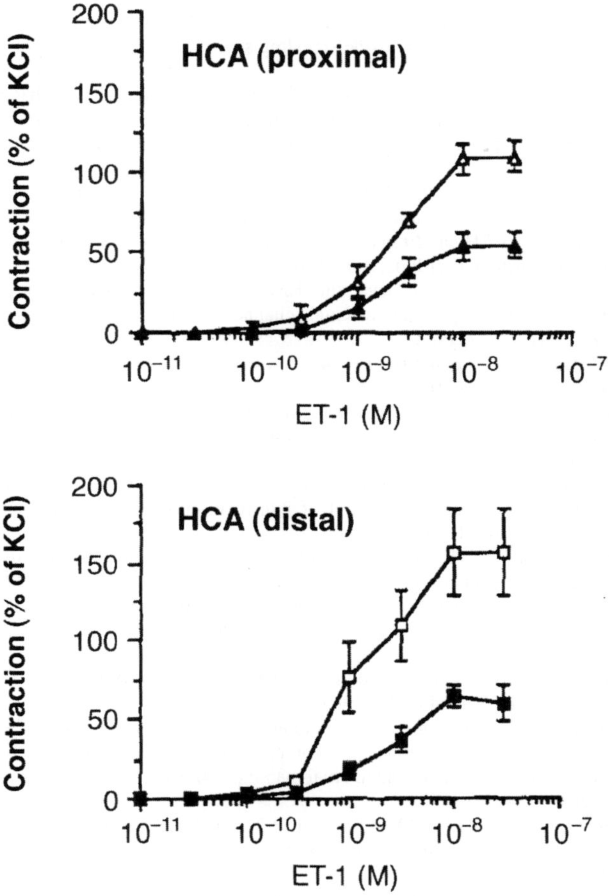

Figure 9. Effect of nisoldipine on concentration-response curve to endothelin-1 (ET-1) of proximal and distal human coronary arteries (HCA). After incubation in nisoldipine 1 μM (solid symbols) or solvent for 90 min (open symbols), the concentration response curve was measured in various rings; modified from [2].

tricle, the rate sequence was lacidipine > amlodipine > felodipine > lercanidipine = nitrendipine, indicating that comparison between drugs require appropriate experimental conditions in order to validate the IC50s ratio.

References

1 Angelico P, Guarneri L, Leonardi A and Testa R. Vascular-selective effect of lercanidipine and other 1,4-dihydropyridines in isolated rabbit tissues. *J Pharm Pharmacol* 51: 709–714, 1999

2 Balligand JL and Godfraind T. Effect of nisoldipine on contractions evoked by endothelin-1 in human isolated distal and proximal coronary arteries and veins. *J Cardiovasc Pharmacol* 24:

618–625, 1994
3 Balligand JL, Kelly RA, Marsden PA, Smith TW and Michel T. Control of cardiac muscle cell function by an endogenous nitric oxide signaling system. *Proc Natl Acad Sci USA* 90: 347–351, 1993
4 Bénardeau A and Ertel EA. Selective block of myocardial T-type calcium channels by mibefradil: A comparison with the 1,4-dihydropyridine amlodipine. In: *Low-voltage-activated T-type Ca channels.*, edited by Tsien RW, Clozel JP and Nargeot J. Chester,UK: Adis International, 1998, p. 386–394
5 Bers DM and Perez-Reyes E. Ca channels in cardiac myocytes: structure and function in Ca influx and intracellular Ca release. *Cardiovasc Res* 42: 339–360, 1999
6 Bohm M, Schwinger RH and Erdmann E. Different cardiodepressant potency of various calcium antagonists in human myocardium. *Am J Cardiol* 65: 1039–1041, 1990
7 Boyd RA, Giacomini JC and Giacomini KM. Species differences in the negative inotropic response of 1,4-dihydropyridine calcium channel blockers in myocardium. *J Cardiovasc Pharmacol* 12: 650–657, 1988
8 Christen MO. Action of pinaverium bromide, a calcium-antagonist, on gastrointestinal motility disorders. *Gen Pharmacol* 21: 821–825, 1990
9 De Paoli P, Cerbai E, Koidl B, Kirchengast M, Sartiani L and Mugelli A. Selectivity of different calcium antagonists on T- and L-type calcium currents in guinea-pig ventricular myocytes. *Pharmacol Res* 46: 491–497, 2002
10 Feron O, Octave JN, Christen MO and Godfraind T. Quantification of two splicing events in the L-type calcium channel alpha-1 subunit of intestinal smooth muscle and other tissues. *Eur J Biochem* 222: 195–202, 1994
11 Finet M, Godfraind T and Khoury G. The positive inotropic action of the nifedipine analogue, Bay K 8644, in guinea-pig and rat isolated cardiac preparations. *Br J Pharmacol* 86: 27–32, 1985
12 Furukawa T, Nukada T, Suzuki K, Fujita Y, Mori Y, Nishimura M and Yamanaka M. Voltage and pH dependent block of cloned N-type Ca^{2+} channels by amlodipine. *Br J Pharmacol* 121: 1136–1140, 1997
13 Godfraind T. Actions of nifedipine on calcium fluxes and contraction in isolated rat arteries. *J Pharmacol Exp Ther* 224: 443–450, 1983
14 Godfraind T. Calcium antagonists and vasodilatation. *Pharmacol Ther* 64: 37–75, 1994
15 Godfraind T, Dessy C and Salomone S. A comparison of the potency of selective L-calcium channel blockers in human coronary and internal mammary arteries exposed to serotonin. *J Pharmacol Exp Ther* 263: 112–122, 1992
16 Godfraind T, Egleme C, Finet M and Jaumin P. The actions of nifedipine and nisoldipine on the contractile activity of human coronary arteries and human cardiac tissue *in vitro*. *Pharmacol Toxicol* 61: 79–84, 1987
17 Godfraind T, Kaba A and Polster P. Differences in sensitivity of arterial smooth muscles to inhibition of their contractile response to depolarization by potassium. *Arch Int Pharmacodyn Ther* 172: 235–239, 1968
18 Godfraind T, Miller R and Wibo M. Calcium antagonism and calcium entry blockade. *Pharmacol Rev* 38: 321–416, 1986
19 Godfraind T, Morel N and Wibo M. The heterogeneity of calcium movements in cardiac and vascular smooth muscle cells. *Scand J Clin Lab Invest Suppl* 180: 29–39, 1986
20 Godfraind T and Polster P. [Comparative study of drugs inhibiting the contractile response of isolated vessels of human and animal origin]. *Therapie* 23: 1209–1220, 1968
21 Godfraind T and Salomone S. Calcium antagonists and endothelial function: focus on nitric oxide and endothelin. *Cardiovasc Drugs Ther* 10: 439–446, 1996
22 Godfraind T, Salomone S, Dessy C, Verhelst B, Dion R and Schoevaerts JC. Selectivity scale of calcium antagonists in the human cardiovascular system based on *in vitro* studies. *J Cardiovasc Pharmacol* 20 Suppl 5: S34–41, 1992
23 Grace AA and Camm AJ. Voltage-gated calcium-channels and antiarrhythmic drug action. *Cardiovasc Res* 45: 43–51, 2000
24 Hatano N, Ohya S, Muraki K, Giles W and Imaizumi Y. Dihydropyridine Ca^{2+} channel antagonists and agonists block Kv4.2, Kv4.3 and Kv1.4 K^{+}-channels expressed in HEK293 cells. *Br J Pharmacol* 139: 533–544, 2003
25 Karaki H. Ca^{2+} localization and sensitivity in vascular smooth muscle. *Trends Pharmacol Sci* 10: 320–325, 1989
26 Kass RS, Arena JP and Chin S. Block of L-type calcium channels by charged dihydropyridines.

Sensitivity to side of application and calcium. *J Gen Physiol* 98: 63–75, 1991
27 Kazda S, Garthoff B, Meyer H, Schlossmann K, Stoepel K, Towart R, Vater W and Wehinger E. Pharmacology of a new calcium antagonistic compound, isobutyl methyl 1,4-dihydro-2,6-dimethyl-4(2-nitrophenyl)-3,5-pyridinedicarboxylate (Nisoldipine, Bay k 5552). *Arzneimittelforschung* 30: 2144–2162, 1980
28 Maier LS and Bers DM. Calcium, calmodulin, and calcium-calmodulin kinase II: heartbeat to heartbeat and beyond. *J Mol Cell Cardiol* 34: 919–939, 2002
29 Morel N, Buryi V, Feron O, Gomez JP, Christen MO and Godfraind T. The action of calcium channel blockers on recombinant L-type calcium channel alpha1-subunits. *Br J Pharmacol* 125: 1005–1012, 1998
30 Nishimura J, Khalil RA, Drenth JP and van Breemen C. Evidence for increased myofilament Ca^{2+} sensitivity in norepinephrine-activated vascular smooth muscle. *Am J Physiol* 259: H2–8, 1990
31 Rousseau MF, Melin J, Benedict CR, Ahn S, Raphael D, Bornemann M and Pouleur H. Effects of nisoldipine therapy on myocardial perfusion and neuro-hormonal status in patients with severe ischaemic left ventricular dysfunction. *Eur Heart J* 15: 957–964, 1994
32 Salomone S, Silva CL, Morel N and Godfraind T. Facilitation of the vasorelaxant action of calcium antagonists by basal nitric oxide in depolarized artery. *Naunyn Schmiedebergs Arch Pharmacol* 354: 505–512, 1996
33 Sarsero D, Fujiwara T, Molenaar P and Angus JA. Human vascular to cardiac tissue selectivity of L- and T-type calcium channel antagonists. *Br J Pharmacol* 125: 109–119, 1998
34 Spedding M, Fraser S, Clarke B and Patmore L. Factors modifying the tissue selectivity of calcium-antagonists. *J Neural Transm Suppl* 31: 5–16, 1990
35 Terland O and Flatmark T. Drug-induced parkinsonism: cinnarizine and flunarizine are potent uncouplers of the vacuolar H^+-ATPase in catecholamine storage vesicles. *Neuropharmacology* 38: 879–882, 1999
36 Triggle DJ. The pharmacology of ion channels: with particular reference to voltage-gated Ca^{2+} channels. *Eur J Pharmacol* 375: 311–325, 1999
37 Uneyama H, Takahara A, Dohmoto H, Yoshimoto R, Inoue K and Akaike N. Blockade of N-type Ca^{2+} current by cilnidipine (FRC-8653) in acutely dissociated rat sympathetic neurones. *Br J Pharmacol* 122: 37–42, 1997
38 Uneyama H, Uchida H, Konda T, Yoshimoto R and Akaike N. Selectivity of dihydropyridines for cardiac L-type and sympathetic N-type Ca^{2+} channels. *Eur J Pharmacol* 373: 93–100, 1999
39 Welling A, Kwan YW, Bosse E, Flockerzi V, Hofmann F and Kass RS. Subunit-dependent modulation of recombinant L-type calcium channels. Molecular basis for dihydropyridine tissue selectivity. *Circ Res* 73: 974–980, 1993
39a Welling A, Ludwig A, Zimmer S, Klugbauer N, Flockerzi V and Hofmann F. Alternatively spliced IS6 segments of the alpha 1C gene determine the tissue-specific dihydropyridine sensitivity of cardiac and vascular smooth muscle L-type Ca^{2+} channels. *Circ Res* 81: 526–532, 1997
40 Wibo M, Bravo G and Godfraind T. Postnatal maturation of excitation-contraction coupling in rat ventricle in relation to the subcellular localization and surface density of 1,4-dihydropyridine and ryanodine receptors. *Circ Res* 68: 662–673, 1991
41 Wibo M, DeRoth L and Godfraind T. Pharmacologic relevance of dihydropyridine binding sites in membranes from rat aorta: kinetic and equilibrium studies. *Circ Res* 62: 91–96, 1988
42 Xu B, Xiao-hong L, Lin G, Queen L and Ferro A. Amlodipine, but not verapamil or nifedipine, dilates rabbit femoral artery largely through a nitric oxide- and kinin-dependent mechanism. *Br J Pharmacol* 136: 375–382, 2002
43 Yatani A, Kunze DL and Brown AM. Effects of dihydropyridine calcium channel modulators on cardiac sodium channels. *Am J Physiol* 254: H140–147, 1988

Calcium Channel Blockers
T. Godfraind

Acute haemodynamic effects of calcium channel blockers

The present chapter considers the acute haemodynamic effects of calcium channel blockers. Although those agents are used in therapy for long-term (even life-long) treatment, it is of interest to examine the acute haemodynamic changes evoked when those agents are administered at pharmacologically active doses. Such a study allows comparing the various CCBs from a functional point of view considering potency, pharmacokinetics and tissue selectivity. The examples taken in this section are illustrative of the actions of CCBs in general, even if all drugs have not been examined. Owing the complexity of haemodynamic reflexes and the tissue selectivity of CCBs at the level of the various vascular beds, it may be anticipated that those drugs may exhibit variations in action according to the vascular bed or the species so far considered. Because of the importance of CCBs for the therapy of coronary diseases, hypertension and stroke, their action has been studied in coronary, renal and cerebral circulations.

The intravenous injection of calcium antagonists produces a hypotensive effect more pronounced in hypertensive than in normotensive animals. In conscious rats, Ishii et al. [11] have observed that a similar decrease of blood pressure was evoked by nifedipine at doses much lower in SHR than in WKY (see also Tab. 1). Knorr and Garthoff [15] have compared the activity of nitrendipine and hydralazine on the blood pressure of SHR and WKY. They have observed that the vasodilator hydralazine was equipotent in both strains, but that nitrendipine evoked a much lesser reduction of blood pressure in WKY than in SHR, an observation consistent with recent clinical studies in humans. Together with haemodynamic observations [13], these studies indicate that calcium antagonists have an activity profile different from classical arteriolar vasodilators. Indeed, it has been reported that during chronic administration of

Table 1. Comparison of the antihypertensive effects of orally-administered cilnidipine, nifedipine, or nicardipine in normotensive and hypertensive rats: ED20 values in mg/kg. Data from [24]

Drug	Normotensive	SHR	Renal hypertensive	DOCA-salt hypertensive
Cilnidipine	9.4	2.3	1.9	2.5
Nifedipine	7.7	2.0	1.4	2.2
Nicardipine	5.7	2.0	1.6	1.5

a calcium antagonist, the decrease of blood pressure is observed without modification of the cardiac frequency [5].

Taylor et al. [22] have studied the response of various arterial territories following the administration of increasing intravenous doses of nitrendipine. There is a progressive reduction of blood pressure, reaching a maximum effect at 50% of initial value. There is an associated reduction in resistance and an increase of blood flow in the femoral and mesenteric territories. They reported a noticeable difference between the femoral and mesenteric beds, since the sensitivity to low doses is greater in the mesenteric bed, with the maximum effect occurring in the femoral circulation. Their results show that calcium antagonists are arteriolar dilatators with differing activities in different circulation beds. Their greatest effect appears in the coronary bed. It is important to note that no significant haemodynamic effects have been reported in the venous circulation.

Systemic haemodynamics

Examination of the action of CCBs on haemodynamics has been performed in animal studies with most of the compounds, once they were identified *in vitro*. Because, an extensive analysis of the published literature would be beyond the scope of this book, we have selected among published articles, those illustrating the various aspects of action of CCBs.

Examination of the haemodynamic effects of CCBs in the unanesthetized dog indicated that the coronary circulation was more influenced that the peripheral one (Fig. 1) they also illustrated that acute response to IV administration evoked major sympathetic reflexes characterized by an increased cardiac rhythm. The selective action on arteries has been widely illustrated, Figure 2 is from a human study, it shows that the vasodilatory action does occur mainly on the arterial side with a modest effect on the venous side. This illustration, coming from a human study after sublingual administration of nifedipine, has been chosen for the convincing evidence that the venous tone remained unchanged when the arterial parameters indicated a vigorous vasodilatation. It is worth to mention that ACE inhibitors dilate to the same extent the arterial and the venous beds. Further observations made after intravenous injection exemplify the differential response to CCBs of various regional beds, such a differentiation is also related to the molecular structure of the CCB, as this is illustrated below.

Haemodynamic responses to a given CCB are usually compared with reactions to other vasodilators such as hydralazine or to other CCBs. Such approaches validate the significance of *in vitro* studies dealing with potency and tissue selectivity. This mode of comparison is illustrated by a recent analysis of the action of cilnidipine [24]. Intravenous administration of cilnidipine, nifedipine, or nicardipine dose dependently decreased the mean blood pressure in conscious spontaneously hypertensive rats (SHRs). The doses causing a

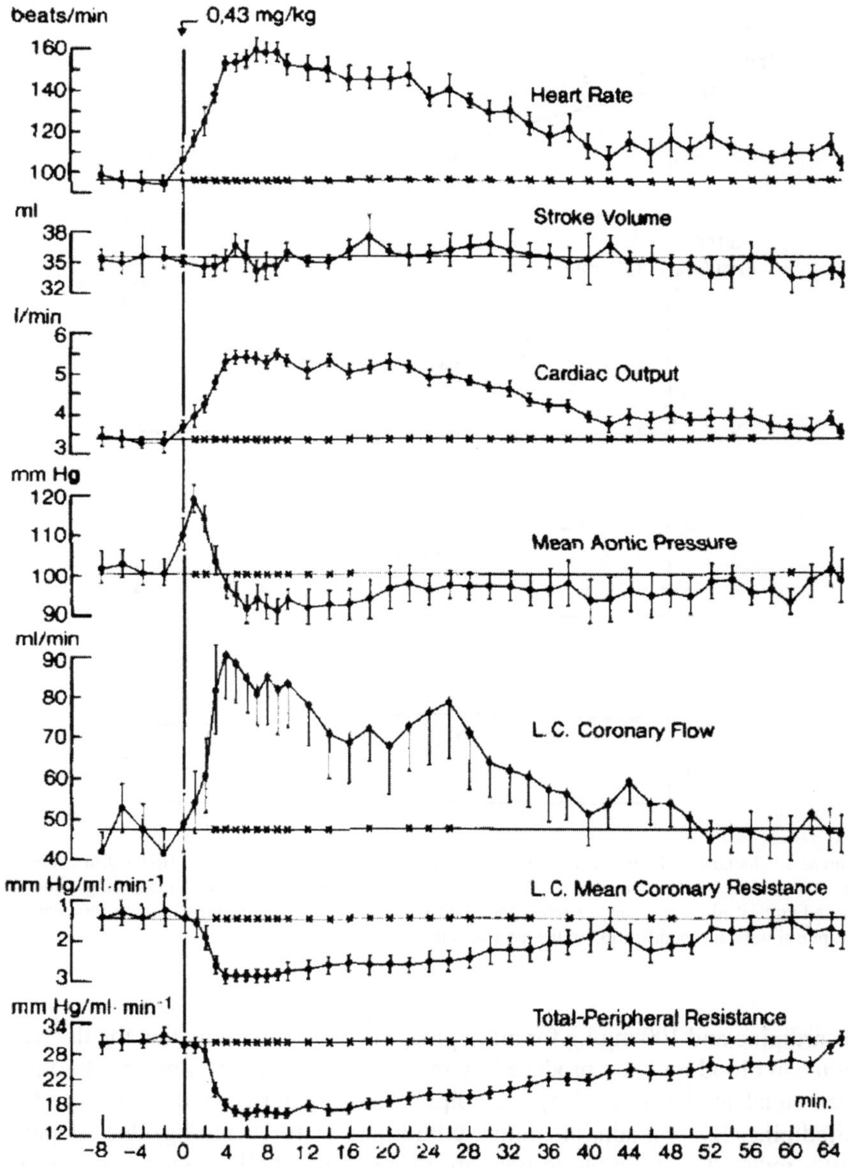

Figure 1. Effects of intravenous (*i.v.*) injection of nifedipine on haemodynamic parameters in the unanesthetized dog (n = 10). Modified from [14] The *i.v.* injection of nifedipine was followed by an important vasodilatation with an increase in cardiac output and heart rate. Note the important increase in coronary flow.

reduction in mean blood pressure of about 25 mmHg were 10 mg/kg for cilnidipine and nicardipine and 30 mg/kg for nifedipine. The doses causing a 45 mmHg reduction in mean blood pressure were 30 mg/kg for cilnidipine and

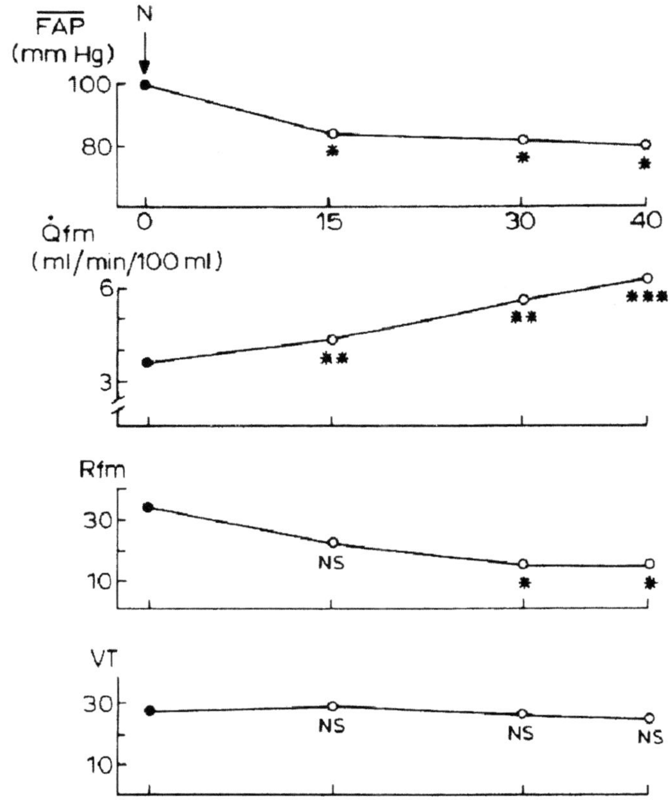

Figure 2. Changes in the mean femoral arterial pressure (FAP), forearm blood flow (Qfm), forearm resistance (Rfm) and venous tone (VT) after administration of nifedipine in human beings; control: closed circles; nifedipine: open circles. Modified from [17]. Note that venous tone was unchanged, despite significant modification in the arterial side.

nicardipine and 100 mg/kg for nifedipine. These results show that the decrease in mean blood pressure produced by intravenous administration of cilnidipine was equal to that caused by nicardipine and greater than that produced by nifedipine. By oral administration, cilnidipine (1 to 10 mg/kg) dose dependently reduced systolic blood pressure in conscious SHRs, renal hypertensive rats (RHRs), and DOCA-salt hypertensive rats (DHRs). In each hypertensive model, the maximal reduction in systolic blood pressure was observed 3 h after administration of the drug. In normotensive rats (NTRs), oral administration of cilnidipine, even at a high dose of 100 mg/kg, produced only a mild dose-dependent decrease in systolic blood pressure. The ED 20 values of cilnidipine in SHRs, RHRs, DHRs, and NTRs are listed in Table 1. In anesthetized dogs, intravenous administration of cilnidipine produced a dose-dependent decrease in mean arterial blood pressure and a slight increase in heart rate. A marked tachycardia, which was observed after administration of either nifedipine or nicardipine, was not observed even at high doses of cilnidipine. The ED 40 values (doses causing a 40% reduction in mean blood pressure) for cilnidipine, nifedipine, and nicardipine were 24.3, 20.1, and 23.3 mg/kg, respectively. These results indicate that in dogs, cilnidipine had almost the same hypotensive activity as nifedipine or nicardipine. The antihypertensive activity of cilnidipine in rats and dogs is characterized by a particular slow onset and long-lasting time course of action. In conscious SHRs, the effect of cilnidipine at 30 mg/kg reached a maximum at 1.7 min after intravenous administration, whereas the peak effects of nifedipine (100 mg/kg) and nicardipine (30 mg/kg), at doses causing a similar maximal decrease, were observed at 0.6 and 0.8 min after intravenous administration, respectively. The half-life of the hypotensive effect was 20.4 min for cilnidipine (30 mg/kg, *i.v.*) and 6 to 8 min for nifedipine (100 mg/kg, *i.v.*) and nicardipine (30 mg/kg, *i.v.*). In anesthetized dogs, similar hypotensive time courses were obtained after intravenous administration of cilnidipine, nifedipine, or nicardipine. The effects of 30 mg/kg (approximately the ED 40 values) of the three drugs reached their peak at 1.8, 0.7, and 0.9 min, respectively. The onset of cilnidipine action was about twice as slow as that of nifedipine or nicardipine, while the duration of its hypotensive effect was twice as long as that of the other two drugs. Thus, it appears that cilnidipine has a slow onset and long-lasting action *in vivo*. Such studies are interesting for the comparison of drugs potency, but they do not give information on the possible variation of action according to the vascular bed so far considered. Indeed, intravenously-administered CCBs induce a dose-related reduction in systemic and coronary vascular resistances, with concomitant decrease in arterial blood pressure and increase in coronary blood flow. Studies have often indicated differences in sensitivity among various vascular beds or between vessel tone and cardiac contractility. For instance for lercanidipine [21], the hypotensive ED25 values were equal to 6.1 micrograms/kg and 4.2 micrograms/kg for the decrease of mean blood pressure and of total peripheral resistances, respectively. The ED50 values on the coronary bed were equal to 4.8 micrograms/kg and 7.8 micrograms/kg for respectively the increase of coronary blood flow and the decrease in coronary vascular resistances. The authors have measured the time course of the haemodynamic effects after the administration of 5 micrograms/kg, a value close to the ED50 for the coronary bed. They observed that the onset of the vasodilatation was slow and that this activity was long-lasting: the peak effects on mean blood pressure and coronary blood flow occurred 20 and 30 minutes after the administration, respectively, and the effects on coronary resistances was still significant 150 min after the administration. The cardiac contractility was illustrated by measuring the contractile index dP/dtmax and dP/dt/P. In the dose-response study, dP/dtmax was practically not affected. In the time course study, dP/dtmax was not modified after administration of 5 micrograms/kg, and dP/dt/P showed a slight but long-lasting increase. The stability of the cardiac contractility was unlikely due to an activation of sympathetic reflex as a result of the vasodilatation, since the authors could not observe any change in heart rate with the dose of 5 micrograms/kg. A reflex increase in heart rate was observed after the administration of doses as high as 10 and 30 micrograms/kg. According to the authors, those haemodynamic investigations confirmed *in vivo* the high vascular selectivity of lercanidipine found *in vitro*.

Regional responses

Variations in regional sensitivity to the vasodilatation effects of CCBs could be anticipated from the observation of their vascular selectivity reported during *in vitro* studies on vessels isolated from various vascular beds. *In vivo* studies indicate that variations in regional sensitivity may be found in various models, including resting unanesthetized dogs. How this regional selectivity could influence the therapeutic action is a matter of further analysis, when the use of CCBs in pathology will be considered.

Coronary circulation

In early studies, CCBs appeared to be highly active on the coronary circulation as shown by the large increase in coronary flow following the injection of nifedipine, illustrated in Figure 1. CCBs reduce myocardial oxygen consumption; in such a situation, the physiological regulation should have diminished coronary blood flow through the metabolic autoregulation. Exposure to CCBs has counteracted this autoregulation, maintaining a significant increase of coronary blood flow. This effect of CCBs is the result of the dilatation of resistance vessels in the coronary bed, which overcomes the coronary vasoconstriction due to a decrease in myocardial oxygen consumption (for references, see [3]).

Mesenteric and renal beds

Janssen et al. [12] have compared in rats the regional specific haemodynamic effects of barnidipine with those obtained with its racemic mixture and with amlodipine. Male adult spontaneously hypertensive rats (SHR) were instrumented with Doppler flow probes and catheters to measure renal (RVR), mesenteric (MVR) and hindquarter (HQVR) vascular resistance changes. One week after surgery, barnidipine, its racemic mixture, and amlodipine were intravenously administered at three doses causing comparable reductions in mean arterial pressure (MAP). At doses of 3, 10 and 30 μg/kg barnidipine reduced MAP (±SEM) by 8 ± 2, 26 ± 3 and 45 ± 4 mmHg ($n = 10$). Equipotent effects on MAP were achieved by the racemic mixture of barnidipine at 10, 30 and 100 μg/kg, and by amlodipine at doses of 100, 300 and

1000 μg/kg. Following the 3 μg/kg and 10 μg/kg dose, barnidipine reduced MVR (% ± SEM) by 4 ± 4 and 19 ± 4, and RVR by 8 ± 2 and 15 ± 4, respectively. In contrast, HQVR remained unaltered. Similar data were obtained for the racemic mixture of barnidipine and for amlodipine, although for the latter the changes in RVR were half of those found after barnidipine. After the highest doses of barnidipine, its racemic mixture as well as amlodipine, HQVR fell more than 25% whereas RVR and MVR remained unaltered. By contrast to short-acting CCBs such as nifedipine and isradipine, which reduced mainly HQVR and did not reduce RVR, the three long-term acting CCBs preferentially dilated the mesenteric and renal vascular bed. The authors concluded that in view of the elevation of RVR in essential hypertension, the reduction of RVR might contribute to the long-term antihypertensive effects of barnidipine and of amlodipine. In their discussion they made also interesting considerations about the different responses observed in the various vascular beds so far studied. The doses of barnidipine, of its racemic mixture and of amlodipine were titrated to result in equipotent reductions of blood pressure. This was achieved using a dose range for barnidipine that was a factor 3 lower than for its racemic mixture and even a factor 30 lower than for amlodipine. In studies on isolated small mesenteric arteries, however, barnidipine was about a factor 20 more potent than its racemic mixture and a factor 200 more potent than amlodipine. The *in vivo* counteracting physiological control systems account most likely for such differences in potency. Following the cumulative intravenous injections of all three agents, arterial pressure decreased dose-dependently in more or less a linear fashion. However, the regional vascular effects that underlay this pharmacodynamic response did not show such linear dose-effect relationship. At the lowest and intermediate dose, barnidipine, its racemic mixture and amlodipine preferentially dilated the mesenteric and renal arteriolar bed. Vascular resistance of the hindquarter bed did not change significantly. Only after the highest dose of the three CCBs a profound dilatation of the muscular hindquarter vascular bed occurred, whereas renal and mesenteric resistances were not further reduced. Among players in the concert of physiological and pharmacological mechanisms that contribute to this differential regional response to the three CCBs, it seems that baroreflex is an important factor that determines the regional distribution of blood flow after injection of the CCBs. In normal conditions in rats, blood flow through the muscular hindquarter vascular bed is predominantly under autonomic control, whereas in the renal and mesenteric circulation autoregulatory mechanisms prevail. Therefore, after doses of barnidipine and amlodipine that caused gradual and moderate blood pressure changes, the reduction in hindquarter resistance could have been masked by a baroreflex-mediated neurogenic vasoconstriction. Thus, the effect of a given CCB might depend upon its rate of action. For instance, as shown by [18], fast and short-acting CCBs such as nifedipine and isradipine preferentially dilate the hindquarter vascular bed, without change in RVR. The difference in the regional haemodynamic response between nifedipine and isradipine on the one hand, and barnidipine and amlodipine on the other hand, may depend upon the degree of activation of the baroreflexes. The unloading of baroreceptor afferents is a dynamic process and depends on the time course of the pressure fall. When blood pressure is reduced too fast or too far, a neurogenic constriction may occur in various vascular beds as a reflex to the blood pressure fall. A major factor to be considered is the ability of the peripheral organs to autoregulate their blood flow in the presence of variations in blood pressure. For instance, the kidney is known to be able to keep its blood flow constant when perfusion pressure changes. In Janssen et al. [12] study, renal and mesenteric blood flows were unchanged with barnidipine 3 and 10 despite that blood pressure fell by about 25 mmHg. Nevertheless, these authors observed a decrease in renal and mesenteric vascular resistance maintaining the blood flow at its control level despite the fall in blood pressure. Besides those regulatory factors, the tissue selectivity of CCBs may also influence the difference in responsiveness observed between the vascular beds. In addition, activation of the renin-angiotensin system by low blood pressure could elevate the tissue level of angiotensin II, which may partly antagonize the effect of CCBs. From *in vitro* experiments on isolated arterial segments, it is known that the vasorelaxant effects of dihydropyridines depend on the level of precontraction. Therefore, it can be assumed that also in an *in vivo* situation, differences in the initial vascular resistance are of importance. Particularly in the SHR in which sympathetic tone to the renal arterioles is thought to be elevated, the relaxing effect of calcium entry blockade may become less visible than in normotensive animals.

Cerebral blood flow

Cerebral blood flow (CBF) is unique in that it is constant in the face of changing blood flow and pressure. Change in blood flow resulting from increase in cardiac output has consequences in tissue perfusion according to the vascular bed. For instance physical exercise producing a three-fold increase in cardiac output leads to a 10-fold increase in blood flow to skeletal muscle, halves renal blood flow, but does not modify CBF. Although the percentage distribution of cardiac output increases in skeletal muscle (21–71%), and decreases substantially in the kidney (19–3%), the change in the brain is far less (13–5%) [26]. This has been shown in several studies with antihypertensive drugs: pharmacological agents can have pronounced effects on CBF. Differences in the mechanisms and sites of action of the various antihypertensive drugs leads to each category producing a characteristic pattern of vasodilatation and redistribution of cardiac output, at least acutely. As discussed by Atkinson and Capdeville [2], antihypertensive drugs can be divided into three categories, in the first of which are found those that decrease CBF. This first category can be further subdivided into drugs which interfere with noradrenergic vascular tone such as ganglion blocking agents, centrally acting hypertensive drugs like clonidine, alpha adrenoreceptor blocking agents such as prazosin and various vasodilators such as diazoxide, sodium nitroprusside and nitroglycerin. A second group is composed of drugs that have minor effects on CBF. Antagonists of the vascular 5-HT2 receptor such as ketanserin, markedly increase cardiac output but produce very little change in CBF, blood flow being distributed mainly to the gut, kidneys and skeletal muscles. Likewise beta-blockers such as atenolol, have apparently no significant effect on CBF. Although other reports suggest that beta-blockers may slightly lower CBF. ACEI do not modify basal CBF. A third category of antihypertensive drugs is composed of those that increase CBF, and amongst these are to be found the CCBs. The increase in cardiac output produced by CCBs, such as the dihydropyridine felodipine, for example, is accompanied by a marked increase in CBF, similar to that observed in coronary blood flow, and far above that seen in other organs such as the kidney, the gut and the skeletal muscles [4]. This pharmacological profile is shared with other vasodilators such as potassium channel activators and hydralazine, but, generally, the cerebrovascular dilator effects of dihydropyridine CCB were found to be more pronounced than those of other vasodilators.

Hara et al. [9] have examined the effects of lomerizine, a CCB of the piperazine group on cerebral cortical blood flow (CBF) in anaesthetized rats by laser Doppler flowmetry and on vertebral blood flow in anaesthetized beagle dogs with an electromagnetic flowmeter. They have observed that lomerizine (1.25–10 mg/kg, p.o.) dose-dependently increased CBF in rats without affecting blood pressure (BP) or heart rate (HR) (Fig. 3). They have measured the plasma concentration of lomerizine (free base) in anaesthetized rats at 30 and 60 min after the initial administration of 5 mg/kg, p.o., times at which there was a significant increase in CBF. The values obtained for Cmax and Tmax were 27.6 ng/mL and 90 min, respectively. Lomerizine has been shown to displace specific ^{3}H-nitrendipine binding to guinea-pig cortex and dog aortic membranes with an IC50 of 86 nmol/L and a Ki of 340 nmol/L, respectively. This indicates that plasma levels so far observed were significant as far as concerned their functional efficacy. Effects recorded in dogs were consistant with observations made in rats and just reported above. Indeed, lomerizine (2.5 and 5 mg/kg, intraduodenally) dose-dependently increased vertebral blood flow in dogs without significantly changing BP or HR. With 10-mg/kg intraduodenal lomerizine, vertebral blood flow remained elevated from 20 to 240 min after administration despite a concomitant decrease of BP occurring from 20 to 120 min (Fig. 4). This confirms the concept reported above that CCBs might oppose the vasoconstrictive reflex in cerebral vessels, which is physiologically activated in response to a fall in blood pressure. It is worth to mention that all authors have not reported such remarkable effects of CCBs on cerebral blood flow (for ref see [2]). This may be due to experimental conditions including pharmacokinetic characteristics of the CCB considered, animal species, technique used to evaluate cerebral blood flow and to produce anesthesia.

Such studies point to the complexity of the response of various vascular beds to a pharmacological intervention directed on the L-type Ca channels, a response that can be modified not only by the rate of action of the considered

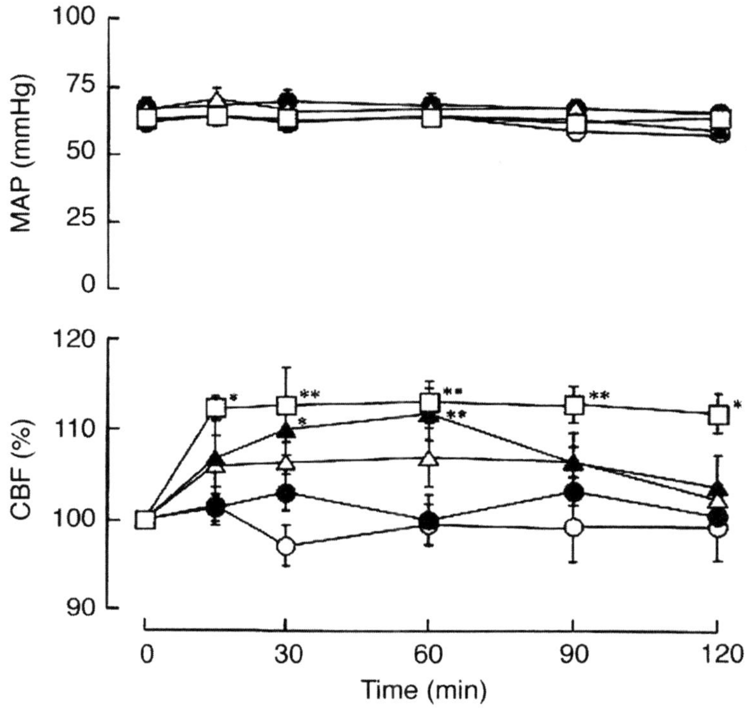

Figure 3. Effects of lomerizine dihydrochloride on mean arterial blood pressure (MAP) (upper panel) and on cerebral cortical blood flow (CBF; measured by laser Doppler flowmetry) (lower panel) in urethane-anaesthetized rats. (from Hara et al. [9]; modified). Each data point represents the mean ± SEM for nine rats. Base values for cerebral CBF were estimated before the administration of the various doses of lomerizine and of the placebo: vehicle (distilled water; open circles); 1.25 mg/kg, p.o., lomerizine (closed circles); 2.5 mg/kg, p.o., lomerizine (open triangles); 5 mg/kg, p.o., lomerizine (closed triangles); 10 mg/kg, p.o., lomerizine (open squares) $^*P < 0.05$, $^{**}P < 0.01$ compared with vehicle. The probe was fixed using adhesive agent to the surface of the thin dura mater, which is close to the cortex. Measurements made in this way represent the blood flow in the superficial vessels below the probe. The output of the equipment gives relative, rather than absolute values. Cerebral blood flow was measured for at least 120 min after drug administration. Note that the effects here measured do not give indication on blood circulation within the intracerebral circulation.

drug but also by factors associated with the pathophysiological situation, which will be examined in another section of this book.

Regional response and differences between CCBs

Studies on anesthetized dogs may also help to characterize differences between molecules, considering not only their potency and the time course of their effect, as this is reported above, but also their specificity of action on a given vascular bed. A recent study dealing with renal haemodynamic does

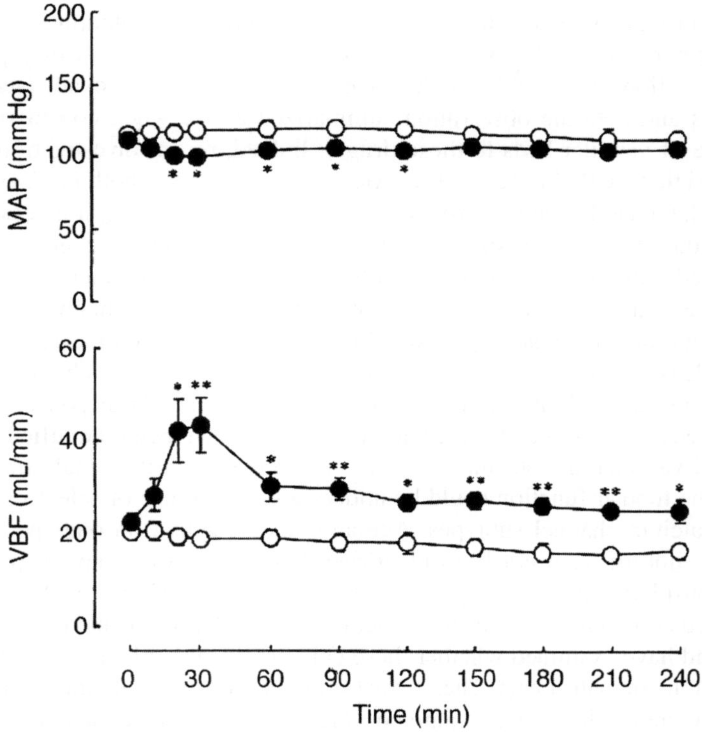

Figure 4. Effect of of lomerizine dihydrochloride in pentobarbital-anaesthetized dogs. Changes in mean arterial blood pressure (MAP, upper panel) and vertebral blood flow (VBF, lower panel) after intraduodenal administration of 10 mg/kg. (from Hara et al. [9]; modified). Each data point represents the mean ± SEM for five dogs. *$P < 0.05$, **$P < 0.01$ compared with vehicle (open circles, lomerizine: closed circles). Note that despite fall in blood pressure, blood flow in cerebral artery was not reduced, as expected from physiological reflex, but was increased due the effect of the CCB.

illustrate this possibility with a comparison between various drugs acting on renal blood flow and on natriuresis, which also provides the opportunity to clarify the mechanisms involved in an effect important for the treatment of hypertension. Although they are potent vasodilators, calcium channel blockers do not cause sodium retention, an undesired effect that is observed with the use of other vasodilators, including α-blockers, hydralazine and minoxidil. Indeed, long-term therapy with calcium antagonists produces no alterations in circulating blood volume. Rather, calcium channel blockers increase sodium excretion in the face of hypotension when administered acutely to patients and experimental animals with hypertension (see [13]). It has been postulated that the mechanisms involved in the natriuresis evoked by calcium channel blockers are associated with various processes such as: changes in renal haemodynamics, direct effects on renal tubules and either activation or suppression of vasoactive substances. Although calcium channel blockers exert their action mainly through the blockade of L-type voltage-dependent calcium channels in vascular smooth muscles, several lines of evidence suggest that they possess multiple actions that could be independent of this channel blockade (see other Chapters and note the observation summarized above when considering the response of vascular beds to those drugs). Indeed, recent investigations have indicated that CCBs increase nitric oxide (NO) production both *in vitro* and *in vivo* [16]. Given that NO contributes to renal sodium handling, it is reasonable to speculate that natriuresis induced by calcium channel blockers might be associated with their interaction with NO. Another possible factor is the role of T-type channels in the renal response. Some calcium channel blockers, including efonidipine, are reported to block at similar concentration T-type, as well as L-type calcium channels, whereas some other calcium channel blockers, including nifedipine, inhibit L-type calcium channels at concentrations much lower than T-type. T-type calcium channels have been identified in cardiac and vascular smooth muscle cells [6], their role in the renal circulation and in the tubular function could be understood by the use of selective blockers to calcium channel subtypes. Actually, agents active on one specific Ca channel subtype have not been identified, but information may be provided when considering the ratio of potency of different drugs. Honda et al. [10] have compared compounds with different actions on renal afferent and efferent arterioles and have examined whether these calcium channel blockers exert divergent actions on natriuresis. Their effect on renal arterioles obviously depends upon the molecule so far examined (Fig. 5). The intravenous infusion of nifedipine (L-type blocker), efonidipine (L/T-type blocker) or mibefradil (predominant T-type blocker) into anaesthetized dogs elicited similar, albeit modest, reductions in blood pressure. Nifedipine (1 $\mu g \cdot min^{-1} \cdot kg^{-1}$) increased renal plasma flow (RPF) by 23 ± 6% ($P < 0.05$) and glomerular filtration rate (GFR) by 25 ± 5% ($P < 0.05$). Efonidipine (0.33 $\mu g \cdot min^{-1} \cdot kg^{-1}$) elevated RPF by 18 ± 6% ($P < 0.05$), and increased GFR by 17 ± 8%, but this was not statistically significant. These drugs exerted contrasting actions on the filtration fraction (FF), with an increase being elicited by nifedipine, whereas efonidipine had no effect. Furthermore, mibefradil (0.01 ± 1 $\mu g \cdot min^{-1} \cdot kg^{-1}$) slightly elevated RPF (between 5 ± 3% and 8 ± 3%), but failed to alter GFR, resulting in a decrease in FF. Nifedipine slightly increased urinary sodium excretion (UNaV): a 29 ± 16% increase of UNaV was observed with 1 $\mu g \cdot min^{-1} \cdot kg^{-1}$ and fractional sodium excretion (FENa) increased by 18 ± 14%. Efonidipine (0.33 $\mu g \cdot min^{-1} \cdot kg^{-1}$), which had a lower effect than nifedipine (1 $\mu g \cdot min^{-1} \cdot kg^{-1}$) on RBF and GFR, elicited marked elevations in UNa V (110·38%; $P < 0.05$) and FENa (102·44%; $P < 0.05$). Mibefradil (1 $\mu g \cdot min^{-1} \cdot kg^{-1}$) exerted a moderate natriuretic action [UNa V: +60 ± 32% (P ¯0.1): FENa: +67 ± 20% ($P < 0.05$)]. The urinary nitrate/nitrite excretion was dose-dependent but it showed no differences between the various calcium channel blockers, indicating that they had similar action on NO production and that this action could not account for the differences observed between drugs in their renal haemodynamic and natriuretic actions which are illustrated by

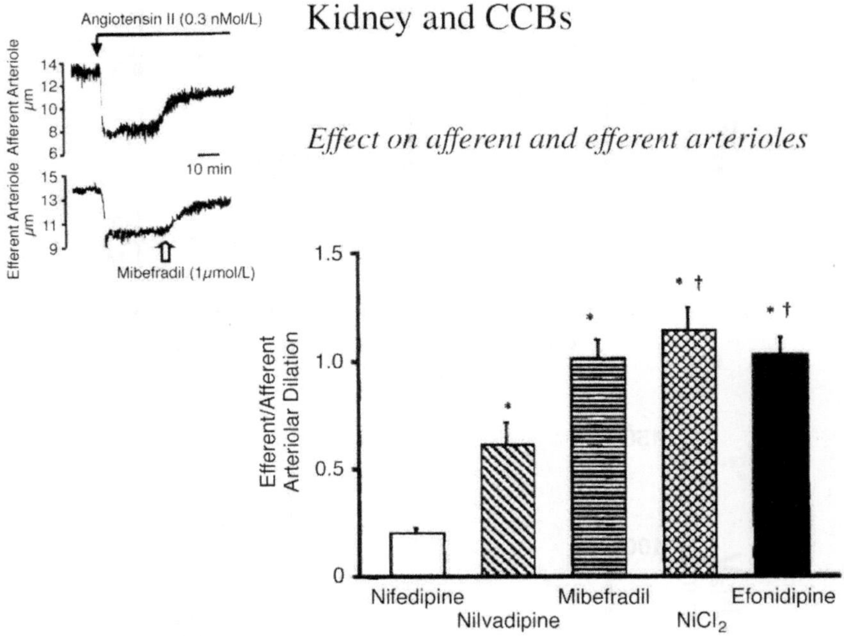

Figure 5. The action of CCBs on kidney perfused with Krebs-Ringer at a perfusion pressure of at 80 mm Hg in the renal artery; their effect on afferent and efferent arterioles. Modified from Ozawa et al. [19]. Upper panel: Experimental representative tracing illustrating the reversal by mibefradil of Ang II-induced constriction of renal arterioles. Note that mibefradil reversed the Ang II-induced vasoconstriction of both afferent and efferent arterioles. In control experiment, Ang II-evoked vasoconstriction of both afferent and efferent arterioles persisted for at least 60 minutes. Lower panel: Further illustration of the selectivity of action of CCBs; their heterogeneity as renal vasodilators. Nifedipine (1 μmol/L), nilvadipine (1 μmol/L), mibefradil (1 μmol/L), $NiCl_2$ (100 μmol/L), and efonidipine (1 μmol/L) administered during Ang II-induced afferent and efferent arteriolar constriction. The ratio of efferent/afferent arteriolar vasodilation is indicated for each CCB, showing differences between drugs.

Figure 6. According to the authors, the natriuretic action of calcium channel blockers could be related to the inhibition of tubular sodium reabsorption associated with the increased post-glomerular blood flow, an effect highly related to the chemical structure of the CCB considered.

Although differences in natriuresis do not appear to be related to a difference in enhanced NO production by CCBs, a role for interaction of CCBs with NO, illustrated by various experiments *in vitro* [7], is also obvious *in vivo*. It has been shown *in vitro* that amlodipine increases NO levels in coronary vessels and aorta via bradykinin-dependent mechanisms (see page 188). Based on their observation that benidipine, a long-acting Ca channel blocker increases cardiac NO levels in ischaemic canine hearts, Asanuma et al. [1] have examined the action of this CCB on reperfusion after injury of coronary arteries. In open chest dogs, the left anterior descending coronary artery was perfused

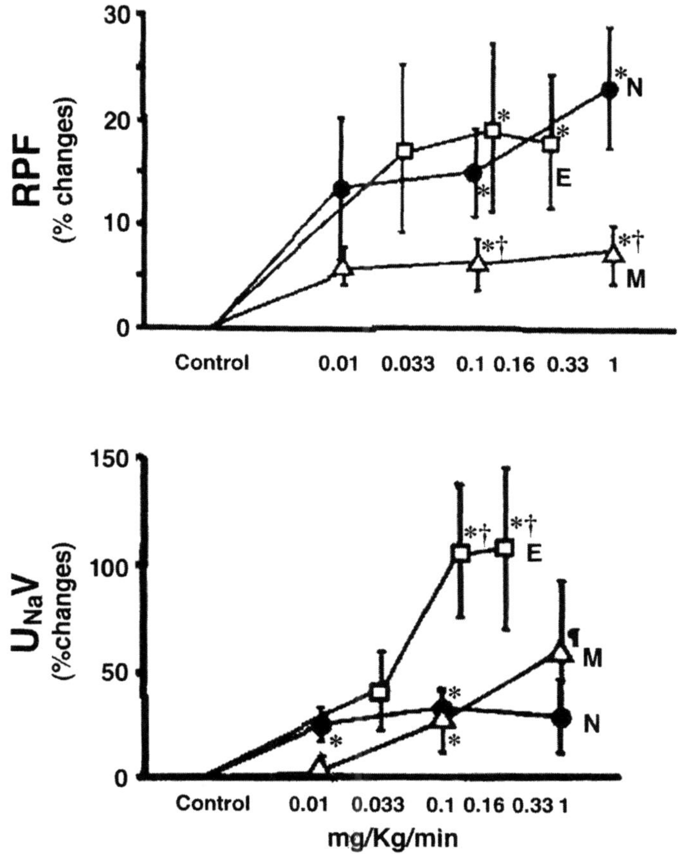

Figure 6. The action of CCBs: N = nifedipine, E = efonidipine, M = mibefradil on RPF (renal plasma flow) and on UnaV (urinary sodium excretion). From Honda et al. [10], (modified) Note dissimilarities between drugs as far as renal plasma flow and urinary sodium excretion are concerned. After the administration of 0.1 µg/min/kg nifedipine, RPF was increased by 15 ± 4% and by 23 ± 6% at a dose of 1 µg/min/kg. Similarly, efonidipine caused marked rises in RPF, with increments of 20 ± 8% and 18 ± 6% at doses of 0.16 and 0.33 µg/min/kg respectively. In contrast, mibefradil elicited modest increments in RPF at 0.1 µg/min/kg and even at 1 µg/min/kg. On the other hand, as this is illustrated in this Figure, nifedipine caused only slight increase of urinary sodium excretion: increments of 32 ± 8% and 25 ± 7% at 0.1 and 1 µg/min/kg respectively. In striking contrast, efonidipine markedly enhanced natriuresis: $U_{Na}V$ was increased by 108 ± 31% and 110 ± 38% at doses of 0.16 and 0.33 µg/min/kg, respectively. Mibefradil exerted a mild natriuretic action: 27 ± 15% at 0.1 µg/min/kg and 60 ± 32% at 1 µg/min/kg, intermediate between that seen with lower nifedipine and efonidipine. Thus this experiment illustrates clearly a dissociation between the action of CCBs on renal plasma flow and on urinary sodium excretion.

with blood through a bypass tube and was occluded for 90 min followed by 6 hours of reperfusion. Infarct size was assessed by TTC staining at 6 hours of reperfusion. When benidipine at doses of 50, 100, and 200 ng/kg/min was infused via the bypass tube between 10 min prior to the onset of ischaemia and after 60 min of reperfusion, systemic blood pressure did not change significantly. Infarct size decreased with the administration of benidipine (50, 100, and 200 ng/kg/min) when compared to the untreated condition (24.8 ± 2.5, 17.3 ± 3.1, and 16.5 ± 2.0 *versus* 43.4 ± 5.6%, respectively), this was associated with the increased release of NO and bradykinin in the coronary venous blood upon reperfusion. The limitation of the infarct size by benidipine was completely blunted by either L-NAME, which inhibits the production of NO by NO-synthase or by HOE140 (icatibant), which antagonizes the action of bradykinine. The protective action of benidipine in this acute ischaemic model involves obviously NO, but this not rules out the role of other actions due to calcium channel blockade, such as the reduction of the heart wall stress associated with the arterial vasodilatation. Again, this confirms the complexity of the *in vivo* action of drugs even if a specific target has been identified for their action.

In the former experimental models, we have considered normal animals, hypertensive ones and animals with coronary insufficiency. Another major pathological event is cardiac insufficiency, a situation where the sympathic system is highly activated. Although there is no real specific antagonist for the L or T-type Ca channels that regulate the function of the cardiovascular system, it has been recently proposed that CCBs more selective for T-type than L-type Ca channels could be efficient in treating cardiac insufficiency. It is known that mibefradil, the prototype of T-type selective CCBs, has been withdrawn from therapy for incompatibility with other drugs, which does not preclude any theoretical consideration related to its action in various pathologies. Because T-type selective CCBs are more selective for inhibiting contractile activity in vascular than in cardiac tissue, it has been hypothesized, by analogy with was done with vascular-selective dihydropyridines like nisoldipine, that they could be used in left ventricular insufficiency. From clinical data it is known that in patients with LV ejection fraction of 40%, *i.v.* mibefradil is associated with a near 30% increase in plasma norepinephrine concentration but this increase is, in general, well within the limits of the analytical method used and considerably lower than that seen with *i.v.* infusion of other CCBs. Despite the marked vasodilator and anti-ischaemic actions of existing calcium channel blockers, their use in the treatment of patients with chronic heart failure (HF) remains highly controversial. Shimoyama et al. [20] compared the short-term haemodynamic effects of *i.v.* mibefradil, a predominant T-type calcium channel blocker with only partial L-type calcium channel antagonism, and diltiazem, a selective L-type calcium channel antagonist (which has been shown to have a vascular selectivity similar to nifedipine, see page 120) in dogs with chronic HF. Each of three interventions namely, mibefradil, diltiazem and normal saline (as placebo control), were studied in random order (six days between each drug intervention), in each of eight dogs with chronic HF produced by multiple intracoronary microembolizations. Intravenous mibefradil and diltiazem were administered as a 100 mg/kg bolus followed by a continuous infusion of 6 and 4 mg/kg/min, respectively, for 15 min. Equal volumes of normal saline were administered in an identical fashion. In all instances, haemodynamic parameters were obtained at baseline and at 5, 10, 15, 30 and 60 min after bolus drug administration. Left ventriculograms were obtained at baseline, and at 15 and 60 min after bolus drug administration. Saline infusion had no effects on haemodynamic or angiographic indexes of left ventricular (LV) function. At 15 min, mibefradil caused significant increases of LV stroke volume and LV ejection fraction compared to baseline (40. 6 5 *versus* 31. 6 3 ml, $P < 0.05$ and 41. 61 *versus* 28. 6 1%, $P < 0.05$, respectively). In contrast, at 15 min, diltiazem produced no significant changes of LV stroke volume or ejection fraction compared to baseline despite reducing mean aortic pressure to the same extent as mibefradil. Short-term *i.v.* mibefradil improves LV function in dogs with chronic HF. According to the authors, the beneficial effects of mibefradil compared to diltiazem may be a consequence of vascular selectivity of this T-type calcium channel selective blocker, resulting in a vasodilatory response that is free of negative inotropy. Similar data have so far be obtained with nisoldipine compared to a non-vascular-specific CCB.

Thus in various situations, haemodynamic studies point to major differences between CCBs, not only in potency but also in selectivity of action. This emphasizes the observation that even drugs having a specific molecular target, may behave differently *in vivo*, because of the uneven distribution of this target among organs, which become important sites of action in some pathophysiological situations. This hypothesis is examined throughout the chapters of this book.

The action of catecholamines illustrates the complexity of regional responses

The regional variation of response to CCBs might be at least partly related to the regional variation in receptors for diverse endogenous vasoconstrictors and vasodilatators, which might influence the blood flow through of the various vascular beds. As reviewed by Guimares and Moura [8], there is a regional variation in the distribution of vascular adrenoceptors and the response to cathecholamines of the various vascular beds is complex. In view of the observations that the relaxing action of CCBs may depend upon the previous tone and because action of vasodilators may be synergistic, it is of importance to examine how the various beds respond to catecholamines. For many years, it has been accepted, at least in humans, that splanchnic and skeletal muscle vascular beds dilate to adrenaline because β-adrenoceptors predominate in their vessels, whereas adrenaline consistently reduces renal and skin blood flow, because in renal and skin vessels α-adrenoceptors are predominant. The cerebral and coronary arteries are of particular importance in the whole of the vascular system, because of the vital functions of the organs they supply. The cerebral circulation of many species has an abundant and dense sympathetic innervation. However, the response of the cerebral vasculature to sympathetic nerve activity is comparatively small. In humans, the influence of sympathetic innervation on the tone of cerebral vasculature is weak and reflects not only a low density of innervation, but also a reduced number of α-adrenoceptors. The sympathetic neurogenic control of cerebral arteries decreases with decreasing diameter of the vessel and the contraction of human pial arteries is very weak in response to nerve stimulation [25]. The maximum vasoconstriction to noradrenaline in the middle meningeal artery reaches 34% of the maximum to KCl and in the pial artery it reaches only about 10%. Furthermore, cerebral arteries of the rat and pig do not contain functional α-adrenoceptors, an indication that some information from animal studies could not be simply extrapolated to human. There is also evidence that the population of postjunctional β-adrenoceptors is not important in cerebral arteries. However, a small number does not necessarily mean a lack of influence of the sympathetic nerves on the cerebral circulation, which may be exerted through a cross-talk between sympathetic nerves and other neuronal systems. For instance, the nicotine-induced relaxation in the porcine basilar artery appears to result from the activation of nicotinic receptors on the presynaptic adrenergic nerve terminals causing a release of noradrenaline that activates β1-adrenoceptors located on nitroergic nerves and promotes the release of NO [23a]. Another effect mediated by adenoceptors is that observed in segments of rabbit middle cerebral arteries, where the activation of endothelial α2-adrenoceptor causes a reduction in endothelin-1 production and promotes vascular relaxation [23].

In the coronary circulation, the relative amount of α-and β-adrenoceptors and the relative functional role they play also does not fit into the general pattern of the vascular beds. In the pig, the small coronary vessels exhibit little or no α-adrenoceptor-mediated activity, and the large coronary artery contains α1-adrenoceptors, mainly of the α_{1A}-subtype, but the functional importance of their vasoconstrictive effect is unclear. In the coronary artery of the dog, the functional role of α-adrenoceptors varies between undetectable and of little expression. In vessels with spontaneous tone, isoprenaline causes concentration-dependent relaxations, whereas noradrenaline and adrenaline cause either contraction (of small magnitude) or relaxation. However, after the tone had been elevated by phenylephrine, both adrenaline and noradrenaline cause concentration-dependent relaxations that is lower than that caused by isoprenaline. In coronary arteries, β1-adrenoceptors are largely predominant by contrast to the mesenteric, splenic, and pulmonary arteries, where β2-adrenoceptors predominate. In dog, the number of β-adrenoceptor-mediated responses of epicardial coronary arteries is inversely related to the size of the vessel. In the splanchnic vascular bed of the dog, α-adrenoceptor-mediated effects always predominate over β-adrenoceptor-mediated responses when adrenaline is used as agonist. It is hypothesized that β-adrenoceptors are associated only with arterioles and precapillary sphincters. In the hindlimb of the dog adrenaline, despite reaching arterioles and precapillary sphincters, causes concentration-dependent increases of the perfusion pressure, showing that α-adrenoceptor-mediated vasopressor effect predominates also in this vascular bed [8].

The vascular response to adrenoceptors stimulation may be affected in many diseases, either due to alteration of the vessel or of control and/or number of the receptors. Additionally, measurement of cardiovascular parameters in animal models for diseases may be the result of multifactor systems. Their interpretation is far more complex than results from *in vitro* experiments. According to Guimares and Moura, the determination of maximum responses of the blood pressure to pressor agents is often impossible; hence, it is hazardous to provide a full and satisfactory description of an enhanced vasopressor response as being due to a parallel shift of the dose-response curve to the left, to an increase of the maximum response, or to both? The analytical description of the effect of any agent preventing this change in responsiveness is also elusive.

As a consequence of such a complexity illustrated by limitations of attempts to delineate from haemodynamic studies the role played by adrenoceptors in various diseases, it may be anticipated that drugs like CCBs, which interact with processes responsible for vascular tone involving catecholamines or other autocoids, may exhibit variations in action according to the vascular bed or the animal model so far considered.

References

1 Asanuma H, Kitakaze M, Node K, Takashima S, Sakata Y, Asakura M, Sanada S, Shinozaki Y, Mori H, Tada M et al. Benidipine, a long-acting Ca channel blocker, limits infarct size via bradykinin- and NO-dependent mechanisms in canine hearts. *Cardiovasc Drugs Ther* 15: 225–231, 2001

2 Atkinson J and Capdeville C. *Hypertension, antihypertensive treatment and cerebrovascular disease.* Southborough: TransMedica Europe Limited, 1990

3 Berdeaux A, Drieu La Rochelle C and Richard V. *Calcium antagonists and the coronary circulation.* Southborough: TransMedica Europe Limited, 1990

4 Bolt GR and Saxena PR. Acute systemic and regional hemodynamic effects of felodipine, a new calcium antagonist, in conscious renal hypertensive rabbits. *J Cardiovasc Pharmacol* 6: 707–712, 1984

5 Frohlich ED. Hemodynamic effects of diltiazem in the spontaneously hypertensive rat and in human hypertension. In: *Essential Hypertension; Calcium Mechanisms and Treatment.* Aoki, K (Ed), p 191-218. Springer, Berlin, Heidelberg, New York, 1986

6 Godfraind T. Calcium antagonists and vasodilatation. *Pharmacol Ther* 64: 37–75, 1994

7 Godfraind T and Salomone S. Calcium antagonists and endothelial function: focus on nitric oxide and endothelin. *Cardiovasc Drugs Ther* 10: 439–446, 1996

8 Guimaraes S and Moura D. Vascular adrenoceptors: an update. *Pharmacol Rev* 53: 319–356, 2001

9 Hara H, Shimazawa M, Sasaoka M, Yamada C, Iwakura Y, Sakai T, Maeda Y, Yamaguchi T, Sukamoto T and Hashimoto M. Selective effects of lomerizine, a novel diphenylmethylpiperazine Ca^{2+} channel blocker, on cerebral blood flow in rats and dogs. *Clin Exp Pharmacol Physiol* 26: 870–876, 1999

10 Honda M, Hayashi K, Matsuda H, Kubota E, Tokuyama H, Okubo K, Ozawa Y and Saruta T. Divergent natriuretic action of calcium channel antagonists in mongrel dogs: renal haemodynamics as a determinant of natriuresis. *Clin Sci (Lond)* 101: 421–427, 2001

11 Ishii H, Itoh K and Nose T. Different antihypertensive effects of nifedipine in conscious experimental hypertensive and normotensive rats. *Eur J Pharmacol* 64: 21–29, 1980

12 Janssen BJ, Kam KL and Smits JF. Preferential renal and mesenteric vasodilation induced by barnidipine and amlodipine in spontaneously hypertensive rats. *Naunyn Schmiedebergs Arch Pharmacol* 364: 414–421, 2001

13 Kazda S and Knorr A. *Calcium antagonists. In: Pharmacology of Antihypertensive Therapeutics. Ganten, D. and Mulrow, P.J. (Ed), p 301–375.* Berlin, Heidelberg, New York, London, Paris, Tokyo, Hong Kong: Springer Verlag, 1990

14 Kirchheim H and Gross R. *Hemodynamic Effects of Adalat in the Unanesthetized Dog*. Berlin-Heidelberg-New york: Springer-Verlag, 1975

15 Knorr A and Garthoff B. Differential influence of the calcium antagonist nitrendipine and the vasodilator hydralazine on normal and elevated blood pressure. *Arch Int Pharmacodyn Ther* 269: 316–322, 1984

16 Krenek P, Salomone S, Kyselovic J, Wibo M, Morel N and Godfraind T. Lacidipine prevents endothelial dysfunction in salt-loaded stroke-prone hypertensive rats. *Hypertension* 37: 1124–1128, 2001

17 Merillon JP, Morgant C, Zygelman M, Abadie E, Charlier P and Gourgon R. *Comparison of the hemodynamic and coronary effects of three vasodilator drugs: dipyridamole, nifedipine and glyceryl trinitrate*. Amsterdam-Oxford-Princeton: Excerpta Medica, 1980

18 Nievelstein HM, Van Essen H, Tijssen CM, Smits JF and Struyker Boudier HA. Systemic and regional hemodynamic actions of calcium entry blockers in conscious spontaneously hypertensive rats. *Eur J Pharmacol* 113: 187–198, 1985

19 Ozawa Y, Hayashi K, Nagahama T, Fujiwara K, Wakino S and Saruta T. Renal afferent and efferent arteriolar dilation by nilvadipine: studies in the isolated perfused hydronephrotic kidney. *J Cardiovasc Pharmacol* 33: 243–247, 1999

20 Shimoyama H, Sabbah HN, Tanimura M, Borzak S and Goldstein S. Short-term hemodynamic effects of mibefradil in dogs with chronic heart failure: comparison with diltiazem. *J Pharmacol Exp Ther* 285: 746–752, 1998

21 Sironi G, Montagna E, Greto L, Leonardi A and Testa R. Haemodynamic effects of lercanidipine in anaesthetized open-chest dogs. *Arzneimittelforschung* 46: 256–261, 1996

22 Taylor DG, Shoemaker S and Kowalski TE. *Effects of Nitrendipine on Organ Vasculature and Baroreceptor Reflexes*. Baltimore-Munich: Urban and Schwarzenberg, 1984

23 Thorin E, Shreeve SM, Thorin-Trescases N and Bevan JA. Reversal of endothelin-1 release by stimulation of endothelial alpha2-adrenoceptor contributes to cerebral vasorelaxation. *Hypertension* 30: 830–836, 1997

23a Toda N and Okamura T. The pharmacology of nitric oxide in the peripheral nervous system of blood vessels. *Pharmacol Rev* 55: 271–324, 2003

24 Uneyama H, Uchida H, Konda T and Yosimoto R. Cilnidipine: preclinical profile and clinical evaluation. *Cardiovascular Drug Reviews* 17: 341–357, 1999

25 Van Riper DA and Bevan JA. Selective variation of agonist and neurally mediated vasoconstriction with rabbit middle cerebral artery branch order. *J Pharmacol Exp Ther* 257: 879–886, 1991

26 Wade OL and Bishop JM. *Cardiac Output and Regional Blood Flow*. Oxford: Blackwell, 1962

Calcium channels and regulation of vascular tone in hypertension

The intravenous injection of calcium antagonists produces a hypotensive effect more pronounced in hypertensive than in normotensive animals. In conscious rats, Ishii et al. [17] have observed that a similar decrease of blood pressure was evoked by nifedipine at doses much lower in SHR than in WKY. Knorr and Garthoff [22] have compared the activity of nitrendipine and hydralazine on the blood pressure of SHR and WKY. They have reported that the vasodilator hydralazine was equipotent in both strains, but that nitrendipine evoked a much lesser reduction of blood pressure in WKY than in SHR, an observation consistent with clinical studies in humans [21, 25] and confirmed with lacidipine and amlodipine [11]. Godfraind and colleagues [12, 26] have measured the tissular concentration of amlodipine and nisoldipine at dosages which significantly reduced blood pressure in hypertensive (SHR) rats, but did not change the blood pressure of normotensive (WKY) rats. As shown on Table 1, the tissular concentration of the drugs was similar in both strains. Together with other haemodynamic observations [14], these studies indicate that calcium antagonists have an activity profile different from classical arteriolar vasodilators. Indeed, it has been reported that during chronic administration of a calcium antagonist, the decrease of blood pressure is observed without modification of the cardiac frequency [31]. It has been shown that vascular smooth muscle from hypertensive animals are hypersensitive to vasoconstrictors [5, 6, 10, 14, 20, 27, 31]. Their hyper-reactivity has been suggested to arise either from change in receptor affinity or in receptor number, or in the transduction mech-

Table 1. Dihydropyridine free tissular concentration in hypertensive and normotensive rats after chronic treatment by nisoldipine (80 mg/kg/day p.o.) or amlodipine (10 mg/kg/day p.o.)

Drug	Nisoldipine		Amlodipine	
	Decrease in BP (mm Hg)	Free tissular concentration	Decrease in BP (mm Hg)	Free tissular concentration
SHR	79 ± 5.8	15–75 pM[a]	35 ± 6.9	4–6 nM[b]
WKY	N.S.	15–75 pM[a]	N.S.	3–5 nM[b]

[a] estimated from the inhibition of the specific binding of $^{3}H(+)$ isradipine in heart membrane (nisoldipine).
[b] Estimated from the displacement of concentration-contraction curve of Bay K8644 in aortic rings. Data recalculated from [12, 26].

anisms of the receptor. In addition, several reports have demonstrated abnormalities of Ca^{2+} handling in vascular smooth muscle cells (SMCs) of hypertensive animals which, regarding the important role played by Ca^{2+} in the regulation of vascular tone, could be responsible for marked change in vessel reactivity [23, 29]. It is generally accepted that abnormalities of resistance arteries may play a role in the pathogenesis and pathophysiology of hypertension in experimental animals and humans. Most authors consider that a fundamental cause of increased peripheral resistance is a decrease in lumen diameter. Vascular tone, which results from the contractile activity of vascular smooth muscle cells in the walls of small arteries and arterioles, is the major determinant of the resistance to blood flow through the circulation. It plays an important role in the regulation of blood pressure and the distribution of blood flow between and within the tissues and organs of the body. Regulation of the contractile activity of vascular smooth muscle cells in the systemic circulation is dependent on a complex interplay of vasodilator and vasoconstrictor stimuli from circulating hormones, neurotransmitters, endothelium-derived factors and blood pressure. All of these signals are integrated by vascular muscle cells to determine the activity of the contractile apparatus of the muscle cells and hence resistance of a blood vessel. Ion channels play a central role in this process. As already discussed above, calcium influx through channels in the plasma membrane and calcium release from intracellular stores are the major source of activator Ca^{2+}. In addition, the movement of ions through ion channels determines membrane potential. Potassium channels are the dominant ion conductive pathways in vascular muscle cell, their activity contributes to determination and regulation of membrane potential and thereby to vascular tone. Opening of potassium channels results in diffusion of this cation out of the cells leading to membrane hyperpolarization; closure of K channels has the opposite effect. Thus the activity of K channels regulates the function of Ca channels. In vascular muscles, different classes of K channels have been identified, including ATP-sensitive K (K_{ATP}) channels, large-conductance Ca^{2+}- activated K (BK_{Ca}) channels, voltage-activated K (K_V) channels, and inward rectifier K (K_{IR}) channels. Expression of BK_{Ca} channels in vascular smooth muscle membranes is increased during hypertension and has been proposed to occur as a negative feedback response to the loss of K_V channels. The increase of reactivity to vasoconstrictors that is observed in hypertension [3, 4, 7, 18, 24, 26] might be related to both up-regulation of Ca channels and K_V channel loss.

The vascular changes that produce decreased lumen size may be structural, mechanical, and functional. In hypertension, the change in structure of resistance arteries involves a combination of processes usually termed eutrophic remodeling and hypertrophic remodeling [16], in cerebral vessels of spontaneously hypertensive salt-sensitive rats, this remodeling is extensive after salt load, see page 169, Figure 5 [2]. When considering the vessel wall, one cannot miss the role of endothelium. Indeed as reported by Vanhoutte [32], abnormal release of relaxing and contracting factors from endothelial cells may contribute to the vascular abnormalities in hypertension. The endothelium controls the tone of the underlying vascular smooth muscle by releasing relaxing and contracting factors. The former include prostacyclin, nitric oxide (NO) and endothelium-derived hyperpolarizing factor (EDHF), and the latter endoperoxides, thromboxane A2, superoxide anions and endothelin. In most types of hypertension, endothelium-dependent relaxations are curtailed, because of a reduced production of endothelium-derived NO and/or action EDHF. Figure 1 illustrates those modifications as observed in rat basilar artery [30]. In essential hypertension, endothelium-dependent relaxations are reduced also because of the endothelium-dependent production of vasoconstrictor prostanoids (endoperoxides and, in some cases, thromboxane A2). The endothelial dysfunction observed in hypertensive blood vessels is likely to contribute to the alteration of the cardiovascular system. Interaction of CCBs with the release and the function of endothelium-derived relaxing factors (NO and EDHF) may contribute to their therapeutic effects, in addition to their direct short- and

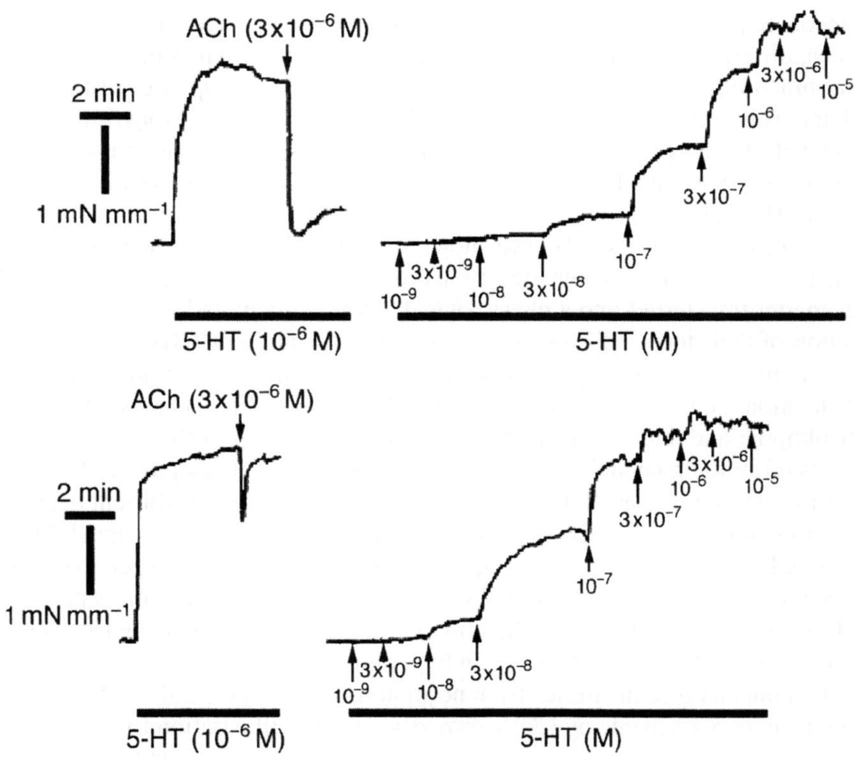

Figure 1. Response of rat isolated basilar artery to acetylcholine (Ach) and serotonin (5-HT). Upper panel: basilar artery isolated from normotensive WKY rat Left: artery precontracted by 5-HT and relaxed by Ach; right: artery exposed to increasing concentrations of 5-HT. Lower panel: basilar artery isolated from hypertensive SHRSP rat Left: artery precontracted by 5-HT and relaxed by Ach; right: artery exposed to increasing concentrations of 5-HT. Note the differences in responses between WKY and SHRSP, indicating a reduced production of NO in SHRSP. Modified from [30].

long-term actions on vascular smooth muscle cells. Functional abnormalities of vessels may be caused or influenced by the over-expression of extracellular matrix components, such as collagen and elastin, and by changes in cell-extracellular fibrillar attachment sites, such as adhesion molecules like integrins [15, 16]. Finally, extrinsic factors related mainly to the activation of the sympathetic nervous system are also operating in hypertension disease [8, 9, 19].

Due to the complexity of the various mechanisms involved we shall only address in this section the immediate interaction of CCBs with hypertensive vessels.

Different observations suggest that voltage-dependent Ca^{2+} channels could be altered in vessels from hypertensive rats. The first argument for the implication of a change in Ca^{2+} channels in hypertension is the blood pressure lowering effect of Ca^{2+} antagonists, which is stronger in hypertensive than in normotensive subjects, as already mentioned above [21, 25]. Indeed, when compared to vessels isolated from normotensive WKY rats, changes are occurring in the functional responses to Ca^{2+} channels modulation in arteries from spontaneously hypertensive rats (SHR). Seeking for the cause of those modifications, different hypothesis have been tested, including a defect in the endothelial function. The existence of a change in the receptor properties of the Ca^{2+} channels has been tested by measuring the binding of a dihydropyridine Ca^{2+} channel blocker [26]. The up-regulation of α_{1c} subunits of calcium channels has been documented in mesenteric arteries and in skeletal muscle arteries from SHR [28].

In vitro experiments [12] have shown that arteries of spontaneously hypertensive rat (SHR), precontracted by exposure to 100 mM KCl solution and thereafter transferred into a physiological solution, exhibited long lasting elevation of their tone. This tone was suppressed by adding CCBs on the top of the contraction, indicating its calcium dependency. It was not found after preincubation of the arteries with the dihydropyridine Ca^{2+} channel blockers nisoldipine and amlodipine, and was absent in aortas from SHR treated with doses of amlodipine and nisoldipine that inhibited the development of hypertension. The amplitude of this post-contraction tone, which was absent in arteries from normotensive rats, was related to the age of the rat, being much higher in older than in younger rats (Fig. 2). Furthermore, after prolonged exposure (hours) of mesenteric arteries in physiological solution, SHR arteries presented an increase in tone and a rhythmic contractile activity not seen in WKY arteries, indicating that arteries from hypertensive animals were controlled by factors unperceived in arteries from normotensive ones [12, 26]. Such a rhythmic activity abolishable by CCBs provides a further illustration for the activity of Ca channels in hypertensive vessels that has been attributed to alterations of dihydropyridine-sensitive Ca channels in SHR vessels [28, 29].

Several reports [1, 14] have shown that arteries isolated from hypertensive rats present an increased sensitivity to the Ca^{2+} channel activator Bay K 8644 which is known to produce a contraction of vascular smooth muscles by increasing the probability of opening of voltage-operated Ca^{2+} channels [13].

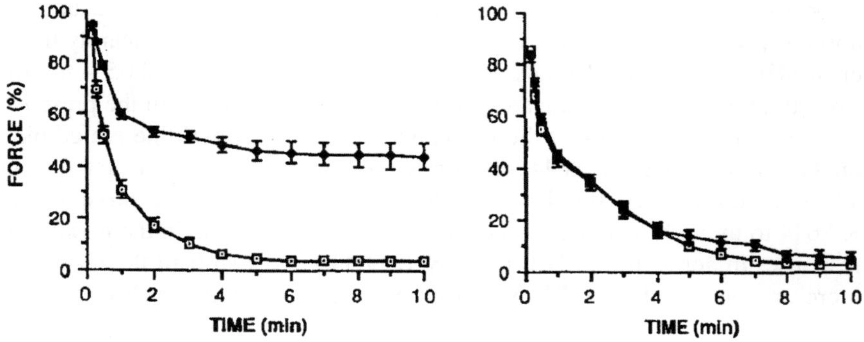

Figure 2. Post-contraction tone in rat mesenteric arteries isolated from rats untreated (left) and treated (right) by nisoldipine 80 mg/kg/day (*per os*). Open symbols: normotensive WKY, closed symbols: hypertensive SHR. Note that this tone was absent in SHR treated with nisoldipine, showing its sensitivity to CCBs. Modified from [12].

This selective responsiveness of arteries from hypertensive rats is illustrated in Figure 3, which shows that mesenteric arteries from 20 week old normotensive WKY and SHR, in the presence of Nω-nitro-L-arginine (L-NNA – 100 μM) to block the synthesis of nitric oxide, were more sensitive to Bay K 8644 compared to preparations from WKY; pD2 values (negative log value of the molar concentration producing 50% of the maximum response) of Bay K 8644 were equal to 8.2 ± 0.07 (n = 7) and 7.62 ± 0.13 (n = 6; $P < 0.05$) in SHR and WKY,

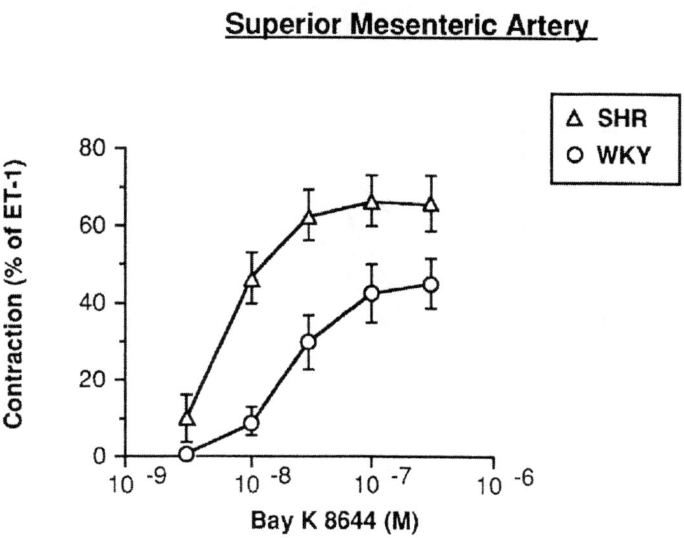

Figure 3. Response of arteries isolated from SHR and WKY to the calcium channel activator Bay K 8644, showing the increased responsiveness of SHR arteries. Modified from [26].

respectively. The concentration-response curves to Bay K 8644 measured in aortic rings of the same rats gave pD2 value of Bay K 8644 significantly higher in SHR (8.06 ± 0.07) compared to WKY (7.67 ± 0.09) ($P < 0.05$ – $n = 6$). The effect of an *in vitro* incubation of the isolated artery rings in the presence of various concentrations of the Ca antagonistic dihydropyridine amlodipine on the response to Bay K 8644 is illustrated in Figure 4. In aortas isolated from WKY, amlodipine (1–10 nM) shifted the concentration-response curve of Bay K 8644 to the right without producing a significant decrease in the maximum response. In aortas from SHR, the Bay K 8644 curves shift to the right was more pronounced than in WKY and the maximum response to Bay K 8644

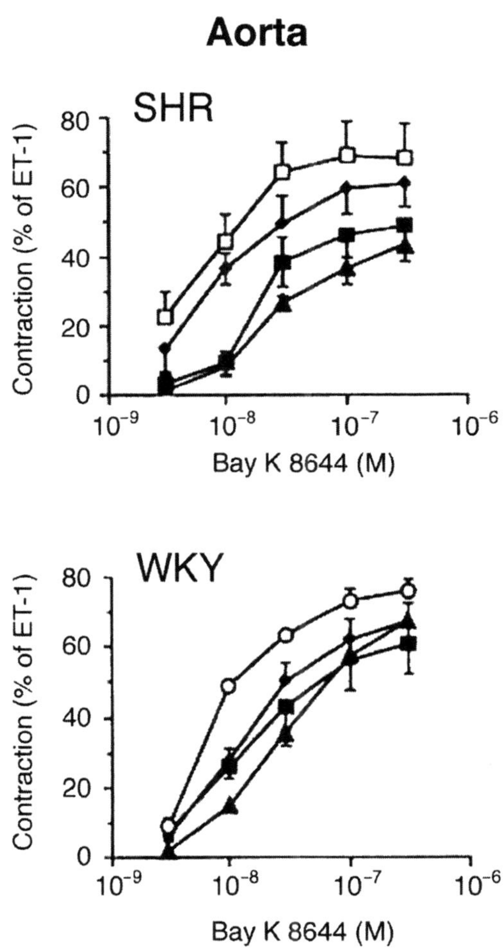

Figure 4. Action of amlodipine on the contractile response of rat aorta isolated from SHR and WKY to the calcium channel activator Bay K 8644. Note the difference in antagonism by amlodipine (1, 3, 10 nM) between SHR and WKY. Modified from [26].

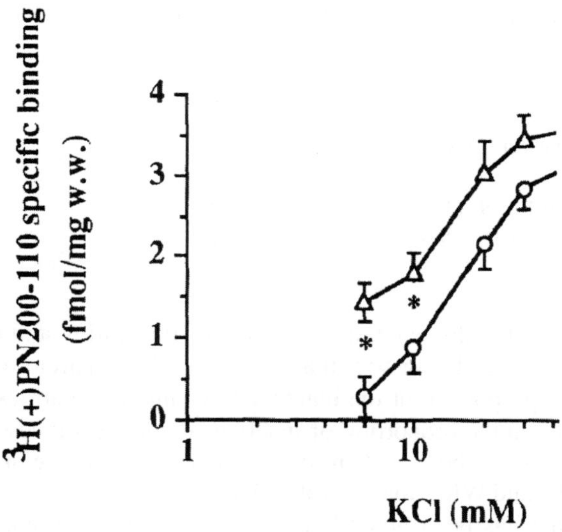

Figure 5. Specific binding of +isradipine (+PN 200-110) in intact aorta isolated from WKY (○) and SHR (△) bathed in physiological solutions at various KCl concentrations shown on the abcissa. Modified from [26].

was significantly depressed. When analyzed with a model of non-competitive antagonism experimental data yielded the following K_B values for amlodipine equal to 3.9 ± 0.7 nM and 1.3 ± 0.3 nM ($P < 0.05$), in WKY and SHR aortas, respectively. Thus, amlodipine is a more potent inhibitor of the Bay K 8644 induced contraction in SHR than in WKY arteries [26].

Pratt et al. [28] have recently shown that arteries from SHR expressed higher levels of α_{1C} subunit mRNA and protein than WKY arteries. Their data provide the evidence that the α_{1C} subunit mRNA and protein are up-regulated in SHR arteries. This increased number of L-type Ca2 channel pores is likely associated with the generation of abnormal vascular tone described above.

Study of DHPs specific binding in segments of intact aortas and mesenteric arteries preserves the cellular factors that regulate the activity of Ca^{2+} channels. The binding of amlodipine was voltage-dependent, according to the modulated receptor model, which shows that the binding affinity of dihydropyridine Ca^{2+} antagonists is varying with the state of the Ca^{2+} channel, the inactivated state of the channel in arteries exposed to high KCl presenting a higher affinity than the resting state of the channel. As illustrates by Figure 5, for KCl concentrations below 20 mM, the specific binding of amlodipine was significantly higher in aorta from SHR compared to WKY ($P < 0.05$). This difference may be related to a higher proportion of inactivated channels in SHR aortas. According to the equation:

$$1/K_{app} = h/K_R + (1 - h)/K_I$$

Table 2. Resting membrane potential (RMP) of SHR and WKY aortic smooth muscle cells (data from [26])

Rat group	RMP (mV)	
	Without L-NNA	With L-NNA
SHR	–40.4 ± 0.9 (13/3)	–36.2 ± 1.9 (8/3)
WKY	–52.2 ± 0.6 (14/3)	–49.2 ± 0.9 (14/3)

where K_R and K_I are the dissociation constants for the resting and inactivated channel, respectively, K_R being >>> than K_I, Kapp the apparent dissociation constant and h the proportion of the inactivated channels. In aortas bathed in physiological solution the proportion of inactivated channels is less than 10% in WKY and amounts to about 30% in SHR [26]. This difference in binding of DHP between SHR and WKY may be related to the difference in resting membrane potential that has been noted between SHR and WKY aortic smooth muscle cells (SMCs), SHR aortic SMCs being depolarized by about 10 mV compared to WKY aortic SMCs (Tab. 2).

From experimental data summarized above, it is obvious that CCBs have a specific interaction with hypertensive vessels, which provides a rationale for explaining why their antihypertensive action is higher in hypertensive than in normotensive subjects. This indicates that calcium channel blockers may be considered as specific antihypertensive agents and not as simple vasodilator agents, a hypothesis that is reinforced when examining their long-term effects (see pages 161–179).

References

1 Aoki K and Asano M. Effects of Bay K 8644 and nifedipine on femoral arteries of spontaneously hypertensive rats. *Br J Pharmacol* 88: 221–230, 1986

2 Arribas SM, Costa R, Salomone S, Morel N, Godfraind T and McGrath JC. Functional reduction and associated cellular rearrangement in SHRSP rat basilar arteries are affected by salt load and calcium antagonist treatment. *J Cereb Blood Flow MeTab.* 19: 517–527, 1999

3 Asano M, Matsuda T, Hayakawa M, Ito KM and Ito K. Increased resting Ca^{2+} maintains the myogenic tone and activates K^+ channels in arteries from young spontaneously hypertensive rats. *Eur J Pharmacol* 247: 295–304, 1993

4 Asano M, Nomura Y, Ito K, Uyama Y, Imaizumi Y and Watanabe M. Increased function of voltage-dependent Ca^{2+} channels and Ca^{2+}-activated K^+ channels in resting state of femoral arteries from spontaneously hypertensive rats at prehypertensive stage. *J Pharmacol Exp Ther* 275: 775–783, 1995

5 Bodin P, Travo C, Stoclet JC and Travo P. High sensitivity of hypertensive aortic myocytes to norepinephrine and angiotensin. *Am J Physiol* 264: C441–445, 1993

6 Boonen HC and De Mey JG. Increased calcium sensitivity in isolated resistance arteries from spontaneously hypertensive rats: effects of dihydropyridines. *Eur J Pharmacol* 179: 403–412, 1990

7 Cox RH and Rusch NJ. New expression profiles of voltage-gated ion channels in arteries exposed to high blood pressure. *Microcirculation* 9: 243–257, 2002

8 Esler M. The sympathetic system and hypertension. *Am J Hypertens* 13: 99S-105S, 2000
9 Folkow B. Physiological aspects of primary hypertension. *Physiol Rev* 62: 347–504, 1982
10 Fouda AK, Capdeville C, Henrion D, Thorin-Trescases N, Thorin E and Atkinson J. Differences between the *in vitro* vasoconstrictor responses of the tail artery to potassium and norepinephrine between spontaneously hypertensive, renovascular hypertensive, and various strains of normotensive rats. *J Pharmacol Methods* 25: 61–68, 1991
11 Frohlich ED. Hemodynamic effects of diltiazem in the spontaneously hypertensive rat and in human hypertension. In: *Essential Hypertension; Calcium Mechanisms and Treatment.* Aoki, K (Ed), p 191–218. Springer, Berlin, Heidelberg, New York, 1986
12 Godfraind T, Kazda S and Wibo M. Effects of a chronic treatment by nisoldipine, a calcium antagonistic dihydropyridine, on arteries of spontaneously hypertensive rats. *Circ Res* 68: 674–682, 1991
13 Hess P, Lansman JB and Tsien RW. Different modes of Ca channel gating behaviour favoured by dihydropyridine Ca agonists and antagonists. *Nature* 311: 538–544, 1984
14 Holloway ET and Bohr DF. Reactivity of vascular smooth muscle in hypertensive rats. *Circ Res* 33: 678–685, 1973
15 Intengan HD and Schiffrin EL. Structure and mechanical properties of resistance arteries in hypertension: role of adhesion molecules and extracellular matrix determinants. *Hypertension* 36: 312–318, 2000
16 Intengan HD and Schiffrin EL. Vascular remodeling in hypertension: roles of apoptosis, inflammation, and fibrosis. *Hypertension* 38: 581–587, 2001
17 Ishii H, Itoh K and Nose T. Different antihypertensive effects of nifedipine in conscious experimental hypertensive and normotensive rats. *Eur J Pharmacol* 64: 21–29, 1980
18 Jackson WF. Ion channels and vascular tone. *Hypertension* 35: 173–178, 2000
19 Janssen BJ, van Essen H, Vervoort-Peters LH, Struyker-Boudier HA and Smits JF. Role of afferent renal nerves in spontaneous hypertension in rats. *Hypertension* 13: 327–333, 1989
20 Kam KL, Hendriks MG, Pijl AJ, van Marle J, van Veen HA, Pfaffendorf M and van Zwieten PA. Contractile responses to various stimuli in isolated resistance vessels from simultaneously hypertensive and streptozotocin-diabetic rats. *J Cardiovasc Pharmacol* 27: 167–175, 1996
21 Kazda S and Knorr A. *Calcium antagonists. In: Pharmacology of Antihypertensive Therapeutics. Ganten, D. and Mulrow, P.J. (Ed), p 301–375.* Berlin, Heidelberg, New York, London, Paris, Tokyo, Hong Kong: Springer Verlag, 1990
22 Knorr A and Garthoff B. Differential influence of the calcium antagonist nitrendipine and the vasodilator hydralazine on normal and elevated blood pressure. *Arch Int Pharmacodyn Ther* 269: 316–322, 1984
23 Kwan CY. Dysfunction of calcium handling by smooth muscle in hypertension. *Can J Physiol Pharmacol* 63: 366–374, 1985
24 Liu Y, Pleyte K, Knaus HG and Rusch NJ. Increased expression of Ca^{2+}-sensitive K^+ channels in aorta of hypertensive rats. *Hypertension* 30: 1403–1409, 1997
25 MacGregor GA, Rotellar C, Markandu ND, Smith SJ and Saguella GA. Contrasting effects of nifedipine, captopril and propranolol in normotensive and hypertensive subjects. *J Cardiovasc Pharmacol* 4: S358–S362, 1982
26 Morel N and Godfraind T. Selective interaction of the calcium antagonist amlodipine with calcium channels in arteries of spontaneously hypertensive rats. *J Cardiovasc Pharmacol* 24: 524–533, 1994
27 Oster L, Chillon JM, Henrion D, Capdeville C, Burlet C and Atkinson J. *In vitro* vasoconstriction induced by calcium in renovascular hypertensive or old rats. *Life Sci* 47: 1227–1234, 1990
28 Pratt PF, Bonnet S, Ludwig LM, Bonnet P and Rusch NJ. Up-regulation of L-type Ca^{2+} channels in mesenteric and skeletal arteries of SHR. *Hypertension* 40: 214–219, 2002
29 Sada T, Koike H, Ikeda M, Sato K, Ozaki H and Karaki H. Cytosolic free calcium of aorta in hypertensive rats. Chronic inhibition of angiotensin converting enzyme. *Hypertension* 16: 245–251, 1990
30 Salomone S, Morel N and Godfraind T. Role of nitric oxide in the contractile response to 5-hydroxytryptamine of the basilar artery from Wistar Kyoto and stroke-prone rats. *Br J Pharmacol* 121: 1051–1058, 1997
31 Thompson LP, Bruner CA, Lamb FS, King CM and Webb RC. Calcium influx and vascular reactivity in systemic hypertension. *Am J Cardiol* 59: 29A-34A, 1987
32 Vanhoutte PM. Endothelial dysfunction in hypertension. *J Hypertens Suppl* 14: S83–93, 1996

Long-term effects of calcium antagonists

In short-term studies, calcium antagonists lower arterial pressure by decreasing total peripheral resistance. As a consequence, the expected physiological response should be reflex tachycardia, increased cardiac output accompanying an increase of plasma catecholamines and of plasma renin activity. This response to abrupt vasodilatation, which can paradoxically elicit angina and even acute myocardial infarction, has been reported in early clinical trials with short-acting compounds [58]. These acute haemodynamic and neuroendocrine changes are not observed with the long-acting formulations and the long acting compounds. Most calcium antagonists diminish automaticity of the sinus node, slow conduction in the atrioventricular node, and have little, if any, effect on the automaticity of the myocytes. The classical dihydropyridines generally have less effect on automaticity and cardiac conduction than non-dihydropyridines. The negative inotropic effect is most profound with non-dihydropyridines and is greatly reduced or absent with newer dihydropyridines, such as isradipine, felodipine, amlodipine, nisoldipine, cilnidipine. Long-acting calcium antagonists generally improve myocardial oxygenation by unloading the heart, increasing coronary blood flow, and reducing myocardial oxygen consumption. Thus, calcium antagonists have a variety of beneficial effects in patients with hypertensive heart disease: they reduce left ventricular hypertrophy and its sequelae, such as ventricular dysrhythmias, impaired filling and contractility, and myocardial ischaemia [37].

The most obvious consequence of the blockade of calcium channels in vascular smooth muscle is the decrease in blood pressure. As discussed above (see page 151), for a given dosage, this decrease is more pronounced in hypertensive than in normotensive, an observation made in both rats and humans, an indication for a specific action of calcium channel blockers as antihypertensive and not simply vasodilator agents. Potential mechanisms involved in their particular action on elevated blood pressure have been considered in the former chapter.

Recently, Frohlich [18] reported that clinical studies have demonstrated a dramatically reduced morbidity and mortality from strokes and coronary heart disease (CHD) with the introduction of the pharmacotherapy of hypertension over the past four decades. The reduction of strokes could be, at least in part, related to the control of elevated blood pressure; but, according to a recent meta-analysis, all drugs used to control blood pressure are not equivalent in this respect [56]. Because, cardiac and renal failure continue to increase unrelentingly, this raises the question that simple reduction of blood pressure could not be the main outcome for the prevention of the fatal consequences of hypertension. Indeed, regional circulations are not strictly pressure-dependent. Local factors may play an important role in controlling tissue perfusion and pathophysiological companions of the elevated blood presure may be activated within the major target organs during hypertensive disease.

Several experimental models have allowed identification of various families of vasodilator drugs including powerful vasodilators such as hydralazine, β-adrenergic agents, ACE inhibitors and calcium antagonists. They have also been used in order to mimic human disease and to characterize pathophysiological pathways and pharmacotherapeutic interventions. Among those models, spontaneously hypertensive rats (SHR), salt-sensitive rats (stroke prone rats (SHRSP), Dahl rats, DOCA-salt rats) and L-NAME-exposed rats have been the most investigated. The best studied organ targets were heart, arteries and kidneys. A typical feature of the cardiovascular system in hypertension is the tissue remodeling macroscopically characterized by hypertrophy of heart and arteries. Cardiovascular remodeling has been observed in angiotensin II-infused rats. Angiotensin II perfusion enhances endothelin-1 (ET-1) tissues levels. ET-1 is produced within the vascular wall and plays a critical role in vascular hypertrophy in many models of hypertension, such as deoxycorticosterone acetate (DOCA)-salt rats or stroke-prone spontaneously hypertensive rats. Indeed, in (DOCA)-salt rats in which ET-1 plays a vasoconstrictor role, ET-1 was over-expressed in the vessel wall, and systolic blood pressure (SBP) was lowered by endothelin receptor antagonists. Moreover, in these experimental models, treatment with ET-1 receptor antagonists evoked regression of vascular growth and inflammation and improved endothelial dysfunction. ET-1 production by endothelial cells can be activated by many other factors, such as insulin or thrombin, through c-*jun* fixation on the activator protein-1 site of the prepro-ET-1 promoter. Those factors might also be operating in the pathologies co-existing with cardiac and renal failure (see [52]).

The endothelin family comprises three 21-amino-peptides: ET-1, ET-2 and ET-3. These peptides are expressed in various tissues and cells. Endothelial cells predominantly produce ET-1 that is also produced by cardiac myocytes, vascular smooth muscle cells, macrophages etc. ET-1 and ET-2 are expressed in the kidney. ET-3 is expressed in the intestine and in adrenal gland [35].

ET-1 is considered as the major cardiovascular peptide. It is a powerful vasoconstrictor. At preconstricting levels, it enhances the response to other vasoconstrictors [14, 20]. Therefore, even minor changes in its local concentration may alter the vascular tone by an interaction with the action of other vasoconstrictors. Furthermore, ET-1 can permanently alter the cardiovascular system through its mitogenic [24] and trophic properties [22]. Sequence analysis of ET-1 cDNA showed that ET-1 is produced from a precursor named preproendothelin. This precursor is cleaved by an endopeptidase to give big-ET-1. Big ET-1 is converted in ET-1 by an endothelin-converting enzyme (ECE). Most of this conversion is occurring in two types of vesicles. According to Russell and Davenport [47] two distinct exocytic pathways are involved in the transport of ET-1 to the cell surface. ET-1 is stored in Weibel-Palade bodies with other vasoactive compounds and is released at the cell surface following an appropriate stimulus; this constitutes the regulated pathway. ET-1 is also stored into secretory vesicles and continuously released by a cAMP-independent constitutive pathway contributing to the maintenance of normal physiological tone. Release of ET-1 via the regulated pathway is activated in response to vascular injury.

ET-1 has a paracrine and autocrine effect by acting through two types of receptors: ET_A and ET_B. ET_A receptors are located in vascular smooth muscle cells, in cardiomyocytes, in lung and in brain. ET_B receptors have been identified on the vascular endothelium, in brain, lung, intestine and kidney. The activation of ET_A receptors is responsible for contraction. The activation of ET_B receptors located on endothelium releases NO and counterbalances the contractile effect.

The involvement of ET-1 in pathology has been suspected early after the discovery of this peptide. This has been demonstrated by the experimental study of the newly-developed antagonists. The antihypertensive efficacy of endothelin antagonists appears to depend upon the model of hypertension. In hypertension with over-expression of endothelin such as DOCA-salt, angiotensin II-induced, SHRSP and Dahl rats, there is a consistent reduction of SBP observed in animals exposed to the antagonists. In hypertension models without over-expression of ET-1 such as SHR or L-NAME hypertension, the effect is inconsistent. The L-NAME model is interesting because, in acute studies an effect of those antagonists was observed, but not in chronic studies. This is surprising in view of the demonstration that NO inhibits ET-1 release and function *in vitro.*

In cultured neonatal cardiac myocytes, ET-I induces hypertrophy, while other stimuli such as mechanical stretch or angiotensin II (Ang II) may evoke hypertrophic growth by increasing ET-1 biosynthesis. ET-1 has also been shown to play an important role in some *in vivo* models of cardiac hypertrophy, ET-1 receptor antagonists prevent, at least transiently, left ventricular (LV) hypertrophy evoked by suprarenal aortic banding or norepinephrine infusion. ET-1 receptor blockade has been reported to attenuate hypertension and cardiac hypertrophy in stroke-prone spontaneously hypertensive rats (SHRSP) fed a high-salt diet, in uninephrectomized rats receiving deoxycorticosterone acetate and a high-salt diet and in rats infused with Ang II [38, 53]. The hypertrophic action of ET-1 might involve the CaMK/HDAC/MEF2 pathway. Calcium/calmodulin-dependent protein kinase (CaMK) has been reported to activate the cardiac hypertrophic response [17]. For instance, the CaMK inhibitor KN-62 blocks hypertrophy evoked by endothelin-1 in cultured cardiomyocytes. CaMK would act by relieving the repression exerted by histone deacetylases (HDAC) on the transcription factor MEF2 (myocyte-enhancer factor 2). This factor is also activated by calcineurin and, provided that derepression by CaMK is present, by p38 MAPK. Thus, MEF2, which is required for normal postnatal cardiac growth, may serve as a common endpoint for diverse hypertrophic signaling pathways. More recently, the role played by

CaMK in the regulation of HDAC has been disputed [64] but the analysis of Hdac9–/– mice confirms that HDAC serves as a focal point for hypertrophic pathways by acting as a stress-signal-responsive repressor of cardiac growth.

As shown by early investigators, long-term administration of CCBs such as nifedipine to spontaneously hypertensive rats (SHR) induced substantial regression of established LV hypertrophy and improved LV function [39]. Regression of hypertrophy could also be obtained with a variety of other antihypertensive drugs and was, therefore, entirely attributed to normalization of blood pressure and LV systolic load. Thereafter, long-term administration of nisoldipine was shown to protect SHR not only against the development of hypertension and cardiac hypertrophy but also again fibrosis, and, eventually, cardiac failure [8, 28, 57]. Similar cardio- and vasculo-protective effects of other CCBs, at hypotensive doses, have been reported in various models. This included: amlodipine, [2, 27, 32, 60, 63], diltiazem [61], felodipine [59], lacidipine [32] nilvadipine [41]. As demonstrated in most of the recent studies, protection against, or regression of cardiac hypertrophy and fibrosis is accompanied by reduction of alterations in myocardial gene expression, such as re-expression of the cardiac fetal gene program or increased expression of collagen genes (Fig. 1).

Even if the role of blood pressure reduction in protection against end organ damage appears indisputable, it has been proposed that additional mechanisms, unrelated to their haemodynamic actions, could contribute to the tissue

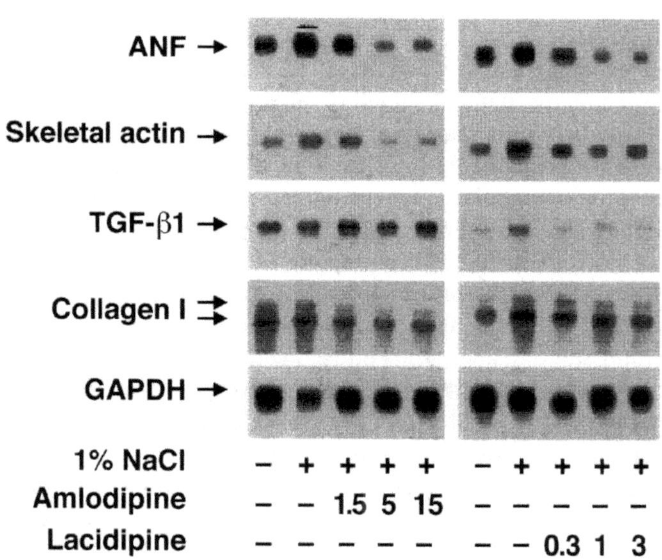

Figure 1. Effect of amlodipine and lacidipine on LV mRNA levels in SHRSP exposed to salt-load. 1% NaCl refers to salt given (+) or not given (–) in drinking water, during six weeks. Subgroups from salt-loaded rats were treated with either amlodipine or lacidipine (mg/k/day indicated on the figure). Modified from data from Kyselovic et al. [32].

protective effects of CCBs. This concept was supported initially by studies on the effect of nimodipine in stroke-prone SHR (SHRSP), a strain that spontaneously develops brain infarction at 10–12 months. Salt-loading of five-month-old SHRSP did not increase the hypertension but drastically accelerated the development of reno- and cerebro-vascular lesions and the occurrence of death. Simultaneous treatment with nimodipine at doses that did not decrease blood pressure prevented the deleterious consequences of salt-loading on vascular damage and mortality [25]. In younger SHRSP, prolonged administration of the long-acting calcium antagonist lacidipine at low doses in parallel with increased dietary salt, protected against stroke and mortality (Fig. 2), cardiac hypertrophy and vascular alterations (Fig. 3) in the absence of marked reduction of blood pressure [11, 31, 32]. Lacidipine treatment prevented not only the salt-dependent increase in cardiac mass, but also salt-dependent increases in various gene products (including: skeletal α-actin, β-myosin heavy chain and type I collagen [33]. In Dahl salt-sensitive rats fed a high-salt diet, a subdepressor dose of benidipine ameliorated LV hypertrophy and fibrosis and remodeling of coronary arterioles [30]. Comparable results were obtained with a subdepressor dose of cilnidipine in the DOCA-salt model of hypertension [29]. Lercanidipine at nonhypotensive doses induced significant nephroprotective effects in SHR [49]. However, in SHR treated with a low, non-hypotensive dose of lacidipine, the progression of LV hypertrophy was not prevented, even though structural alterations were found to be reduced at the level of mesenteric resistance vessels [46]. This indicates that experi-

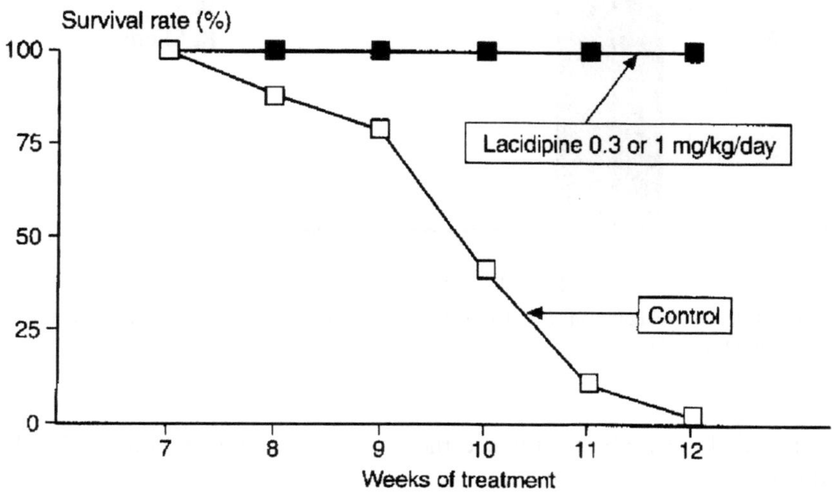

Figure 2. Survival rate in SHRSPs groups exposed to salt-load with or without lacidipine. Salt-load accelerated mortality as a result of salt-induced stroke and renal lesions. Rats exposed to salt-load without lacidipine died within 12 weeks of salt-rich diet, whereas all animals survived during the same period when exposed to salt-load with lacidipine at 0.3 and 1 mg/kg once a day. Modified from Cristofori et al. [11].

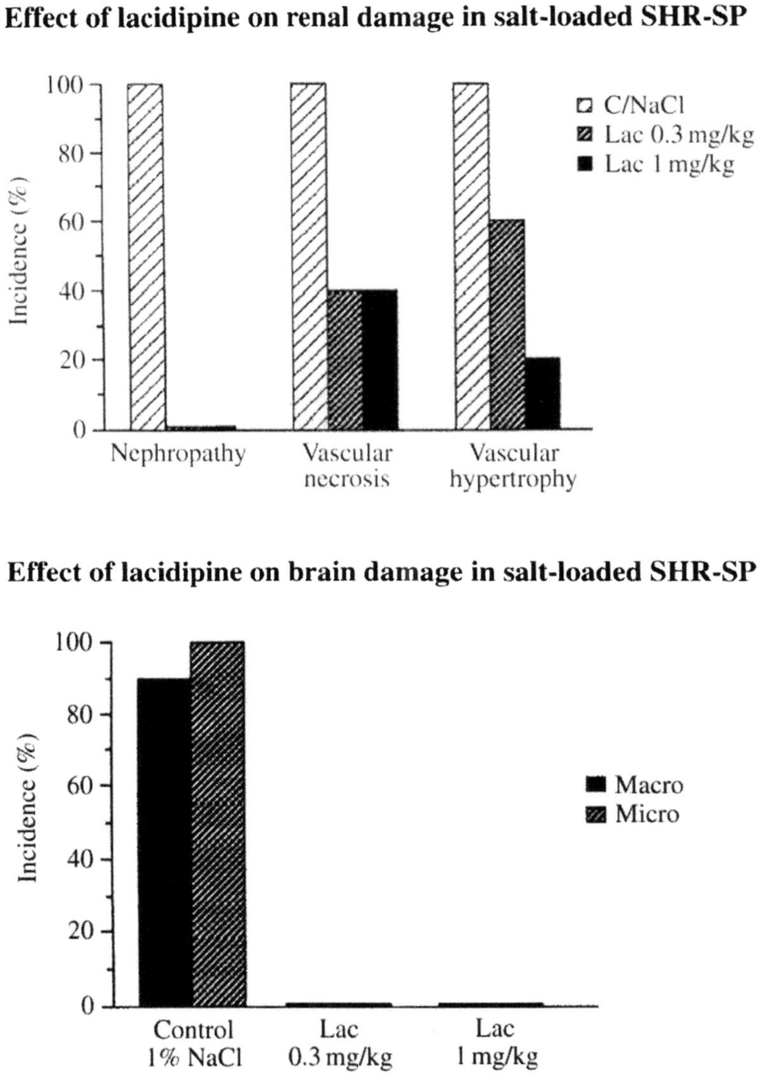

Figure 3. Effect of lacidipine on renal and brain damages in SHRSP exposed to salt-load, modified from Cristofori et al. [11].

mental conditions might influence the evaluation of this action unrelated to reduction of blood pressure.

If CCBs are endowed with cardio- and vasculo-protective properties unrelated to their capacity to lower blood pressure, one may anticipate that their efficacy to prevent or regress cardiovascular remodeling for a given reduction of blood pressure could differ from that of other classes of antihypertensive drugs. Indeed, CCBs, as well as ACE inhibitors [26] are more effective than

hydralazine, a vasodilator with a different, ill-defined mechanism of action, to prevent end-organ damage, at least in some models. Rats fed a high-fructose diet develop hypertension, cardiac hypertrophy and cardiac and renal fibrosis; although both hydralazine and lacidipine reversed the increase in blood pressure, only lacidipine was effective in reducing renal and cardiac damage [10]. In SHR, at equally hypotensive doses, CCBs (lercanidipine, manidipine and nicardipine) were more effective than hydralazine to reduce renal alterations and albuminuria [49]. In rats with renovascular hypertension and hypertensive heart disease, nifedipine, but not labetalol, was found to induce regression of myocardial fibrosis, whereas both drugs were equipotent on blood pressure. On the other hand, comparable effects on cardiovascular remodeling have been reported for CCBs and ACE inhibitors in various models (amlodipine *versus* benazepril, SHR [2, 7]; amlodipine *versus* enalapril, SHRSP [27]; lacidipine *versus* ramipril, experimental diabetes [9]; nifedipine *versus* zofenopril, renovascular hypertension [7]). However, occasionally, CCBs were reported to be less active than ACE inhibitors or angiotensin receptor blockers. For example, in aged SHR (65 wk), enalapril was more effective than felodipine in reducing LV and aortic mass indices, LV hydroxyproline concentration (fibrosis) and improving coronary haemodynamics [59].

Analysis of a typical model: end-organ protection in SHRSP, a rat strain sensitive to salt

Long-term effects: cardiac remodeling

The long-term effects have been studied in various hypertensive rat models. Recently, we have used the SHRSP (stroke-prone spontaneously hypertensive rat), a rat strain sensitive to high-salt diet, in which some CCBs, such as nimodipine, nifedipine and lacidipine, prevent salt-dependent end-organ damages including stroke, cardiovascular hypertrophy and renal failure [31–33].

We have examined the action of high-salt diet on blood pressure and heart weight of SHRSP treated or not treated with lacidipine, a long-acting CCB. Salt-load during seven weeks induces a slight increase in systolic blood pressure. Lacidipine has been given orally at dosages of 0.3 and 1 mg/kg per day, which do not lower blood pressure in WKY, normotensive rats. The regimen of 0.3 mg may be considered as a threshold dose on the blood pressure of SHRSP exposed to salt load, whereas 1 mg reduces significantly but does not correct the elevated blood pressure. Salt-loading induces significant cardiac hypertrophy in SHRSP, and this increase is totally prevented by lacidipine. In view of the potential role of endothelin-1 (ET-1) and transforming growth factor β1 (TGF-β1) in cardiovascular hypertrophy and fibrosis, we have investigated the levels of preproET-1 and TGF-β1 gene transcripts in the heart of SHRSP. These levels are significantly augmented by salt-loading and concomitant lacidipine treatment prevents salt-related preproET-1 gene over-

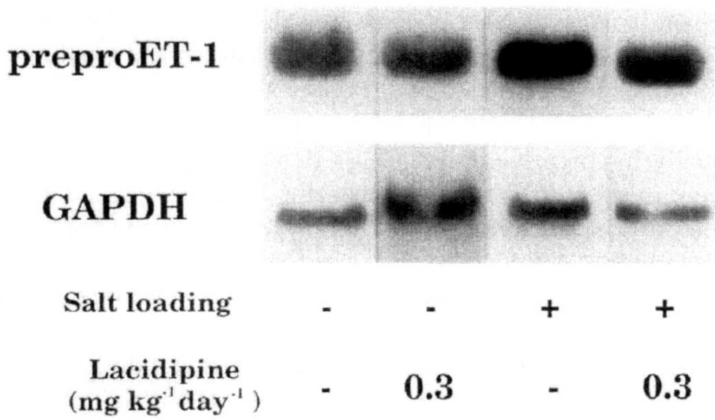

Figure 4. Effect of lacidipine on LV preproET-1 mRNA levels in SHRSP exposed to salt-load. 1% NaCl refers to salt given (+) or not given (–) in drinking water, during six weeks. Subgroups from salt-loaded rats were treated with lacidipine 0.3 mg/k/day, modified from data from Feron et al. [15].

expression (Fig. 4), as well as TGF-β1 gene over-expression [32]. A protective action of lacidipine on left ventricular hypertrophy and preproET-1 over-expression has also been observed in another, more acute model of hypertension induced by aortic constriction [36].

To elucidate whether the regulation of contractile proteins gene expression could be modulated by salt-loading in SHRSP and influenced by lacidipine, the mRNA levels of cardiac genes associated with hypertrophy and remodeling (α- and β-MHC, skeletal and cardiac α-actin, TGF-β1 and collagen type I) were estimated by Northern blot analysis on LV samples. Salt-loading increased those levels, and this increase was prevented by amlodipine and lacidipine (Fig. 1). This indicates that the reprogramming of foetal genes, which accompanies cardiac hypertrophy related to ANF, can be prevented by CCBs. Another feature of cardiac remodeling in hypertension is the extension of myocardial fibrosis. Cardiac fibrosis is a major determinant of diastolic stiffness, a negative factor added to altered relaxation of hypertrophied cardiomyocytes, which could precipitate cardiac failure. The mRNA level of type 1 collagen was increased by salt-loading and the treatment with lacidipine and amlodipine prevented this salt-dependent change (Fig. 1). Since these two dosage regimens do have different influence on blood pressure, 0.3 mg being a threshold dose, this observation illustrates further that lacidipine has effects on gene transcripts that are independent of the action on blood pressure.

Vascular remodeling

Salt-loading of SHRSP induces structural and functional alterations in arteries, mostly studied in cerebral arteries. Figure 5 shows that the normal orientation

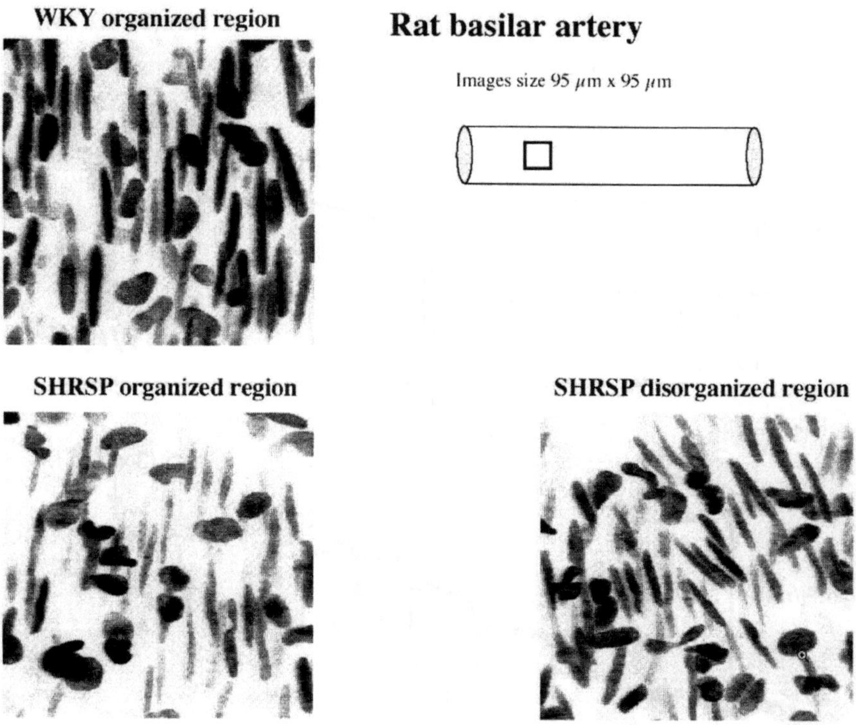

Figure 5. Orientation of the smooth muscle cells (SMC) identified by their elongated-shape nuclei in the three layers of the media of the basilar artery of normotensive Wistar Kyoto rats (WKY) and in hypertensive SHRSP exposed to salt, showing the reduction of the numbers of SMC in hypertensive and their disorganization sections were perpendicular to the longitudinal axis of the vessel (schematized on the upper right of the figure); modified from Arribas et al. [3].

of smooth muscle cells is modified in arteries from rats exposed to high-salt diet. We observed that this disorientation was prevented by lacidipine [3]. Structural changes are accompanied by functional changes characterized by increased threshold sensitivity to the action of vasoconstrictors despite a large reduction of the mechanical force developed by the arteries. This is illustrated in Figure 6 for serotonin, the most important regulator of cerebral vessels tone. This figure also shows that vessel isolated from rat treated with lacidipine had lost this high sensitivity to serotonin and regained contractile force. This high sensitivity to vasoconstrictors is reduced *in vitro* by treating the vessel with bosentan, an endothelin antagonist [50]. This indicates that there is an important production of endothelin in this vessel and that this production is reaching a functionally active level. As shown by Figure 7, the abundance of the mRNA of preproET-1 is increased in the aorta from SHRSP exposed to salt-load, an effect prevented by treatment with lacidipine [31]. Figure 7 also shows that lacidipine stimulates the activation of the gene of endothelial NO synthase (eNOS), the enzyme producing the vasorelaxant agent nitric oxide (NO).

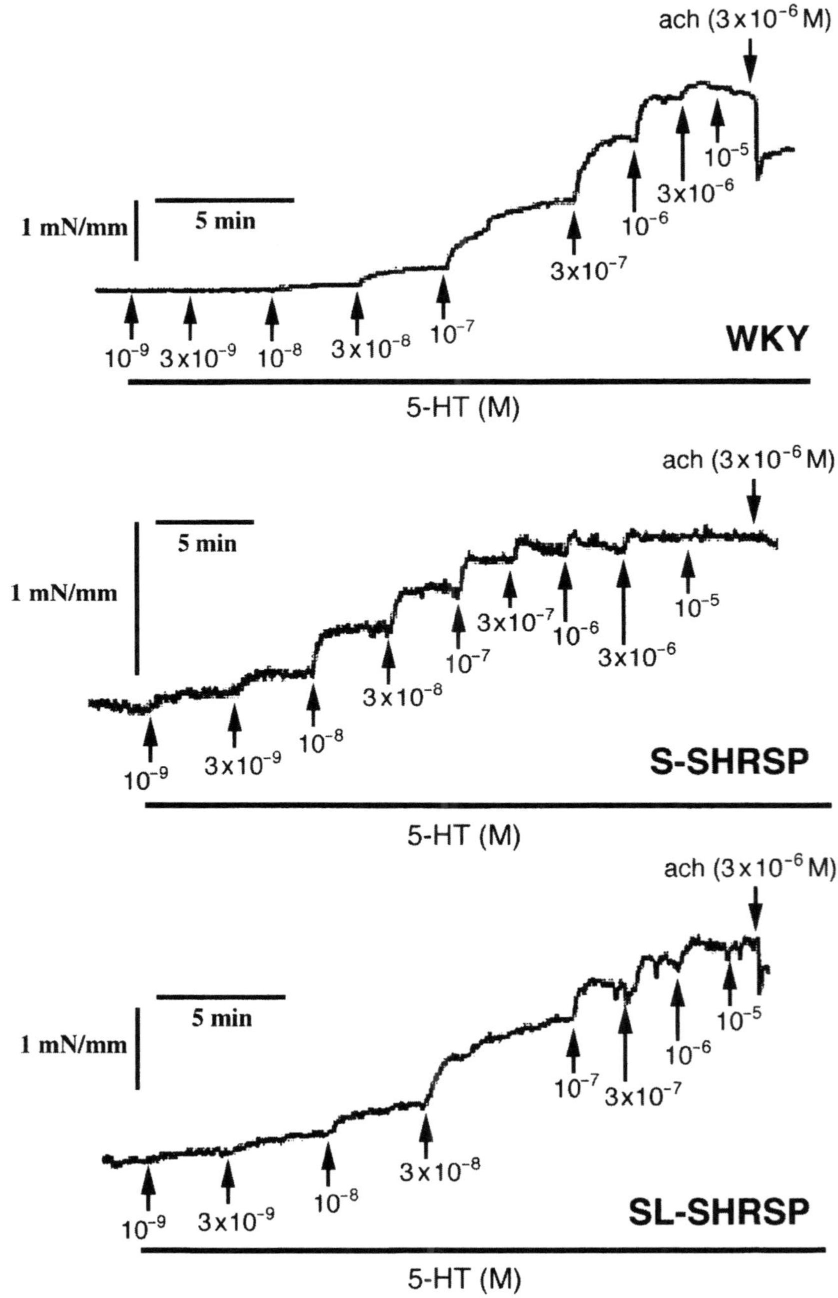

Figure 6. Response of basilar artery isolated from Wistar Kyoto (WKY), from SHRSP exposed during six weeks to salt-load without (S-SHRSP) or with lacidipine (SL-SHRSP). Note that the increased sensitivity to serotonin (5HT) and the decreased contractile force induced by salt-load were prevented by lacidipine, modified from Godfraind and Salomone [21].

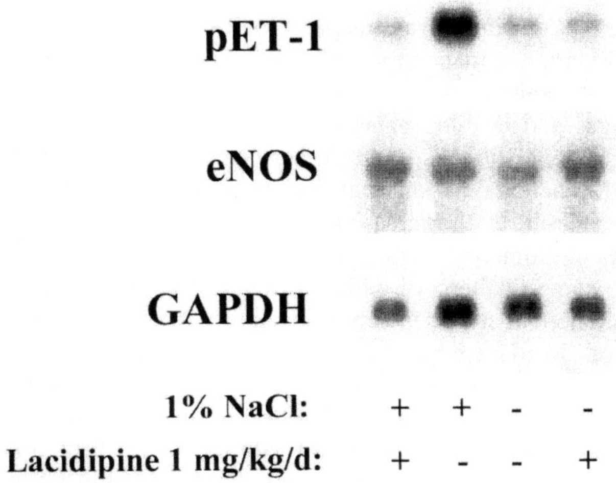

Figure 7. Typical autoradiograms of Northern blot analysis of mRNA levels in aortic tissue from SHRSP. Nacl refers to salt given (+) or not given (–) in drinking water for six weeks; modified from Krenek et al. [31].

Simultaneously, the weak vasorelaxation in response to acetylcholine, observed in SHRSP exposed to high-salt diet, is greatly augmented in arteries isolated from SHRSP exposed to high-salt diet and treated by lacidipine (Fig. 8). This could account for improvement of organ perfusion that is reduced in hypertension.

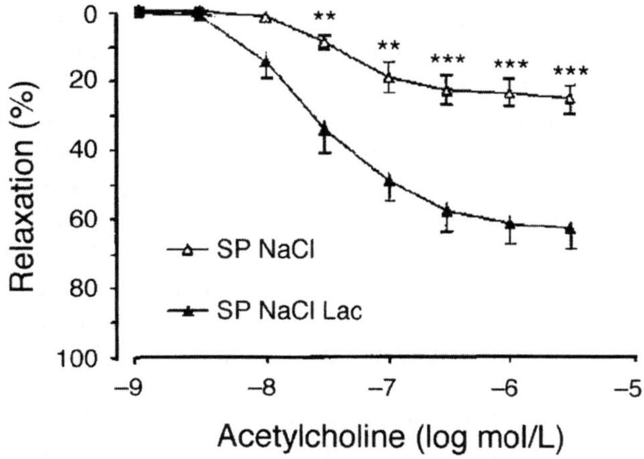

Figure 8. Concentration-relaxation curves to acetylcholine of aortic rings isolated from SHRSP and precontracted by norepinephrine. Rats were exposed to salt in the drinking water for six weeks, being treated (Lac) or not with lacidipine, modified from Krenek et al. [31].

Renal protection

Kidney failure is occurring in various pathologies including hypertension and diabetes. The kidney is a main target of hypertension. In both human essential hypertension and spontaneously hypertensive rats (SHR), the kidneys undergo vascular changes and develop areas of ischaemic cortical atrophy that are accompanied by renal fibrosis with glomerular lesions and tubular changes associated with functional impairment evidenced by hypoperfusion, elevation of glomerular pressure with increased glomerular filtration rate, proteinuria, and other signs of glomerular injury. The action of CCBs has been much disputed because some of them vasodilate afferent, but not efferent arterioles. This causes glomerular hypertension associated with progression of the disease, instead of affording renal protection. Recent evidence has shown that novel compounds endowed of long-acting action such as lercanidipine, manidipine and efonidipine, vasodilate both afferent and efferent arterioles and have a renal protective effect also reported with lacidipine. Experimental studies have enrolled various animal models susceptible of suffering from kidney failure, including hypertensive and diabetic rats. [11, 16, 43, 48, 62].

Diabetic nephropathy is characterized by persistent proteinuria, hypertension, and declining renal function, defined as a reduction in glomerular filtration rate (GFR). Approximately 30% of patients with insulin-dependent diabetes develop kidney disease and this is associated with excess mortality. Metabolic control is essential in preventing diabetic nephropathy and improved glycaemic control has led to a decrease in the incidence of diabetic kidney disease in the Western world. Furthermore, antihypertensive treatment with angiotensin-converting enzyme (ACE) inhibitors has proven effective in preventing or postponing the development of overt nephropathy and end-stage renal failure in patients with diabetes. CCBs may also be effective in the treatment of diabetic kidney disease, but controversy exists whether nondihydropyrine (nDHP) CCBs and dihydropyridine (DHP) CCBs are equally effective [1, 4, 5, 34, 44, 45, 54, 55].

Several animal models have been utilized in order to test the potential protection afforded by CCBs. Diabetes has been induced by streptozotocyn (STZ) and the animals have been studied after a period of three or six months [42]. CBBs are usually given after three or six months for a short period. Reduction of pathological parameters has been observed with some CCBs after three but not six months. For instance, according to Nielsen et al., after three months of untreated diabetes, nitrendipine treatment for six weeks significantly reduced urinary albumin excretion (UAE; $P < 0.05$) and glomerular hypertrophy. Nitrendipine also prevented an increase in systemic blood pressure compared with untreated diabetes. However, there was no detectable effect when nitrendipine was given after six months of untreated diabetes.

In SHR, long-term treatment with different 1,4-DHPs at doses that decreased blood pressure to a similar extent showed that the long-acting CCBs lercanidipine and manidipine were more effective than nicardipine in countering glomerular injury and the luminal narrowing of efferent arterioles, whereas the three drugs similarly vasodilated the afferent arteriole [48]. This suggests a causal link between vasodilation of the efferent arteriole and nephroprotection, more especially as these properties are also shared by ACE inhibitors.

Earliest studies failed to demonstrate the beneficial action of calcium antagonists on renal impairment. The hypothesis was that short-acting calcium antagonists exhibiting a preferential action on the afferent arteriole might produce pressure load on the glomerulus and thereby deteriorate the outcome of chronic renal disease. Studies with long-acting CCBs have shown that some of them could protect kidneys from end-damages observed in hypertension. Saruta et al. [51]have studied the nature of the renal protective effects of calcium channel blockers (Ca blockers) compared to those of the angiotensin-converting enzyme inhibitor (ACEI), enalapril, on the progression of renal injury in 5/6 nephrectomized spontaneously hypertensive rats (SHR) fed a high-salt diet. They studied the effects of various Ca blockers on the glomerular afferent and efferent arterioles using the isolated perfused hydronephrotic kidneys of six-week-old male Sprague-Dawley rats. In the first study, 40 six-week-old male SHRs which underwent 5/6 nephrectomy were equally divided into five groups. One group received no therapy. In two groups, therapy was started at four weeks post-nephrectomy, one with amlodipine and the other with enalapril. In the remaining two groups, amlodipine or enalapril therapy was started at eight weeks postnephrectomy. Amlodipine was more effective than enalapril in reducing proteinuria and glomerulosclerosis in the group that was started on drug therapy eight weeks after surgery. Their results indicated that amlodipine was effective at reducing renal injury in 5/6 nephrectomized SHR, and that it was more effective than ACEI in advanced stages of renal injury. They also reported that at concentrations varying from 10^{-6} down to 10^{-9} M, nifedipine, nicardipine and amlodipine dilated the afferent, but not the efferent arteriole preconstricted with angiotensin II. On the other hand, efonidipine and manidipine clearly dilated angiotensin II-induced constriction of both the afferent and efferent arterioles. According to these authors, the renal protective effect of Ca blockers is not necessarily dependent on the dilation of the efferent arterioles [51]. Further studies with CCBs including efonidipine, lercadipine, manidipine, nilvadipine, mibefradil have shown that they exhibit dilatory action of both afferent and efferent arterioles exposed *in vitro* to angiotensin II. They share a renal microvascular action with angiotensin converting enzyme (ACE) inhibitors. This class of antihypertensive agent possesses unique actions associated with angiotensin II (Ang II) blockade. Angiotensin II increases mesangial matrix formation directly by stimulating its production and indirectly by increasing glomerular capillary pressure through vasoconstriction of the efferent arteriole. The latter action is blunted by ACE inhibitors that cause efferent as well as afferent arteriolar dilation, and the subsequent amelioration of glomerular hypertension. Efonidipine reduced renal injury in subtotally nephrectomized spontaneously hypertensive rats to the same level as that of enalapril, whereas nifedipine (which dilates the afferent arteriole to a much larger extent than the efferent arteriole) failed to halt the progression of renal injury. This observation supports the hypothesis that agents with efferent as well as afferent arteriolar dilator action exert a preventive action on renal injury [23].

That all CCBs do not exhibit the same pattern of vasoselectivity is in line with our previous observations that nisoldipine was much more potent to block serotonin-induced contraction of human coronary artery than of human internal mammary artery (Fig. 8, page 125), whereas diltiazem and verapamil displayed a similar potency in both arteries [19]. It therefore appears that the vascular action of CCBs could play a major role in renal protection, but mechanisms unrelated to L-type Ca currents blockade need to be considered. T-type Ca current blockade appeared to be more beneficial than simple L-type Ca current blockade in DOCA-salt rats. This model has been exposed to mibefradil and amlodipine at dosages equiactive on blood pressure during four to five weeks, increased protein excretion and damaged glomeruli were significantly more reduced with mibefradil than with amlodipine [6]. It could be that the difference between these two CCBs was related to a lower selectivity of amlodipine for T-type currents when compared to mibefradil [13]. However, cilnidipine a N- and L-type Ca channels blocker is also endowed of protective effect on kidney. Zhou and his colleagues have studied the actions of the new dihydropyridine N- and L-type calcium antagonist, cilnidipine, on systemic and renal haemodynamics, glomerular dynamics, renal function, and histopathology in an N-omega-nitro-l-arginine methylester spontaneously hypertensive rat (L-NAME/SHR) model of nephrosclerosis. They have observed that in SHR exposed for three weeks to L-NAME with or without cilnidipine, the CCB significantly reduced mean arterial pressure, total peripheral resistance and renal vascular resistance, while increasing effective renal blood flow and glomerular filtration rate ($P < 0.01$) in L-NAME/SHR. These haemodynamic changes were associated with significantly increased single nephron glomerular filtration rate (SNGFR) and plasma flow (SNPF) and decreased afferent glomerular arteriolar resistances when cilnidipine was used alone, and with increased SNGFR and SNPF, but decreased glomerular capillary pressure, afferent and efferent arteriolar resistances, urinary protein excretion, serum creatinine and uric acid concentrations (at least $P < 0.05$) in L-NAME-exacerbated SHR nephrosclerosis. In addition, glomerular and arteriolar injuries were markedly reversed (both $P < 0.01$), and glomerular apoptosis and cellular proliferation were inhibited and associated with glomerular tuft enlargement and an increase in cell number. Cilnidipine not only prevented but reversed the severe renal haemodynamic and glomerular dynamic changes, including apoptosis and glomerular cellular proliferation, in L-NAME/SHR-exacerbated nephrosclerosis. This dual L-N channel calcium antagonist thus exerted renoprotective effects [65].

In other models of salt-dependent hypertension, CCBs also appear to be highly renoprotective. For instance, in Dahl-S rats and in SHRSP lacidipine reduced kidneys lesions such as tissue necrosis and hypertrophy of arteries observed in animal exposed to salt load. This morphological protection was associated with a prevention of increased urinary protein excretion [12].

It has been proposed that TGF-β1 is a major activator of tissue fibrosis and has complex interactions with the renin-angiotensin system (RAS). Activation of the RAS, which has been reported to occur in salt-loaded SHRSP at the onset of renal and cerebrovascular lesions may amplify the enhanced cardiac production of both TGF-β1 and endothelin-1, a factor endowed of profibrogenic action. TGF-β1 appears therefore to be an appropriate indicator of the importance of kidney fibrosis [40]. Therefore, we investigated the relation between the reduction of blood pressure evoked by two long-acting CCBs and their protective effect against renal damage in salt-loaded SHRSP. The salt-induced renal damage in SHRSP, as measured by urinary protein excretion or lesions of malignant nephrosclerosis, is disproportionate to the corresponding increase in absolute blood pressure. This nephropathy has been shown to be partly prevented by CCBs, e.g., nimodipine, lacidipine and amlodipine at dosages that do not evoke a marked reduction of blood pressure (Fig. 3) [11]. The nephroprotective effect of lacidipine that has been demonstrated by both morphological and functional (urinary protein excretion) methods is consistent with our observation that the increase in kidney levels of TGF-β1 mRNA in salt-loaded SHRSP was prevented by CCBs [32]. Indeed, TGF-β1 is considered as playing a key role in the glomerulosclerosis associated with hypertensive renal disease. A paradoxical PRA increase is observed in salt-loaded SHRSP, it is accompanied by elevated renal levels of renin mRNA, confirming that the physiological down-regulation by salt of renin production by the kidney is lost in those hypertensive rats [32]. Activation of renin production is probably secondary to renal damage that is accelerated by the high dietary salt intake in this strain. Therefore, prevention by low-dose CCBs of the paradoxical PRA increase in salt-loaded SHRSP is likely to be related to a nephroprotective action that is partly independent of the effect on blood pressure. The elevation of TGF-β1 transcripts in the kidney of salt-loaded SHRSP was similarly reduced by amlodipine and lacidipine. Amlodipine or lacidipine were used at three dosage regimens producing similar effects on blood pressure. The lowest dosages of both drugs had nonsignificant effects on blood pressure but inhibited the paradoxical increases in plasma renin activity (PRA and mRNA in kidney that were found in salt-loaded SHRSP. As show in Figure 9, the lowest dosage of lacidipine, which reduced left ventricular hypertrophy and mRNA levels of atrial natriuretic factor and transforming growth factor-β1 (see Fig. 1), restored the physiological down-regulation of renin production by high salt. This again indicates that reduction of blood pressure is not the sole mechanism involved in the prevention of cardiac remodeling by calcium channel blockers and that protection against kidney damage and excessive renin production should contribute to their beneficial cardiovascular effects.

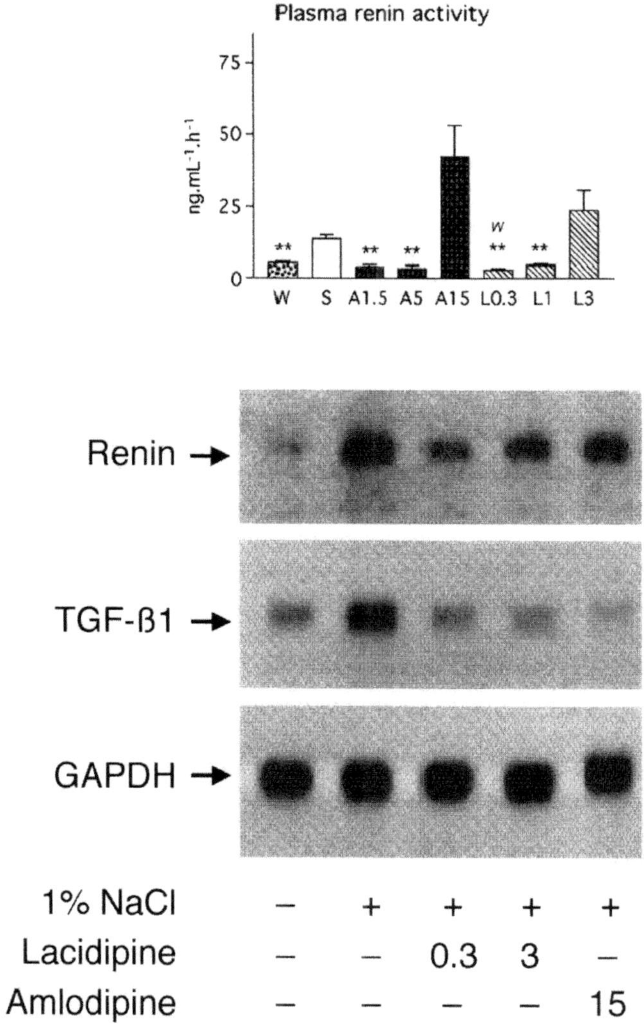

Figure 9. Upper panel. Plasma renin activity in SHRSP: controls (W), exposed to salt (S) with CCBs $mg \cdot kg^{-1} \cdot day^{-1}$: amlodipine, A or lacidipine L. Lower panel. Northern analysis of mRNA levels in kidney tissue. NaCl refers to salt given (+) or not given (–) in drinking water. Data from Kyselovic et al. [32], modified.

References

1 Agodoa LY, Appel L, Bakris GL, Beck G, Bourgoignie J, Briggs JP, Charleston J, Cheek D, Cleveland W, Douglas JG et al. Effect of ramipril vs amlodipine on renal outcomes in hypertensive nephrosclerosis: a randomized controlled trial. *Jama* 285: 2719–2728, 2001

2 Arita M, Horinaka S and Frohlich ED. Biochemical components and myocardial performance after reversal of left ventricular hypertrophy in spontaneously hypertensive rats. *J Hypertens* 11: 951–959, 1993

3 Arribas SM, Costa R, Salomone S, Morel N, Godfraind T and McGrath JC. Functional reduction and associated cellular rearrangement in SHRSP rat basilar arteries are affected by salt load and calcium antagonist treatment. *J Cereb Blood Flow MeTab.* 19: 517–527, 1999
4 Bakris GL, Mangrum A, Copley JB, Vicknair N and Sadler R. Effect of calcium channel or beta-blockade on the progression of diabetic nephropathy in African Americans. *Hypertension* 29: 744–750, 1997
5 Bakris GL, Weir MR, DeQuattro V and McMahon FG. Effects of an ACE inhibitor/calcium antagonist combination on proteinuria in diabetic nephropathy. *Kidney Int* 54: 1283–1289, 1998
6 Baylis C, Qiu C and Engels K. Comparison of L-type and mixed L- and T-type calcium channel blockers on kidney injury caused by deoxycorticosterone-salt hypertension in rats. *Am J Kidney Dis* 38: 1292–1297, 2001
7 Brilla CG. Regression of myocardial fibrosis in hypertensive heart disease: diverse effects of various antihypertensive drugs. *Cardiovasc Res* 46: 324–331, 2000
8 Campbell SE, Turek Z, Rakusan K and Kazda S. Cardiac structural remodelling after treatment of spontaneously hypertensive rats with nifedipine or nisoldipine. *Cardiovasc Res* 27: 1350–1358, 1993
9 Cao Z, Hulthen UL, Allen TJ and Cooper ME. Angiotensin converting enzyme inhibition and calcium antagonism attenuate streptozotocin-diabetes-associated mesenteric vascular hypertrophy independently of their hypotensive action. *J Hypertens* 16: 793–799, 1998
10 Cosenzi A, Bernobich E, Plazzotta N, Seculin P, Odoni G and Bellini G. Lacidipine reduces high blood pressure and the target organ damage induced by high fructose diet in rats. *J Hypertens* 17: 965–971, 1999
11 Cristofori P, Micheli D, Terron A and Gaviraghi G. Lacidipine: experimental evidence of vasculoprotective properties. *J Cardiovasc Pharmacol* 23 Suppl 5: S90–93, 1994
12 Cristofori P, Sbarbati A, Accordini C, Terron A and Micheli D. Protective action of lacidipine in cardiac hypertrophy of the spontaneously hypertensive stroke-prone rat: an ultrastructural study. *J Submicrosc Cytol Pathol* 26: 331–340, 1994
13 De Paoli P, Cerbai E, Koidl B, Kirchengast M, Sartiani L and Mugelli A. Selectivity of different calcium antagonists on T- and L-type calcium currents in guinea-pig ventricular myocytes. *Pharmacol Res* 46: 491–497, 2002
14 Dohi Y, Hahn AW, Boulanger CM, Buhler FR and Luscher TF. Endothelin stimulated by angiotensin II augments contractility of spontaneously hypertensive rat resistance arteries. *Hypertension* 19: 131–137, 1992
15 Feron O, Salomone S and Godfraind T. Inhibition by lacidipine of salt-dependent cardiac hypertrophy and endothelin gene expression in stroke-prone spontaneously hypertensive rats. *Biochem Biophys Res Commun* 210: 219–224, 1995
16 Fleming JT, Parekh N and Steinhausen M. Calcium antagonists preferentially dilate preglomerular vessels of hydronephrotic kidney. *Am J Physiol* 253: F1157–1163, 1987
17 Frey N, McKinsey TA and Olson EN. Decoding calcium signals involved in cardiac growth and function. *Nat Med* 6: 1221–1227, 2000
18 Frohlich ED. Local hemodynamic changes in hypertension: insights for therapeutic preservation of target organs. *Hypertension* 38: 1388–1394, 2001
19 Godfraind T, Dessy C and Salomone S. A comparison of the potency of selective L-calcium channel blockers in human coronary and internal mammary arteries exposed to serotonin. *J Pharmacol Exp Ther* 263: 112–122, 1992
20 Godfraind T, Mennig D, Morel N and Wibo M. Effect of endothelin-1 on calcium channel gating by agonists in vascular smooth muscle. *J Cardiovasc Pharmacol* 13 Suppl 5: S112–117; discussion S123, 1989
21 Godfraind T and Salomone S. New advances in hypertensive treatment with calcium antagonists. *J Cardiovasc Pharmacol* 30 (Suppl.2): S1–S5, 1997
22 Grainger DJ, Witchell CM, Weissberg PL and Metcalfe JC. Mitogens for adult rat aortic vascular smooth muscle cells in serum-free primary culture. *Cardiovasc Res* 28: 1238–1242, 1994
23 Hayashi K, Kumagai H and Saruta T. Effect of efonidipine and ACE inhibitors on proteinuria in human hypertension with renal impairment. *Am J Hypertens* 16: 116–122, 2003
24 Hirata Y, Takagi Y, Fukuda Y and Marumo F. Endothelin is a potent mitogen for rat vascular smooth muscle cells. *Atherosclerosis* 78: 225–228, 1989
25 Kazda S, Grunt M, Hirth C, Preis W and Stasch JP. Calcium antagonism and protection of tissues from calcium damage. *J Hypertens Suppl* 5: S37–42, 1987

26 Kim S, Ohta K, Hamaguchi A, Omura T, Yukimura T, Miura K, Inada Y, Ishimura Y, Chatani F and Iwao H. Angiotensin II type I receptor antagonist inhibits the gene expression of transforming growth factor-beta 1 and extracellular matrix in cardiac and vascular tissues of hypertensive rats. *J Pharmacol Exp Ther* 273: 509–515, 1995
27 Kim S, Ohta K, Hamaguchi A, Yukimura T, Miura K and Iwao H. Effects of an AT1 receptor antagonist, an ACE inhibitor and a calcium channel antagonist on cardiac gene expressions in hypertensive rats. *Br J Pharmacol* 118: 549–556, 1996
28 Knorr A, Kazda S, Neuser D, Stasch JP and Seuter F. Long-term protective effects of nitrendipine in experimental hypertension. *J Cardiovasc Pharmacol* 18 Suppl 5: S1–4, 1991
29 Kobayashi N, Mori Y, Mita S, Nakano S, Kobayashi T, Tsubokou Y and Matsuoka H. Effects of cilnidipine on nitric oxide and endothelin-1 expression and extracellular signal-regulated kinase in hypertensive rats. *Eur J Pharmacol* 422: 149–157, 2001
30 Kobayashi N, Nakano S, Mori Y, Kobayashi T, Tsubokou Y and Matsuoka H. Benidipine inhibits expression of ET-1 and TGF-beta1 in Dahl salt-sensitive hypertensive rats. *Hypertens Res* 24: 241–250, 2001
31 Krenek P, Salomone S, Kyselovic J, Wibo M, Morel N and Godfraind T. Lacidipine prevents endothelial dysfunction in salt-loaded stroke-prone hypertensive rats. *Hypertension* 37: 1124–1128, 2001
32 Kyselovic J, Krenek P, Wibo M and Godfraind T. Effects of amlodipine and lacidipine on cardiac remodelling and renin production in salt-loaded stroke-prone hypertensive rats. *Br J Pharmacol* 134: 1516–1522, 2001
33 Kyselovic J, Morel N, Wibo M and Godfraind T. Prevention of salt-dependent cardiac remodeling and enhanced gene expression in stroke-prone hypertensive rats by the long-acting calcium channel blocker lacidipine. *J Hypertens* 16: 1515–1522, 1998
34 Lewis EJ, Hunsicker LG, Bain RP and Rohde RD. The effect of angiotensin-converting-enzyme inhibition on diabetic nephropathy. The Collaborative Study Group. *N Engl J Med* 329: 1456–1462, 1993
35 Masaki T. The discovery of endothelins. *Cardiovasc Res* 39: 530–533, 1998
36 Massart PE, Donckier J, Kyselovic J, Godfraind T, Heyndrickx GR and Wibo M. Carvedilol and lacidipine prevent cardiac hypertrophy and endothelin-1 gene overexpression after aortic banding. *Hypertension* 34: 1197–1201, 1999
37 Michalewicz L and Messerli FH. Cardiac effects of calcium antagonists in systemic hypertension. *Am J Cardiol* 79: 39–46; discussion 47–38, 1997
38 Moreau P. Endothelin in hypertension: a role for receptor antagonists? *Cardiovasc Res* 39: 534–542, 1998
39 Motz W and Strauer BE. Nifedipine in the long-term management of hypertensive heart disease. *Hypertension* 5: II39–44, 1983
40 Nakamura T, Obata J, Kuroyanagi R Kimura H, Ikeda Y, Takano H, Naito A, Sato T and Yoshida Y. Involvement of angiotensin II in glomerusclerosis of stroke-prone spontaneously hypertensive rats. *Kidney Int Suppl* 55: S109–112, 1996
41 Naruse M, Tanabe A, Seki T, Adachi C, Yoshimoto T, Mishina N, Imaki T, Naruse K, Demura R and Demura H. Effects of two calcium channel blockers on messenger RNA expression of endothelin-1 and nitric oxide synthase in cardiovascular tissue of hypertensive rats. *J Hypertens* 17: 53–60, 1999
42 Nielsen B, Gronbaek H, Osterby R and Flyvbjerg A. Effect of the calcium channel blocker nitrendipine in normotensive and spontaneously hypertensive, diabetic rats on kidney morphology and urinary albumin excretion. *J Hypertens* 17: 973–981, 1999
43 Ozawa Y, Hayashi K, Nagahama T, Fujiwara K, Wakino S and Saruta T. Renal afferent and efferent arteriolar dilation by nilvadipine: studies in the isolated perfused hydronephrotic kidney. *J Cardiovasc Pharmacol* 33: 243–247, 1999
44 Parving HH and Hommel E. Prognosis in diabetic nephropathy. *Bmj* 299: 230–233, 1989
45 Parving HH, Jacobsen P, Rossing K, Smidt UM, Hommel E and Rossing P. Benefits of long-term antihypertensive treatment on prognosis in diabetic nephropathy. *Kidney Int* 49: 1778–1782, 1996
46 Porteri E, Rizzoni D, Castellano M, Bettoni G, Muiesan ML, Salvetti M, Quartaroli M, Gaviraghi G and Rosei EA. Structural changes of small resistance arteries in spontaneously hypertensive rats after treatment with various doses of lacidipine. *J Hypertens* 15: 619–625, 1997
47 Russell FD and Davenport AP. Secretory pathways in endothelin synthesis. *Br J Pharmacol* 126: 391–398, 1999

48 Sabbatini M, Leonardi A, Testa R, Vitaioli L and Amenta F. Effect of calcium antagonists on glomerular arterioles in spontaneously hypertensive rats. *Hypertension* 35: 775–779, 2000
49 Sabbatini M, Vitaioli L, Baldoni E and Amenta F. Nephroprotective effect of treatment with calcium channel blockers in spontaneously hypertensive rats. *J Pharmacol Exp Ther* 294: 948–954, 2000
50 Salomone S, Dessy C, Morel N and Godfraind T. Inhibition by bosentan, an endothelin antagonist, of the hypersensitivity to Ca^{2+} channel activator evoked by salt-loading in basilar artery of stroke-prone spontaneously hypertensive rats. *Life Sci* 59: PL247–253, 1996
51 Saruta T, Kanno Y, Hayashi K and Konishi K. Antihypertensive agents and renal protection: calcium channel blockers. *Kidney Int Suppl* 55: S52–56, 1996
52 Schiffrin EL. Role of endothelin-1 in hypertension and vascular disease. *Am J Hypertens* 14: 83S-89S, 2001
53 Schiffrin EL. State-of-the-Art lecture. Role of endothelin-1 in hypertension. *Hypertension* 34: 876–881, 1999
54 Slataper R, Vicknair N, Sadler R and Bakris GL. Comparative effects of different antihypertensive treatments on progression of diabetic renal disease. *Arch Intern Med* 153: 973–980, 1993
55 Smith AC, Toto R and Bakris GL. Differential effects of calcium channel blockers on size selectivity of proteinuria in diabetic glomerulopathy. *Kidney Int* 54: 889–896, 1998
56 Staessen JA, Wang JG and Thijs L. Cardiovascular protection and blood pressure reduction: a meta-analysis. *Lancet* 358: 1305–1315, 2001
57 Stasch JP, Kazda S, Hirth C and Morich F. Role of nisoldipine on blood pressure, cardiac hypertrophy, and atrial natriuretic peptides in spontaneously hypertensive rats. *Hypertension* 10: 303–307, 1987
58 Stone PH, Muller JE, Turi ZG, Geltman E, Jaffe AS and Braunwald E. Efficacy of nifedipine therapy in patients with refractory angina pectoris: significance of the presence of coronary vasospasm. *Arq Bras Cardiol* 41: 469–476, 1983
59 Susic D, Varagic J and Frohlich ED. Pharmacologic agents on cardiovascular mass, coronary dynamics and collagen in aged spontaneously hypertensive rats. *J Hypertens* 17: 1209–1215, 1999
60 Suzuki M, Yamanaka K, Nabata H and Tachibana M. Long-term effects of amlodipine on organ damage, stroke and life span in stroke prone spontaneously hypertensive rats. *Eur J Pharmacol* 228: 269–274, 1993
61 Takahashi T, Tanikawa S and Takahashi K. Protective effects of CD-832 on organ damage in stroke-prone spontaneously hypertensive rats. *Eur J Pharmacol* 331: 193–198, 1997
62 Tojo A, Kimura K, Matsuoka H and Sugimoto T. Effects of manidipine hydrochloride on the renal microcirculation in spontaneously hypertensive rats. *J Cardiovasc Pharmacol* 20: 895–899, 1992
63 Yamazaki T, Komuro I, Zou Y, Kudoh S, Shiojima I, Mizuno T, Hiroi Y, Nagai R and Yazaki Y. Efficient inhibition of the development of cardiac remodeling by a long-acting calcium antagonist amlodipine. *Hypertension* 31: 32–38, 1998
64 Zhang CL, McKinsey TA, Chang S, Antos CL, Hill JA and Olson EN. Class II histone deacetylases act as signal-responsive repressors of cardiac hypertrophy. *Cell* 110: 479–488, 2002
65 Zhou X, Ono H, Ono Y and Frohlich ED. N- and L-type calcium channel antagonist improves glomerular dynamics, reverses severe nephrosclerosis, and inhibits apoptosis and proliferation in an l-NAME/SHR model. *J Hypertens* 20: 993–1000, 2002

Blood pressure-independent effects of calcium antagonists

The hypothesis that the reduction of elevated blood pressure is not the only mechanism of tissue protection has not reached full acceptance because of poor evidence from clinical studies. In a recent paper, Ruilope and Schiffrin [41] debated the question of whether blood pressure lowering alone is responsible for the benefits accrued from antihypertensive therapy as demonstrated in many multicenter randomized clinical trials with different antihypertensive agents or whether there is evidence that some agents have special properties that result in benefits that go beyond those resulting from lowering blood pressure. The authors pointed out that over the past 30 years, it has been demonstrated that lowering blood pressure in severe forms of hypertension, and more recently in systolic and even mild hypertension, will result in reduced incidence of stroke and slower progression of heart and renal failure. These effects have been easier to demonstrate in sicker patients, because enough end points may be counted in the three to five years that these clinical trials last. However, better prevention by a specific drug, of risk attributable to high blood pressure has not been identified in the much larger group of hypertensive individuals, who have less severe forms of hypertension. With agents such as renin-angiotensin system inhibitors or calcium channel blockers, it has been demonstrated that hypertensive vascular remodeling and endothelial dysfunction may be corrected. However, only specifically designed clinical trials could indicate that benefits beyond blood pressure lowering may be achieved with the use of specific drugs to lower blood pressure. Although some evidence suggests that this may be the case, the question remains for the time being largely unanswered.

Evidence from analytical pharmacology

Analytical pharmacology may provide valuable information for the existence of an action of CCBs beyond blood pressure lowering. However, one should carefully consider the characteristics of the model used, as shown from experiments with cilnidipine. Although it was reported in SHR that cilnidipine reduced LV hypertrophy in the DOCA-salt model of hypertension [22], it has been observed in rat exposed to L-NAME, in order to block NO production, that reduction of the resulting increase in blood pressure by cilnidipine did not prevent cardiac hypertrophy observed in this model [55].

To gain further insight into the mechanism(s) of the cardioprotective action of CCBs, we compared the dose-dependence of their effect on SBP and on cardiac remodeling in salt-loaded SHRSP. As already mentioned above, salt-load induces in this strain an important hypertrophy of heart and vessels. When rats exposed to salt are treated with CCBs, this salt-dependent hypertrophy was prevented. Figure 1 provides a comparison between two long-acting CCBs. It shows the dose-dependence of their effect on SBP and on cardiac remodeling in salt-loaded SHRSP. For a similar effect on SBP, the reduction of the relative LV mass was significantly more important with lacidipine than with amlodipine. At each of the three doses utilized, lacidipine and amlodipine reduced SBP in a comparable manner, but this reduction was not statistically significant with the lowest dose (L0.3 and A1.5). With the exception of amlodipine 1.5 $mg \cdot kg^{-1}$ (A1.5), each drug treatment evoked a significant reduction of LV mass ($P < 0.001$) and the values attained were not significantly different from the LV mass in untreated SHRSP (2.91 ± 0.02 $mg \cdot g^{-1}$ body weight, not shown in Figure 1. However, for a similar level of SBP, the LV mass was lower in the group treated with lacidipine than in the group treated with amlodipine ($P < 0.05$). Increasing the dosage from 1 to 3 $mg \cdot kg^{-1}$ for lacidipine, or from 5 to 15 $mg \cdot kg^{-1}$ for amlodipine, did not decrease LV mass further despite a consistent reduction in SBP. This comparison, illustrating the relation between

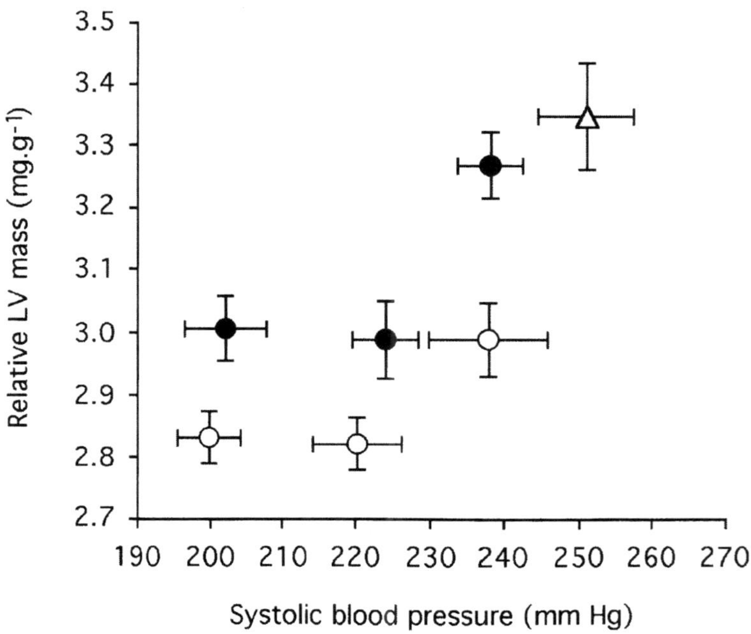

Figure 1. Relation between relative left ventricular mass and systolic blood pressure in salt-loaded SHRSP. Δ: salt-loaded SHRSP, with either ●: amlodipine 1.5, 5 and 15 mg kg^{-1} or ○: lacidipine 0.3, 1 and 3 mg kg^{-1}. Modified from [24].

SBP and the LV relative mass in rats exposed to salt with or without CCB treatment, indicates that the beneficial effect of CCBs on cardiac remodeling could not simply be related to the reduction of SBP [24].

When considering renal protection in SHR, long-term treatment with different 1,4-DHPs, at doses that decreased blood pressure to a similar extent, showed that the long-acting CCBs lercanidipine and manidipine were more effective than nicardipine in countering glomerular injury and the luminal narrowing of efferent arterioles, whereas the three drugs similarly vasodilated the afferent arteriole [43, 44]. This suggests a causal link between vasodilation of the efferent arteriole and nephroprotection. This nephroprotective action, which likely resulted from blockade of L-type Ca channels, is not directly related to the decrease of blood pressure, but is rather in line with our observations on tissue selectivity [13].

Other experimental data supporting the hypothesis for a role of blood pressure-independent effects are coming from studies on the action of CCBs on Ca^{2+} function in isolated myocytes exposed to hypertrophic stimuli, on their interaction with the renin-angiotensin system and the L-arginine-NO pathway, on their inhibitory effect on the translocation of PKC and on their antioxidant properties.

CCBs target cardiac myocytes exposed to hypertrophic stimuli

Cultured cardiac cells are an *in vitro* model allowing to unravel mechanisms involved in the antihypertrophic effects of CCBs that are independent on blood pressure lowering, in those cells that contain L-type Ca channels. Neonatal cardiomyocytes are easier to keep in culture than cardiomyocytes from adult animals, which undergo marked phenotypic changes even after three days in culture. Most of the results have been obtained on primary cultures of neonatal rat cardiomyocytes. These cells do not exhibit the typical rod-shape appearance of adult cells, their myofibrillar organization is poorly developed and they beat spontaneously. Moreover, a large body of evidence indicates that the functional organization of *in situ* cardiomyocytes changes markedly in the postnatal period, especially in the rat. These changes are striking at the level of excitation-contraction coupling, the sarcoplasmic reticulum assuming progressively a larger role in the Ca fluxes involved in contraction and relaxation [28]. As was mentioned above (pages 123, 124), the subcellular distribution of Ca channels differs in neonatal and adult myocytes. The sensitivity of contracting adult heart to CCBs is lesser than that of neonatal hearts. Therefore, when assessing the Ca-dependent pathways potentially implicated in gene transcription, a critical evaluation of the data obtained on neonatal cells should be made before the conclusions drawn from such studies may be extended to adult cardiomyocytes, and, *a fortiori*, to the *in vivo* situation. For example, considering two vasoactive peptides that induce hypertrophy in cultured neonatal cardiomyocytes, Ang II, but not ET-1, failed to elicit $Ca^{2+}{}_i$

responses in freshly isolated adult cardiomyocytes, presumably because the membrane density of AT receptors was much less in adult than in neonatal cells [53].

The most straightforward mechanism of action of CCBs is reduction of L-type calcium entry currents through voltage-operated channels. Subsequent lowering of $Ca^{2+}{}_i$ would be expected to down-regulate important signaling pathways involved in the development of cardiac hypertrophy. Increased cytoplasmic Ca activates calmodulin. The delta isoform of Ca^{2+}/calmodulin-dependent protein kinase II (CaMKII) predominates in the heart. In transgenic (TG) mice that express the nuclear delta (B) isoform of CaMKII, the expressed CaMKIIdelta (B) transgene is restricted to the myocardium and is highly concentrated in the nucleus, indicating the possible translocation of CaCam from the membrane to the nucleus. Cardiac hypertrophy was evidenced by an increased left ventricle to body weight ratio and up-regulation of embryonic and contractile protein genes, including atrial natriuretic factor, beta-myosin heavy chain, and alpha-skeletal actin [64]. Mechanical stretch, which undoubtedly plays a key triggering role in the development of cardiac hypertrophy, increases $Ca^{2+}{}_i$ in neonatal cardiomyocytes, and this increase was partly antagonized by the Ca channel blocker diltiazem at a rather high concentration: 100 μM [42]. This *in vitro* observation suggests that reducing stretch-activated L-type calcium entry currents through voltage-operated channels might attenuate the hypertrophic response to stretch, at least to the extent that this response is dependent on an increase in $Ca^{2+}{}_i$. In this respect, activation of MAP kinase pathway(s), which is involved in the hypertrophic response to mechanical loading, is partially dependent on trans-sarcolemmal influx of Ca^{2+}, half of which is attributable to a nifedipine (10 nM)-sensitive channel [58, 60]. Stretch-induced $Ca^{2+}{}_i$ increase might also depend on activation of the Na^+/H^+ antiporter, resulting in elevation of $Na^+{}_i$ and stimulation of Na^+/Ca^{2+} exchange.

In addition to mechanical stretch, vasoactive substances that are operating *in vivo* (Ang II, α-adrenoceptor agonists, ET-1) and are acting through G-protein coupled receptors cause hypertrophic responses in cultured cardiac myocytes. They activate tyrosine kinase, MAP kinase and 90-kD S6 kinase and enhance the expression of immediate-early genes (c-Fos) and other genes. Activation of these kinases and induction of c-Fos expression by Ang II is critically dependent on $Ca^{2+}{}_i$ [46]. However, L-type Ca entry currents seem not to be required for the stimulation by Ang II and ET-1 of c-Fos expression and cell growth at least in neonatal cardiomyocytes [20, 45]. In contrast, in the same model, CCBs attenuated markedly α-agonist-stimulated protein synthesis and ANF expression [50]. In addition, the hypertrophic response of neonatal cardiomyocytes to serum stimulation was slightly inhibited by nifedipine and enhanced by the L-type channel agonist Bayer K 8644 [25]. Those observations show that blockade of L-type currents in heart is a player in the reduction of cardiac hypertrophy. This indicates why the *in vivo* action of CCBs might not easily be dissociated from the reduction of blood pressure.

Blockade of the renin-angiotensin-aldosterone system

The renin-angiotensin system (RAS) has long been known to play a major role in cardiovascular remodeling induced by hypertension, as evidenced by the beneficial effects of ACE inhibitors and AT_1 receptor blockers [21]. Ang II may act partly by increasing the production of other mediators, including ET-1 [19] a potent inducer of cardiomyocyte hypertrophy, and transforming growth factor-β1 (TGF-β1) [49]. Increased aldosterone levels favor myocardial fibrosis through activation of cardiac aldosterone receptors, independently of haemodynamic factors [61]. As shown by Müller et al. [32], circulating renin can be taken up by the heart and induce local synthesis of Ang II. Thus, increased renin production by the kidney may be expected to contribute to activation of cardiac RAS and to favor cardiac remodeling. Most probably, such a mechanism is operative in the salt-loaded SHRSP model, in which renin production is paradoxically enhanced. Activation of renal renin synthesis seems to be related to salt-induced renal damage [16]. Renal damage occurring in salt-sensitive rats is evidenced by increased urinary protein excretion, lesions of malignant nephrosclerosis and increased gene expression of TGF-β1, a key mediator of glomerulosclerosis [35]. In stroke-prone SHR exposed to salt-load, this nephropathy, and the concomitant elevation of renin production, is prevented by amlodipine and lacidipine at dosages that cause little reduction in blood pressure [10]. The reduction of PRA was accompanied by reduction of the salt-dependent over-expression of ET-1 in both heart and vessels [12, 23] showing that CCBs attenuated the production of two major cardiac hypertrophic factors. Ang II is a potent stimulus not only for cardiomyocyte hypertrophy and gene reprogramming but also for hyperplasia and up-regulation of fibrosis-associated genes in cardiac fibroblasts. Prevention of the activation of the renin-angiotensin-aldosterone system by CCBs may contribute to blood-pressure independent end-organ protection in SHRSP exposed to salt-load. Too high doses of CCBs, however, are able to further stimulate renal renin production in salt-loaded SHRSP, an action that appears to be unrelated to kidney damage [24], but is a branch of reflexes evoked by too low blood pressure.

Blockade of the renin-angiotensin-aldosterone (RAS) system is a powerful therapeutic mechanism illustrated by the actions of ACE inhibitors and angiotensin antagonists. Such an action can be achieved by CCBs. Their action may result either from reduction of the production of renin, as observed in salt-loaded SHRSP, or from ACE inhibition. A direct action on ACE has been shown for amlodipine. It has been reported that the vasodilatory effect of amlodipine might be attributable to an increase in local bradykinin concentration, secondary to inhibition of its breakdown by ACE. Indeed, when examining the ability of amlodipine to cause ACE inhibition in a serum sample, Xu B et al. [57] found that amlodipine can potently inhibit ACE activity, to a similar extent to enalapril, a well-established ACE inhibitor used widely in clinical practice. The kinin- and NO-dependent component of the vasorelaxation induced by amlodipine may indeed relate to its ability to inhibit ACE. NO biosynthesis by the vascular endothelium is generally thought of as beneficial, since NO, quite apart from its vasodilatory properties, exerts anti-atherogenic effects on the vascular wall as reported by Napoli and Ignarro [38]. Thus, one might postulate that a CCB such as amlodipine, which stimulates NO biosynthesis, might exert an additional vasculoprotective effect not shared with another agent which produces a similar degree of vasorelaxation but do not generate NO.

Inhibition of protein kinase C

The protein kinase C (PKC) family comprises three sub-groups of serine/threonine kinases that are differentiated on the basis of their sensitivity to calcium and lipid. Classical PKCs (PKC-α, -β_1, -β_2 and γ) are activated by phosphatidylserine, Ca^{2+} and diacylglycerol (DAG) or its synthetic analog phorbol myrisate acetate (PMA). Novel PKCs (PKC-δ, -ε, -η, -η, -μ) are Ca^{2+}-independent but require DAG. Atypical PKCs (PKC-ζ, -ι, -λ) do not require Ca^{2+} or DAG.

PKCs are involved in various cellular events including muscle contraction, cardiovascular hypertrophy and endothelial permeability. Their activation is observed in various conditions including exposure of tissues to vasoconstrictors, to growth factors and to ischaemia. The translocation of PKC from the soluble to the particulate fraction of cells exposed to appropriate stimuli gives a measure of the activation of the enzyme. It has been reported that CCBs may inhibit PKC translocation. Block and co-workers [2, 3] have used two recombinant PDGF homodimers to determine the roles of each isoform in the activation of phosphatidylinositol turnover in vascular smooth muscle cells (VSMC) isolated from rat thoracic aorta, their mitogenic effect on VSMC, and their vasoconstrictor effect on intact strips of aortic vascular tissue. Three Ca^{2+}-channel blockers, nifedipine, verapamil, and diltiazem, were employed as antagonists for investigating the PDGF-dependent changes mediated by the homodimers. PDGF-BB had a greater efficacy than PDGF-AA on inositol 1,4,5-triphosphate release, on the formation of diacylglycerol, and on Ca^{2+} mobilization, which was also associated with vasoconstrictor activity and effective mitogenicity. PDGF-AA, on the other hand, was more potent than PDGF-BB in stimulating protein kinase C. In all instances, Ca^{2+}-channel blockers inhibited the activation of the phosphatidylinositol turnover by the two homodimers. The results of Block et al. showed that representatives of three chemical groups of calcium antagonists (nifedipine, verapamil, and diltiazem) all inhibited the action of recombinant platelet-derived growth factor in vascular smooth muscle cells and reduced PKC activation. They also observed that calcium antagonists modulate expression of HMG-CoA reductase and LDL-receptor genes stimulated by platelet-derived growth factor. These calcium antagonist-mediated effects on gene expression were observed at pharmacological concentrations that were one to two orders of magnitude lower than those required for inhibition of depolarization-induced opening of voltage-sensitive L-type calcium channels. Similar observations have been made by other groups (see for instance [59]). However, in the above-mentioned studies, the effects of calcium antagonists were investigated in cell types that possess L-type calcium channels, such as vascular smooth muscle cells. *In vivo* studies have confirmed those experiments performed on isolated cells. For instance, when calcium ionophore A23187 or phenylephrine were injected *i.p.*, they induced translocation of protein kinase C (PKC) from the cytosol to the membrane fraction of the rat frontal cortex and hippocampus. The action of A23187 was blocked in a dose-dependent manner by nifedipine and verapamil. The phenylephrine-induced translocation of PKC was blocked by prazosin and in a dose-dependent manner by nifedipine and verapamil. This indicates that the influx of calcium ions through an L-type calcium channel is probably necessary for a full alpha$_1$-adrenoceptor mediated activation and translocation of PKC that can be blocked by CCBs, but under conditions able to cause reduction in blood pressure [52]. Therefore, in order to examine if CCBs may have BP independent effects, studies need to be performed in cells that do not contain L-type Ca channels. In this regard, endothelial cells provide an interesting model to describe actions of CCBs. Hempel et al. [17] have tested the hypothesis that nifedipine can prevent ischaemia-induced endothelial permeability increases by inhibiting protein kinase C (PKC) in cultured porcine endothelial cells. The inhibition of ischaemia-induced permeability by nifedipine seems to be mediated primarily by PKC-α inhibition. In those cells that do not contain L-type Ca channels, nifedipine inhibited both PKC-α and PKC-ζ translocation at very low concentration. The authors have concluded that nifedipine exerts a direct effect on endothelial cell permeability that is independent of calcium channels.

Interaction with the L-arginine-NO pathway

In isolated precontracted rat aorta, the relaxation evoked by CCBs is more pronounced in the presence than in the absence of endothelium [14, 48]. This indicates that NO has a role in the vasodilatation evoked by CCBs. Furthermore, cGMP (which is formed through the action of NO) and verapamil are synergistic to produce vascular muscle relaxation [48]. The facilitation of CCBs action due to the L-arginine-NO pathway may also result from other effects. Brovkovych et al. studied the effect of endothelium-dependent vasorelaxation, the release of NO and superoxide (O_2) in the presence of nifedipine in isolated cultured rabbit endothelial cells. Highly sensitive electrochemical microsensors were placed onto the cell membrane, and the kinetics of NO and superoxide (O_2) were measured simultaneously with time resolutions of 0.1 and 0.05 ms, respectively. Nifedipine at its therapeutical concentrations stimulated NO release and scavenged superoxide (O_2) in endothelial cells. The NO concentration was approximately 50% and 30% of the concentration measured in the presence of receptor-dependent (acetylcholine) and the receptor-independent (Ca^{2+} ionophore A23187) NO synthase (eNOS) agonists, respectively. NO release stimulated by eNOS agonists was followed by the generation of the NO scavenger superoxide. The average rate of NO release by nifedipine was relatively slow, in sharp contrast to the fast rate of NO release by acetylcholine. These experiments illustrate how nifedipine, apart from its well-known Ca^{2+} antagonistic properties in vascular smooth muscle cells, stimulates the release of significant concentration of NO in endothelium and also preserves NO concentration. Thus nifedipine in the nanomolar range stimulates the release of NO from endothelial cells and preserves NO concentration [5]. Zhang and Hintze [65] demonstrated that amlodipine increases nitrite production from healthy canine coronary micro vessels *in vitro*, reflecting an increase in NO biosynthesis that is kinin-dependent. Similar results were obtained in coronary micro-vessels from dogs with pacing-induced heart failure [67]. These same workers subsequently demonstrated in similar fashion that amlodipine can increase nitrite generation in coronary microvessels isolated from failing human hearts at the time of cardiac transplantation [66]. Amlodipine may increase NO generation in the vasculature through an increase in kinin activity [65, 68]. Vaziri and his colleagues observed that administration of felodipine enhances nitric oxide (NO) production and NO synthase (NOS) isotype expressions and activities in rats with chronic renal failure CRF. Having found marked increases in nitric oxide (NO) production and endothelial and inducible NO synthase (eNOS and iNOS) expressions with calcium channel blockade in rats with chronic renal failure, Ding and Vaziri studied whether enhanced NO production with calcium channel blockade is a direct effect of this therapy or a consequence of the associated haemodynamic and humoral changes. They tested the effects of felodipine on nitrate and nitrite (Nox) generation, Ca^{2+}-dependent and -independent NOS activity, and eNOS and iNOS protein masses in proliferating and quiescent rat aortic endothelial cells in culture. Compared with vehicle alone, felodipine significantly increased NOx generation, Ca^{2+}-dependent NOS activity, and eNOS protein mass in proliferating and quiescent endothelial cells. Felodipine did not modify the stimulatory action of 10% fetal calf serum on DNA synthesis (thymidine incorporation) and cell proliferation. Ca^{2+}-independent NOS activity and iNOS protein expression were negligible and unaffected by calcium channel blockade. NOx production and NOS expression were greater in proliferating cells than in quiescent cells. Thus, calcium channel blocker up-regulates endothelial NO production *in vitro*, confirming their previous *in vivo* study. They concluded that their observation indicates that the reductions in cytosolic $[Ca^{2+}]$ and vasodilation with calcium channel blockade are not only due to inhibition of Ca^{2+} entry but also to an NO-cGMP mediated mechanism. There is thus a marked up-regulations of basal and acetylcholine-stimulated NO production and endothelial NOS (eNOS) expression and activity by felodipine in cultured endothelial cells [11,

56]. Krenek et al. [23] have shown that lacidipine restored the loss of endothelium-dependent vascular relaxation in SHRSP exposed to salt-load, an effect likely related to increased eNOS expression. These *in vivo* and *in vitro* studies provided convincing evidence for the up-regulatory action of CCBs. These studies were extended by showing that in cultured human coronary artery endothelial cells, both nifedipine and diltiazem significantly increased NO production and eNOS protein expression and activity, whereas verapamil had no discernible effect on NO system in human coronary artery endothelial cells *in vitro*. This observation was confirmed by Xu et al. [57] who showed that amlodipine increases vascular NO generation in anesthetized rabbit and that the subsequent femoral artery dilatation is sensitive to a kinin antagonist. Additionally, several CCBs have been demonstrated to possess antioxidant and oxygen free radical-scavenging properties (see below and [37, 40, 51]). Superoxide anion can remove NO by combining chemically with it, forming the potent oxidant and cytotoxic radical peroxynitrite. Because of their antioxidant property, CCB may potentially increase NO availability through removal of superoxide anion.

The interaction of CCBs with the over-expression of iNOS has also been studied [47]. iNos produces large quantities of NO, which may be deleterious for the cardiovascular system. There are a number of studies showing that cytokines generated by activated immune cells cause an increase in nitric oxide (NO) via induction of NO synthase (NOS), which results in a direct negative inotropic effect and a modulation of inotropic responsiveness. Increases in inflammatory circulating cytokines have been detected in patients with heart failure and cardiomyopathy, elevated plasma levels of nitrite/nitrate inpatients with heart failure have been reported, and inducible NOS (iNOS) has been found in ventricular tissue from patients with dilated cardiomyopathy [31]. Overproduction of nitric oxide (NO) from inducible nitric oxide synthase (iNOS) is also importantly involved in the pathogenesis of atherosclerosis [7]. Therefore, it is of interest to know the action of CCBs on iNOS expression due to inflammatory agents. In endotoxemia induced by *Salmonella typhosa* lipopolysaccharide (LPS), amlodipine-treatment reduced both the LPS-induced Ca^{2+}-independent NOS activity in homogenates of heart and the expression of iNOS mRNA in aortae (Fig. 2). Amlodipine (10 µM) inhibited nitrite production in macrophage culture challenged with LPS [47]. Chou et al. [7] investigated the effect of amlodipine on nitrite production and iNOS induction both in lipopolysaccharide (LPS) and interferon-gamma (IFN-gamma)-treated rat aortic smooth muscle cells (RASMC). Incubation with amlodipine (0.1–10 microM) for 24 h resulted in a significant and dose-dependent attenuation in medium nitrite as well as iNOS protein expression in LPS/IFN-gamma-treated RASMC. These results suggest that amlodipine may exert vascular beneficial effects by suppressing pro-inflammatory cytokines and free radical generation related to iNOS induction in smooth muscle cells during activation of inflammatory mechanism.

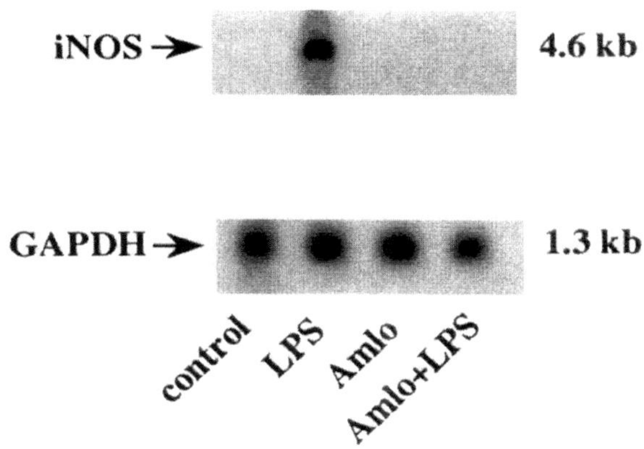

Figure 2. Typical autoradiograms of Northern analysis of mRNA levels in aortic tissue from Wistar rats exposed or not to LPS with or without amlodipine; Modified from Salomone et al. [47].

Antioxidant effects

Oxidative stress describes the injury caused to cells by the oxidizing of macromolecules resulting from increased formation of reactive oxygen species (ROS) and/or decreased antioxidant reserve. Recent works have reported that all types of vascular cells generate ROS. A growing number of reports have provided a critical role for oxidative stress in the pathogenesis of cardiovascular diseases, including hypertension. Oxidant stress contributes to vascular diseases by promoting vascular smooth muscle proliferation, monocyte/macrophage infiltration, vascular tone alteration, and matrix metalloproteinases activation. Recent evidence suggests that hypertension, in particular, is associated with increased vascular oxidant stress. A membrane bound NADH/NADPH oxidase, the major source of reactive oxygen species in blood vessels is activated in rats made hypertensive by prolonged angiotensin II infusion [62]. This increase in superoxide anion production contributes to impaired endothelium-dependent relaxation, the hypertension being ameliorated by treatment with membrane-targeted forms of superoxide dismutase (SOD) which is one of the major cellular defenses against superoxide anion. Hypertrophy of vascular smooth muscle cells caused by angiotensin II is mediated by reactive oxygen species derived mainly from the membrane bound NADH/NADPH oxidase. Similarly, a recombinant heparin-binding SOD acutely lowers blood pressure in spontaneously hypertensive rats [36]. Taken together, these findings indicate that oxidant stress critically contributes to the pathogenesis of hypertension and its related vascular disease [15].

An enhanced production of ROS contributes to the dysregulation of physiological processes, which leads to structural and functional alterations observed in hypertension and atherosclerosis. Enzymatic sources of ROS in the vascular wall playing a functional role in hypertension are NAD(P)H oxidase, NO synthase, xanthine oxidase, and cyclooxygenase. Several experimental observations have shown an enhanced superoxide generation as a result of the activation of vascular NAD(P)H oxidase by shear stress and various factors including angiotensin II, PDGF and TNFα. Two characteristic alterations of the vascular wall in hypertension are endothelial dysfunction and vascular smooth muscle cell (VSMC) hypertrophy. A role for ROS has been proposed in angiotensin II pathological action. ROS are also involved in several signal pathways and in the activation of redox-sensitive transcriptional factors, such as nuclear factor (NF)-κB [18]. It has been shown that angiotensin II activates NF-κB in VSMCs. Furthermore, NF-κB has been implicated in the transcription of a number of vascular genes [4]. Finally, NF-κB seems to play a pivotal role in angiotensin II-stimulated ROS generation and inflammatory mechanisms (see review [26, 27]). Antioxidant mechanisms can be divided into two major classes based on their mode of action: antioxidant enzymes and non-enzymatic antioxidants (scavengers). The class of antioxidants enzymes consists of superoxide dismutase (SOD), catalase and glutathione peroxidase. Dismutation of O_2^- by SOD produces H_2O_2 a more stable ROS, which in turn is converted to H_2O by catalase and glutathione peroxidase. Several authors have described the antioxidant properties of CCBs as being due either to direct scavenging effect or to preservation of the activity of superoxide dismutase. Experimental studies [29] have shown that some CCBs may inhibit oxidative damage to lipids associated with cellular membranes and lipoprotein particles. Under controlled experimental conditions, they may inhibit lipid peroxide formation at concentrations as low as 10.0 nM, independent of calcium channel modulation. This antioxidant activity is found with high lipophilic CCBs when their chemical structure facilitates proton-donating and resonance-stabilization mechanisms that quench the free radical reaction. By inserting to a location in the membrane near polyunsaturated fatty acids at relatively high concentrations, amlodipine and lacidipine are capable of donating protons to lipid peroxide molecules, thereby blocking the peroxidation process. The remaining unpaired free electron associated with the CCB molecule can be stabilized in well-defined resonance structures associated with the dihydropyridine ring. The reaction that describes the antioxidant effects of a dihydropyridine (DHP) CCB is as follows in which LOO* represents a lipid peroxide molecule:

$$LOO^* + DHP \rightarrow LOOH + DHP^*$$

The antioxidant capacity of any chemical compound can be measured *in vitro*. According to Ursini [54], for all dihydropyridines, the rate constant for the interaction with peroxyl radicals is three orders of magnitude lower than that of the vitamin E derivative, and therefore all these molecules must be considered as rather weak antioxidants. However, it is worth considering the binding to specific structures and the partition coefficient to membranes, which provides a local high concentration. Therefore, the actual rate of the interaction with free radicals could be sufficient even though the rate constant of the reac-

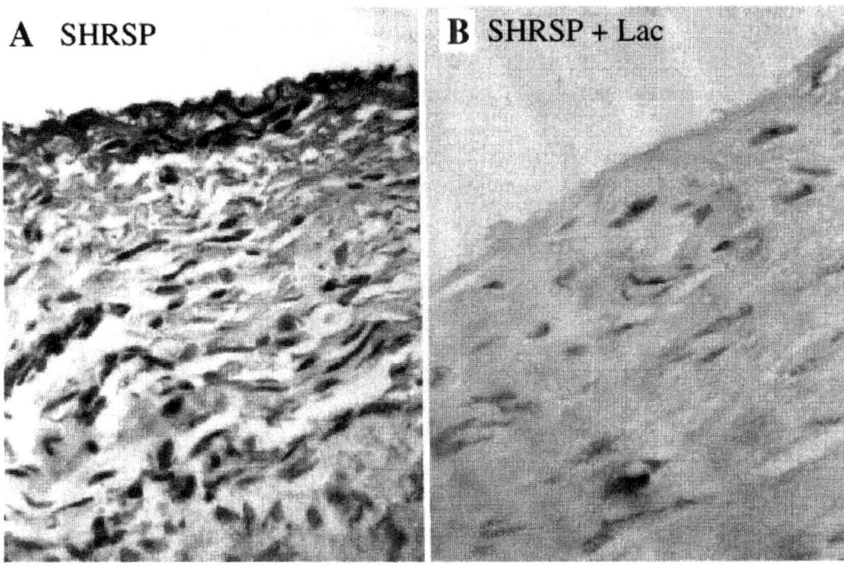

Figure 3. *In vivo* antioxidant capacity of CCBs. Illustration by the action of lacidipine on the abundance of oxidized LDL identified in the arterial intima of rat carotid artery by specific antibodies. Modified from Napoli et al. [39].

tion is lower than that of vitamin E. Indeed, in SHRSP exposed to salt-load and treated with CCBs or vitamin E, Napoli et al. [39] have observed a marked reduction of the presence of oxidation-specific epitopes in carotid and middle cerebral arteries (Fig. 3). This reduction was unrelated to decrease of elevated blood pressure and was similar to the action of vitamine E that was without effect on blood pressure. They have also reported that nifedipine and lacidipine reduced the rate of oxidation of LDL measured in the blood *ex vivo* (Tab. 1).

The antioxidant action of CCBs has been demonstrated in other experimental setup. Berkels et al. [1] have reported that treatment of the endothelium with dihydropyridine calcium antagonists resulted in an increased release in NO that

Table 1. *Ex vivo* peroxidation of LDL [39]

Species	Rate: nmol/(min. mg LDL)
WKY	9.9 ± 1.5*
SHRSP	12.4 ± 1.5
+ Nif (80 mg)	9.1 ± 1.4*
+ Lac (1 mg)	8.8 ± 1.5*
+ Lac (0.3 mg)	9.0 ± 1.5*
+ Vit E (100 IU)	8.4 ± 1.6*

is not due to a modulation of L-type calcium channels, because macrovascular endothelial cells do not express this channel. In their study, they investigated how long-term (48 hours) treatment of porcine endothelial cell cultures with nifedipine resulted in a enhanced NO liberation. With regard to the underlying mechanism, they examined whether nifedipine changed the mRNA and protein levels of the constitutive endothelial NO synthase (NOS) in endothelial cell cultures or exerted an NO protective effect via its antioxidative properties, as revealed in a cell culture model and with native endothelium from porcine coronary arteries. They observed that nifedipine induced a significant time- and concentration-dependent increase in the basal NO liberation that was not due to elevated eNOS mRNA and protein levels. However, at the same concentration, nifedipine significantly reduced the basal and glucose-stimulated formation of reactive oxygen species, indicating therefore that nifedipine might protect released NO from oxidation by ROS. They concluded this increased NO availability may cause part of the vasodilation and might contribute to the antithrombotic, antiproliferative, and antiatherosclerotic effects of dihydropyridine calcium antagonists. Indeed, antioxidants are endowed with antihypertrophic effects both *in vitro* (on cultured neonatal cardiomyocytes [34]) and in some *in vivo* models (in double transgenic rats harboring both human renin and angiotensinogen genes [33]), possibly by opposing ROS-dependent NF-κB activation. It was indeed reported by Cominacini et al. [8] that lacidipine inhibits the activation of the transcription factor NF-κB and the expression of adhesion molecules induced by pro-oxidant signals on endothelial cells. Increasing evidence indicates that activation of the endothelium during inflammation plays a role in the pathogenesis of atherosclerosis and thrombosis and is a pivotal factor in myocardial reperfusion injury, mediating the migration of neutrophils into ischaemic/reperfused myocardium. Recent studies have demonstrated that activated endothelium displays up-regulated levels in a variety of molecules, including growth factors, cytokines, and cell surface adhesion molecules. The up-regulated endothelial cell adhesion molecules act in concert with leukocyte adhesion molecules to co-ordinate the localization of leukocytes to inflamed tissue. The pivotal role of NF-κB activation has been reported in this process. Moreover, antagonizing the vascular nuclear factor-B pathway may modulate the atherosclerotic process. According to Cabrero et al. [6], activation of NF-κB is required for hypertrophic growth of cardiomyocytes. They showed that etomoxir, an irreversible inhibitor of carnitine palmitoyltransferase I (CPT-I) that activates peroxisome proliferator-activated receptor alpha (PPARalpha), induces cardiac hypertrophy via increased cellular oxidative stress and NF-κB activation. Lacidipine, at the doses of 0.3 and 1 mg/kg/d, has been shown to display antioxidant properties in salt-loaded SHRSP (as evidenced, for instance, by the reduction of oxidized LDL in the arterial intima) and to be more effective in this respect than nifedipine [39]. As was observed in other experimental conditions, differences may also been observed among drugs belonging to the 1,4-DHP class. Carvedilol (7.5 mg/kg), a non-selective, vasodilating β-blocker with potent antioxidant properties was, like lacidipine, more effective than labetalol (60 mg/kg) to prevent LV hypertrophy and the activation of the endothelin gene evoked by aortic banding, whereas those drugs did not appreciably reduce mean carotid pressure and similarly blocked the increase in plasma renin activity [30]. However, in contrast to lacidipine, vitamin E did not lower cardiac weight in salt-loaded SHRSP [39], which indicates that, in this model, the antioxidant activity alone was not sufficient to induce an antihypertrophic effect. It therefore appears that inhibitors of NF-κB and antioxidants might have a therapeutic role in cardiac hypertrophy, independently of an action on blood pressure, they also have a therapeutic action in atherosclerosis [9, 63].

References

1 Berkels R, Egink G, Marsen TA, Bartels H, Roesen R and Klaus W. Nifedipine increases endothelial nitric oxide bioavailability by antioxidative mechanisms. *Hypertension* 37: 240–245, 2001
2 Block LH, Emmons LR, Vogt E, Sachinidis A, Vetter W and Hoppe J. Ca^{2+}-channel blockers inhibit the action of recombinant platelet-derived growth factor in vascular smooth muscle cells. *Proc Natl Acad Sci USA* 86: 2388–2392, 1989
3 Block LH, Matthys H, Emmons LR, Perruchoud A, Erne P and Roth M. Ca^{2+}-channel blockers modulate expression of 3-hydroxy-3-methylglutaryl-coenzyme A reductase and low density lipoprotein receptor genes stimulated by platelet-derived growth factor. *Proc Natl Acad Sci USA* 88: 9041–9045, 1991
4 Brasier AR and Li J. Mechanisms for inducible control of angiotensinogen gene transcription. *Hypertension* 27: 465–475, 1996
5 Brovkovych VV, Kalinowski L, Muller-Peddinghaus R and Malinski T. Synergistic antihypertensive effects of nifedipine on endothelium: concurrent release of NO and scavenging of superoxide. *Hypertension* 37: 34–39, 2001
6 Cabrero A, Merlos M, Laguna JC and Carrera MV. Down-regulation of acyl-CoA oxidase gene expression and increased NF-kappaB activity in etomoxir-induced cardiac hypertrophy. *J Lipid Res* 44: 388–398, 2003
7 Chou TC, Yang SP and Pei D. Amlodipine inhibits pro-inflammatory cytokines and free radical production and inducible nitric oxide synthase expression in lipopolysaccharide/interferon-gamma-stimulated cultured vascular smooth muscle cells. *Jpn J Pharmacol* 89: 157–163, 2002
8 Cominacini L, Garbin U, Fratta Pasini A, Paulon T, Davoli A, Campagnola M, Marchi E, Pastorino AM, Gaviraghi G and Lo Cascio V. Lacidipine inhibits the activation of the transcription factor NF-kappaB and the expression of adhesion molecules induced by pro-oxidant signals on endothelial cells. *J Hypertens* 15: 1633–1640, 1997
9 Cristofori P, Lanzoni A, Quartaroli M, Pastorino AM, Zancanaro C, Cominacini L, Gaviraghi G and Turton J. The calcium-channel blocker lacidipine reduces the development of atherosclerotic lesions in the apoE-deficient mouse. *J Hypertens* 18: 1429–1436, 2000
10 Cristofori P, Micheli D, Terron A and Gaviraghi G. Lacidipine: experimental evidence of vasculoprotective properties. *J Cardiovasc Pharmacol* 23 Suppl 5: S90–93, 1994
11 Ding Y and Vaziri ND. Calcium channel blockade enhances nitric oxide synthase expression by cultured endothelial cells. *Hypertension* 32: 718–723, 1998
12 Feron O, Salomone S and Godfraind T. Action of the calcium channel blocker lacidipine on cardiac hypertrophy and endothelin-1 gene expression in stroke-prone hypertensive rats. *Br J Pharmacol* 118: 659–664, 1996
13 Godfraind T, Dessy C and Salomone S. A comparison of the potency of selective L-calcium channel blockers in human coronary and internal mammary arteries exposed to serotonin. *J Pharmacol Exp Ther* 263: 112–122, 1992
14 Godfraind T and Salomone S. Calcium antagonists and endothelial function: focus on nitric oxide and endothelin. *Cardiovasc Drugs Ther* 10: 439–446, 1996
15 Griendling KK, Sorescu D and Ushio-Fukai M. NAD(P)H oxidase: role in cardiovascular biology and disease. *Circ Res* 86: 494–501, 2000

16 Griffin KA, Churchill PC, Picken M, Webb RC, Kurtz TW and Bidani AK. Differential salt-sensitivity in the pathogenesis of renal damage in SHR and stroke prone SHR. *Am J Hypertens* 14: 311–320, 2001

17 Hempel A, Lindschau C, Maasch C, Mahn M, Bychkov R, Noll T, Luft FC and Haller H. Calcium antagonists ameliorate ischemia-induced endothelial cell permeability by inhibiting protein kinase C. *Circulation* 99: 2523–2529, 1999

18 Irani K. Oxidant signaling in vascular cell growth, death, and survival: a review of the roles of reactive oxygen species in smooth muscle and endothelial cell mitogenic and apoptotic signaling. *Circ Res* 87: 179–183, 2000

19 Ito H, Hirata Y, Adachi S, Tanaka M, Tsujino M, Koike A, Nogami A, Murumo F and Hiroe M. Endothelin-1 is an autocrine/paracrine factor in the mechanism of angiotensin II-induced hypertrophy in cultured rat cardiomyocytes. *J Clin Invest* 92: 398–403, 1993

20 Ito H, Hirata Y, Hiroe M, Tsujino M, Adachi S, Takamoto T, Nitta M, Taniguchi K and Marumo F. Endothelin-1 induces hypertrophy with enhanced expression of muscle-specific genes in cultured neonatal rat cardiomyocytes. *Circ Res* 69: 209–215, 1991

21 Kim S and Iwao H. Molecular and cellular mechanisms of angiotensin II-mediated cardiovascular and renal diseases. *Pharmacol Rev* 52: 11–34, 2000

22 Kobayashi N, Mori Y, Mita S, Nakano S, Kobayashi T, Tsubokou Y and Matsuoka H. Effects of cilnidipine on nitric oxide and endothelin-1 expression and extracellular signal-regulated kinase in hypertensive rats. *Eur J Pharmacol* 422: 149–157, 2001

23 Krenek P, Salomone S, Kyselovic J, Wibo M, Morel N and Godfraind T. Lacidipine prevents endothelial dysfunction in salt-loaded stroke-prone hypertensive rats. *Hypertension* 37: 1124–1128, 2001

24 Kyselovic J, Krenek P, Wibo M and Godfraind T. Effects of amlodipine and lacidipine on cardiac remodelling and renin production in salt-loaded stroke-prone hypertensive rats. *Br J Pharmacol* 134: 1516–1522, 2001

25 Lubic SP, Giacomini KM and Giacomini JC. The effects of modulation of calcium influx through the voltage-sensitive calcium channel on cardiomyocyte hypertrophy. *J Mol Cell Cardiol* 27: 917–925, 1995

26 Luft FC. Angiotensin, inflammation, hypertension, and cardiovascular disease. *Curr Hypertens Rep* 3: 61–67, 2001

27 Luft FC. Workshop: mechanisms and cardiovascular damage in hypertension. *Hypertension* 37: 594–598, 2001

28 Mahony L. Regulation of intracellular calcium concentration in the developing heart. *Cardiovasc Res* 31 Spec No: E61–67, 1996

29 Mason RP. Mechanisms of plaque stabilization for the dihydropyridine calcium channel blocker amlodipine: review of the evidence. *Atherosclerosis* 165: 191–199, 2002

30 Massart PE, Donckier J, Kyselovic J, Godfraind T, Heyndrickx GR and Wibo M. Carvedilol and lacidipine prevent cardiac hypertrophy and endothelin-1 gene overexpression after aortic banding. *Hypertension* 34: 1197–1201, 1999

31 Matsumori A. Calcium channel blocker-induced protection against cardiovascular damage. *Int J Cardiol* 62 Suppl 2: S39–46, 1997

32 Müller D, Fischli W, Clozel J, Hilgers KS, Bohlender J, Menard J, Busjahn A, Ganten D, Luft FC. Local angiotensin II generation in the rat heart: role of renin uptake. *Circ Res* 82: 13–20, 1998

33 Muller DN, Dechend R, Mervaala EM, Park JK, Schmidt F, Fiebeler A, Theuer J, Breu V, Ganten D, Haller H and Luft FC. NF-kappaB inhibition ameliorates angiotensin II-induced inflammatory damage in rats. *Hypertension* 35: 193–201, 2000

34 Nakamura K, Fushimi K, Kouchi H, Mihara K, Miyazaki M, Ohe T and Namba M. Inhibitory effects of antioxidants on neonatal rat cardiac myocyte hypertrophy induced by tumor necrosis factor-alpha and angiotensin II. *Circulation* 98: 794–799, 1998

35 Nakamura T, Obata J, Kuroyanagi R, Kimura H, Ikeda Y, Takano H, Naito A, Sato T and Yoshida Y. Involvement of angiotensin II in glomerusclerosis of stroke-prone spontaneously hypertensive rats. *Kidney Int Suppl* 55: S109–112, 1996

36 Nakazono K, Watanabe N, Matsuno K, Sasaki J, Sato T and Inoue M. Does superoxide underlie the pathogenesis of hypertension? *Proc Natl Acad Sci USA* 88: 10045–10048, 1991

37 Napoli C, Chiariello M, Palumbo G and Ambrosio G. Calcium-channel blockers inhibit human low-density lipoprotein oxidation by oxygen radicals. *Cardiovasc Drugs Ther* 10: 417–424, 1996

38 Napoli C and Ignarro LJ. Nitric oxide-releasing drugs. *Annu Rev Pharmacol Toxicol* 43: 97–123,

2003
39 Napoli C, Salomone S, Godfraind T, Palinski W, Capuzzi DM, Palumbo G, D'Armiento FP, Donzelli R, de Nigris F, Capizzi RL et al. 1,4-Dihydropyridine calcium channel blockers inhibit plasma and LDL oxidation and formation of oxidation-specific epitopes in the arterial wall and prolong survival in stroke-prone spontaneously hypertensive rats. *Stroke* 30: 1907–1915, 1999
40 Rojstaczer N and Triggle DJ. Structure-function relationships of calcium antagonists. Effect on oxidative modification of low density lipoprotein. *Biochem Pharmacol* 51: 141–150, 1996
41 Ruilope LM and Schiffrin EL. Blood pressure control and benefits of antihypertensive therapy: does it make a difference which agents we use? *Hypertension* 38: 537–542, 2001
42 Ruwhof C, van Wamel JT, Noordzij LA, Aydin S, Harper JC and van der Laarse A. Mechanical stress stimulates phospholipase C activity and intracellular calcium ion levels in neonatal rat cardiomyocytes. *Cell Calcium* 29: 73–83, 2001
43 Sabbatini M, Leonardi A, Testa R, Tomassoni D, Vitaioli L and Amenta F. Effects of dihydropyridine-type Ca^{2+} antagonists on the renal arterial tree in spontaneously hypertensive rats. *J Cardiovasc Pharmacol* 39: 39–48, 2002
44 Sabbatini M, Vitaioli L, Baldoni E and Amenta F. Nephroprotective effect of treatment with calcium channel blockers in spontaneously hypertensive rats. *J Pharmacol Exp Ther* 294: 948–954, 2000
45 Sadoshima J and Izumo S. Signal transduction pathways of angiotensin II—induced c-fos gene expression in cardiac myocytes *in vitro*. Roles of phospholipid-derived second messengers. *Circ Res* 73: 424–438, 1993
46 Sadoshima J, Qiu Z, Morgan JP and Izumo S. Angiotensin II and other hypertrophic stimuli mediated by G protein-coupled receptors activate tyrosine kinase, mitogen-activated protein kinase, and 90-kD S6 kinase in cardiac myocytes. The critical role of Ca^{2+}-dependent signaling. *Circ Res* 76: 1–15, 1995
47 Salomone S, Morel N and Godfraind T. A therapeutic dosage of amlodipine prevents vascular hyporeactivity induced in rats by lipopolysaccharide. *Naunyn Schmiedebergs Arch Pharmacol* 357: 252–259, 1998
48 Salomone S, Silva CL, Morel N and Godfraind T. Facilitation of the vasorelaxant action of calcium antagonists by basal nitric oxide in depolarized artery. *Naunyn Schmiedebergs Arch Pharmacol* 354: 505–512, 1996
49 Schultz Jel J, Witt SA, Glascock BJ, Nieman ML, Reiser PJ, Nix SL, Kimball TR and Doetschman T. TGF-beta1 mediates the hypertrophic cardiomyocyte growth induced by angiotensin II. *J Clin Invest* 109: 787–796, 2002
50 Sei CA, Irons CE, Sprenkle AB, McDonough PM, Brown JH and Glembotski CC. The alpha-adrenergic stimulation of atrial natriuretic factor expression in cardiac myocytes requires calcium influx, protein kinase C, and calmodulin-regulated pathways. *J Biol Chem* 266: 15910–15916, 1991
51 Sobala G, Menzel EJ and Sinzinger H. Calcium antagonists as inhibitors of *in vitro* low density lipoprotein oxidation and glycation. *Biochem Pharmacol* 61: 373–379, 2001
52 Szmigielski A, Szmigielska H, Zalewska-Kaszubska J and Marczak G. The cooperation between the influx of extracellular calcium and alpha1-adrenoceptor-induced translocation of protein kinase C. *Pharmacol Res* 36: 211–219, 1997
53 Touyz RM, Fareh J, Thibault G, Tolloczko B, Lariviere R and Schiffrin EL. Modulation of Ca^{2+} transients in neonatal and adult rat cardiomyocytes by angiotensin II and endothelin-1. *Am J Physiol* 270: H857–868, 1996
54 Ursini F. Tissue protection by lacidipine: insight from redox behavior. *J Cardiovasc Pharmacol* 30: S28–S30, 1997
55 Varagic J, Susic D and Frohlich ED. Cilnidipine improves spontaneously hypertensive rat coronary hemodynamics without altering cardiovascular mass and collagen. *J Hypertens* 20: 317–322, 2002
56 Wang XQ and Vaziri ND. Erythropoietin depresses nitric oxide synthase expression by human endothelial cells. *Hypertension* 33: 894–899, 1999
57 Xu B, Xiao-hong L, Lin G, Queen L and Ferro A. Amlodipine, but not verapamil or nifedipine, dilates rabbit femoral artery largely through a nitric oxide- and kinin-dependent mechanism. *Br J Pharmacol* 136: 375–382, 2002
58 Yamazaki T, Komuro I, Kudoh S, Zou Y, Nagai R, Aikawa R, Uozumi H and Yazaki Y. Role of ion channels and exchangers in mechanical stretch-induced cardiomyocyte hypertrophy. *Circ Res* 82:

430–437, 1998
59 Yamazaki T, Komuro I, Zou Y, Kudoh S, Shiojima I, Mizuno T, Hiroi Y, Nagai R and Yazaki Y. Efficient inhibition of the development of cardiac remodeling by a long-acting calcium antagonist amlodipine. *Hypertension* 31: 32–38, 1998
60 Yamazaki T, Tobe K, Hoh E, Maemura K, Kaida T, Komuro I, Tamemoto H, Kadowaki T, Nagai R and Yazaki Y. Mechanical loading activates mitogen-activated protein kinase and S6 peptide kinase in cultured rat cardiac myocytes. *J Biol Chem* 268: 12069–12076, 1993
61 Young M, Fullerton M, Dilley R and Funder J. Mineralocorticoids, hypertension, and cardiac fibrosis. *J Clin Invest* 93: 2578–2583, 1994
62 Zalba G, San Jose G, Moreno MU, Fortuno MA, Fortuno A, Beaumont FJ and Diez J. Oxidative stress in arterial hypertension: role of NAD(P)H oxidase. *Hypertension* 38: 1395–1399, 2001
63 Zanchetti A, Bond MG, Hennig M, Neiss A, Mancia G, Dal Palu C, Hansson L, Magnani B, Rahn KH, Reid JL et al. Calcium antagonist lacidipine slows down progression of asymptomatic carotid atherosclerosis: principal results of the European Lacidipine Study on Atherosclerosis (ELSA), a randomized, double-blind, long-term trial. *Circulation* 106: 2422–2427, 2002
64 Zhang T, Johnson EN, Gu Y, Morissette MR, Sah VP, Gigena MS, Belke DD, Dillmann WH, Rogers TB, Schulman H et al. The cardiac-specific nuclear delta(B) isoform of Ca^{2+}/calmodulin-dependent protein kinase II induces hypertrophy and dilated cardiomyopathy associated with increased protein phosphatase 2A activity. *J Biol Chem* 277: 1261–1267, 2002
65 Zhang X and Hintze TH. Amlodipine releases nitric oxide from canine coronary microvessels: an unexpected mechanism of action of a calcium channel-blocking agent. *Circulation* 97: 576–580, 1998
66 Zhang X, Kichuk MR, Mital S, Oz M, Michler R, Nasjletti A, Kaley G and Hintze TH. Amlodipine promotes kinin-mediated nitric oxide production in coronary microvessels of failing human hearts. *Am J Cardiol* 84: 27L-33L, 1999
67 Zhang X, Recchia FA, Bernstein R, Xu X, Nasjletti A and Hintze TH. Kinin-mediated coronary nitric oxide production contributes to the therapeutic action of angiotensin-converting enzyme and neutral endopeptidase inhibitors and amlodipine in the treatment in heart failure. *J Pharmacol Exp Ther* 288: 742–751, 1999
68 Zhang XP, Loke KE, Mital S, Chahwala S and Hintze TH. Paradoxical release of nitric oxide by an L-type calcium channel antagonist, the R+ enantiomer of amlodipine. *J Cardiovasc Pharmacol* 39: 208–214, 2002

From early clinical studies to randomized controlled clinical trials

As already mentioned above, the therapeutic indications of calcium antagonists were supported by considering their vasorelaxant properties, at a time when the current hypothesis was that some cardiovascular pathology resulted from reduced tissue perfusion. In the present chapter the first clinical studies, on which have been justified the clinical indication will be briefly reviewed. Those studies enrolled a limited number of subjects. Their conclusions have been challenged by some authors [28, 87]. The actual clinical use is based on large multicenter clinical trials and have been defined in several guidelines that are not reviewed in this book. In this chapter, we will review studies dealing with the cardiovascular system. We shall address the action of calcium antagonists in cardiac ischaemia (stable effort angina, circadian rhythm of angina and silent ischaemia, angina caused by coronary spasm: vasospastic angina, unstable angina and acute myocardial infarction), their action in cardiac arrhythmias, in hypertension and atherosclerosis.

The action of calcium antagonists in cardiac ischaemia

Chronic stable effort angina

Agents other than nitrates may efficiently treat stable angina. Beta-blockers have preceded calcium antagonists in that respect, therefore several trials have attempted to evaluate the relative efficiency of calcium antagonists by comparison with propranolol as well as their action over placebo. The criteria usually adopted in order to assess the efficacy of the drugs were the following:

1) decrease of nitroglycerin consumption
2) reduction of the frequency of angina episodes
3) prolongation of exercise time
4) increase of work capacity
5) ST recovery time, measuring myocardial ischaemia following exercise by the duration of ST depression
6) degree of ST depression at a defined workload, providing the demonstrated reproducibility of this depression

The action of verapamil

Verapamil, which was synthetized in 1962 [36], was initially described as a coronodilatator. It has therefore been introduced to treat angina, as soon as 1963 by Tschirdewahn and Klepzig [132]. In 1968, it was considered as a beta-blocker [50a, 76], but was later characterized as a calcium antagonist by Fleckenstein et al. [25a]. Several controlled clinical trials have established the efficacy of verapamil over placebo [81].

Most of the controlled clinical trials (CRTs) dealt with comparison of verapamil *versus* propranolol, using as an objective criteria the action on ST-segment depression. Figure 1 illustrates a theoretical exemple of changes in ST segment during and after exercise [43]. The usual procedure was to estimate the duration of a given work on the appearance of conventional electrocardiographic positivity (1 mm ST depression). As reported by de Ponti and Vincenzi [21], the duration of work, expressed in second, increased significantly after verapamil administration and this effect was dose-dependent. Furthermore, after intravenous injection, the effective dose of verapamil was much lower than the dose required per oral route, an indication that the bioavailability of verapamil is reduced *per os*. In pharmacokinetic studies, the bioavailability of verapamil in human was estimated of 22% [24]. This estimate was confirmed in functional studies, when the reduction of ST depression for a given workload was measured in patients treated with various doses of verapamil [43].

Comparison of verapamil with beta-blockers

Comparison with beta-blockers has been performed in controlled studies by measuring the reduction of pain attacks or of nitroglycerin consumption. It appeared that verapamil 360 mg/day was equiactive to propranolol 300 mg/day [25, 26, 46, 53, 61, 100, 101, 126]. Since there is a dose-dependency for both agents, it is obvious that the superiority of one agent against the other cannot be estimated by comparing a single dose of each drug. When other criteria were used, it appeared that if beta-blockers delayed ECG alterations more than angina, verapamil, and nifedipine delayed angina more than ECG alterations, indicating the existence of a qualitative difference between beta-blockers and calcium antagonists [21]. The significance of this observation is still unclear, but it makes obvious that comparison between various agents cannot be based on one single parameter.

The action of nifedipine and diltiazem in stable angina

Nifedipine action has been widely investigated in patients suffering of stable angina. From earlier studies, its action over placebo appeared to be highly significant (see for instance Terry [128], Sherman and Liang [114]). Exercise-induced ST segment depression was reduced after 20 mg nifedipine (sublingual) as Figure 2 illustrates [43]. This effect was also observed after oral administration and it was dose-related [43]. This beneficial response was also evoked after intravenous and intracoronary administration. When given orally at 20 mg three times per day, nifedipine action persisted during prolonged

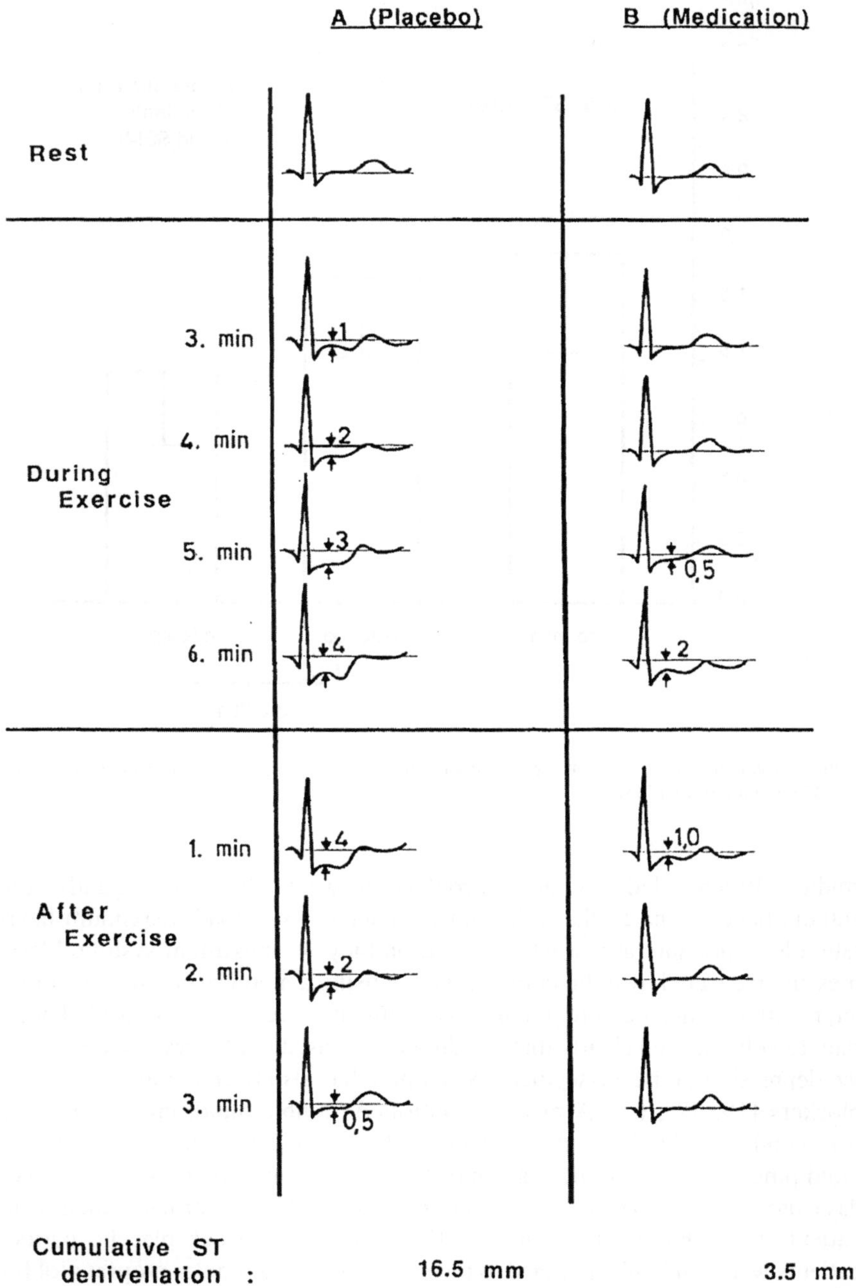

Figure 1. Theoretical illustration of ST-segment depression during exercise and of its recovery after exercise in patients with stable effort angina treated by placebo and effective medication (modified from [43]).

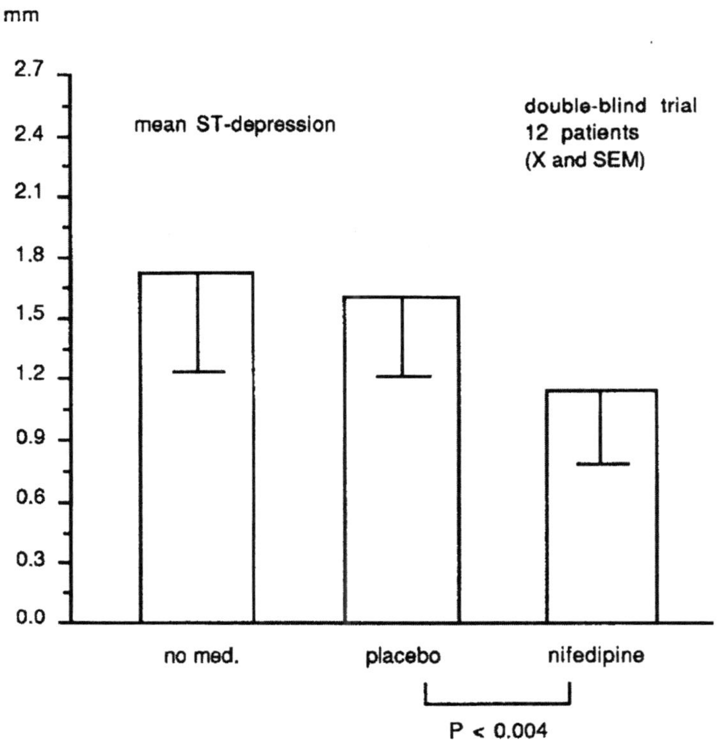

Figure 2. Reduction of ST-segment depression after nifedipine (20 mg sublingual). Double blind trial (n = 12); modified from [43].

studies. When nifedipine and nitroglycerin were given sublingually, the authors have estimated the following parameters: workload, maximum heart rate, blood pressure at rest while seated on bicycle, maximum systolic blood pressure measured by indirect measurement using a mercury column manometer, maximum rate pressure product, ST-segment depression at controlled heart rate. Results showed clearly that nifedipine increased total work and decreased the depression of the ST-segment. Nifedipine has also been compared to beta-blockers [19, 42a, 62]. A placebo-controlled, double-blind, crossover study was conducted by Higginbotham et al. [42a] to determine the effects of nifedipine (60 to 90 mg per day) monotherapy and propranolol (240 mg per day) monotherapy on symptoms, angina threshold, and cardiac function in patients with chronic stable angina. Following a two-week placebo period, patients were randomly assigned to receive either nifedipine or propranolol for a five-week treatment period, after which they crossed over to the alternative regimen. All 21 patients were men with chronic stable angina pectoris, 13 of whom had symptoms both at rest and on exertion. New York Heart Association functional class improved in patients taking either nifedipine or propranolol, and nitroglycerin consumption decreased with both treatments compared with placebo. Nifedipine significantly delayed the onset of chest pain and 1 mm of ST-segment depression during bicycle exercise; increases with propranolol were smaller and not statistically significant. Nine patients had a preferential clinical response to nifedipine compared with six patients to propranolol; this was unrelated to the presence or absence of pain at rest or to any baseline haemodynamic finding. Nifedipine and propranolol were equally effective in relieving exertional ischaemia as shown by improvement in radionuclide ejection fraction at identical workload. Exercise wall motion, assessed by a semi-quantitative wall motion score, also improved with both drugs. Propranolol treatment decreased exercise cardiac output by 14 percent ($p = 0.01$) through its effect on heart rate. In contrast, nifedipine treatment had no negative effect on cardiac output. According to the authors, nifedipine was more effective on several measurements than propranolol when administered as single drug therapy in stable angina and had the advantage of preserving cardiac output during exercise [42].

Dargie et al. have compared the antianginal effects of nifedipine and propranolol, alone or in combination, with those of placebo in a double-blind clinical trial that included 16 patients with chronic stable angina triggered by exertion. A low dose and a high dose of the active drugs were administered (nifedipine, 30 and 60 mg/day; propranolol, 240 and 280 mg/day). Precordial exercise mapping and continuous electrocardiographic recordings were used to assess objective response to therapy, and the patients were asked to keep a diary of episodes of chest pain and consumption of nitroglycerin tablets for subjective appraisal. Both frequency of chest pain and nitroglycerin consumption were significantly reduced by each of the active drugs when compared with placebo, and the combination of nifedipine and propranolol added significantly to the effectiveness. Reductions in area of ischaemia and number of episodes of ST segment depression on 48-hour ambulatory electrocardiographic monitoring corroborated the efficacy of each active treatment with respect to placebo. Nearly 60 percent of all episodes of ST segment depression were painless and responded to the active treatment in the same manner as did the episodes associated with chest pain. Side-effects were mild and all treatments were well tolerated. The objective methods used allowed for clear-cut differentiation of treatment effects with the various regimens. Although the two drugs alone were significantly more effective than placebo, their combination provided an even greater improvement (p less than 0.005), and therefore it appears to be a safe and effective form of treatment for chronic stable angina [19].

However, with large doses of nifedipine, side-effects were found in patients. Earliest observations indicated that short-acting nifedipine may provoke cardiac ischaemia, observations reconfirmed some years later [28]. The proportion of patients who have to experience this chest pain varied according to various studies: between 10% for Stone et al. [122] and less than 1% in a retrospective review of Terry [128] over 3,000 patients. A recent study [87] has bet-

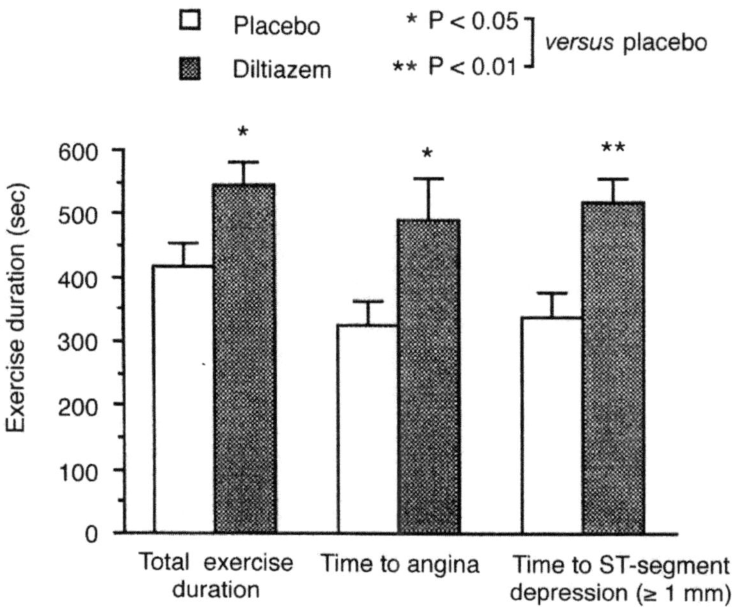

Figure 3. Effect of diltiazem on criteria usually adopted in order to assess the efficacy of drugs in stable angina; modified from [108].

ter quantified the proportion of cardiac ischaemia crisis; this has prompted a revision of the mode of administration of nifedipine, which is nowadays given by oral route in slow releasing (GITS) preparations.

Diltiazem has also been studied in stable angina and compared to placebo and propranolol. Usually, those comparisons used diltiazem 9 mg four times daily, propranolol 60 mg four times daily against placebo. Figure 3 [108] illustrates the significant effect of diltiazem on three parameters: total exercice duration, time to angina, and time to ST-segment depression. According to Schroeder et al. [108], diltiazem decreased the sub-maximal and maximal degree of exercise-induced ST segment depression by over 50% compared to placebo (P less than 0.01 *versus* placebo). Diltiazem resulted in a higher exercise left ventricular ejection fraction compared to placebo, propranolol or the combination of diltiazem or propranolol (all less than P less than 0.05). Sinus bradycardia occurred in patients on the high-dose combination therapy and required dose reduction. This bradycardia also observed with verapamil is likely related to blockade of Ca_v3 channels [123].

Side-effects of verapamil, nifedipine and diltiazem observed during those studies

Drug-induced cardiac ischaemia results from a sympathetic reflex in response to a rapid lowering of blood pressure, which may be due to fast-acting agents.

The more frequent side-effects of nifedipine, verapamil and diltiazem were related to their action on smooth muscles; with verapamil, about 70% of the patients complained of constipation; with nifedipine, the major side-effect was ankle oedema, a side-effect also reported with diltiazem. Due to their potent negative inotropic effect, overdosage of verapamil and diltiazem have been avoided in order not to aggravate symptoms of cardiac insufficency.

The proportion of subjects who had to discontinue one of those three agents due to those side-effects varied between 3 and 5%.

Circadian rhythm of angina and silent ischaemia

Several studies using out-of-hospital ambulatory electrocardiographic STsegment monitoring have shown that several ischaemic episodes are not associated with pain [9, 10]. They exhibit a circadian rhythm with clusters of ischaemic episodes in the early morning hours. ST-segment changes similar to those occurring with pain attacks have been termed silent ischaemia. Patients with silent ischaemia are usually divided into three groups. Those with only silent ischaemia who never have angina and have not had a myocardial infarction, represent a very negligible group of patients identified by chance on Holter monitoring. A second group of patients develop silent ischaemia after a myocardial infarction. The third group comprised those with typical angina pectoris and episodes of silent ischaemia. This third group is the largest one because most angina patients have silent episodes and often more silent than painful episodes. According to Taylor et al. [127] a clear circadian rhythm exists for angina, with the frequency of attacks increasing during the mid-morning and mid-afternoon hours. This pattern is comparable to circadian rhythms previously reported for the incidence of myocardial infarction and sudden cardiac death. The frequency of angina attacks precipitated by physical exertion showed a more pronounced circadian pattern compared to non-exertional angina. Beta-adrenergic blocking agents did not abolish the circadian rhythm of total angina and exertional angina attacks. Figure 4 illustrates this circadian rhythm of angina attack, showing a peak between 10.00 and 12.00 a.m. and a second peak between 2.00 and 3.00 p.m. [127]. Taylor et al. have evaluated the action of amlodipine on the circadian rhythm of angina in a pool data issued from nine multicenter double-blind placebo controlled studies. Placebo and amlodipine did not change the circadian rhythm, but amlodipine reduced significantly the anginal attacks when compared to placebo ($p < 0.0001$). Similar observations were made with nifedipine and other dihydropyridines. For instance, Nesto et al. [77, 78] conducted a randomized, double-blind, crossover study in patients to assess the effect of nifedipine *versus* placebo on total ischaemic activity and circadian distribution of ischaemic episodes. After baseline exercise treadmill testing and 48-hour ambulatory electrocardiographic ST-segment monitoring, patients received either nifedipine (mean dose, 80 mg/day) or placebo administered four times per day, with

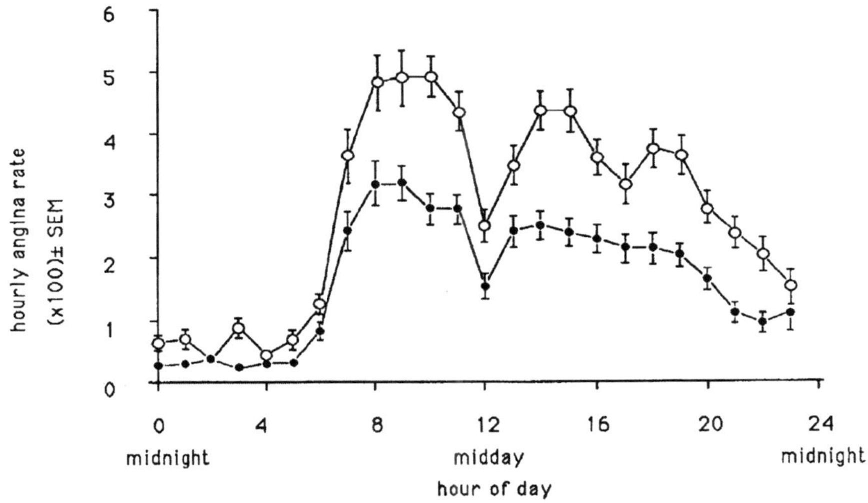

Figure 4. Circadian rhythm of angina in patients treated with placebo (○) and amlodipine (●); modified from [127].

the initial dose taken immediately upon arising in the morning. Patients were maintained on a stable dose of each study drug for seven days, after which they underwent repeat exercise treadmill testing and 48-hour ambulatory electrocardiography. During exercise treadmill testing, greater exercise duration was achieved by patients receiving nifedipine than by those receiving placebo (421 ± 121 *versus* 353 ± 155 seconds, respectively; p less than 0.05). Time to greater than or equal to 1 mm ST depression was significantly greater with nifedipine (282 ± 146 seconds) than at baseline (130 ± 72 seconds, p less than 0.003) and with placebo (150 ± 98 seconds, p less than 0.0005). During ambulatory electrocardiographic monitoring, nifedipine reduced both the total number of ischaemic episodes (18 *versus* 54 at baseline and 63 with placebo; p less than 0.02 for both) and the total duration of ischaemia (260 *versus* 874 at baseline and 927 minutes with placebo; p less than 0.02 for both). The surge of ischaemia between 06:00 and 12:00 noted at baseline and during placebo therapy was nearly abolished during nifedipine treatment. Nifedipine at this dosage, administered in this manner, was effective in reducing total ischaemic activity and prevented morning surges of ischaemic episodes.

Similarly, prolonged treatment during three weeks with nisoldipine at the dose of 10 mg/once daily produced a marked reduction of the duration of episodes with the most remarkable reduction in the early morning hours [96]. In those earliest studies, the long acting agents such as nisoldipine and amlodipine were efficient when administered once daily, when the short acting nifedipine was given three times daily.

Angina caused by coronary spasm: vasospastic angina

Vasospastic angina, also termed variant angina is a clinical entity characterized by angina crisis occurring predominantly at rest and associated with ST-segment elevation during the ischaemic episode (also named Prinzmetal's variant angina). The significance of pain at rest associated with reversible ST-segment elevation has become somewhat ambiguous since the time of the original description, because the response to therapy and the clinical outcome among patients who share this clinical characteristic may likewise be quite varied. Angina pectoris at rest with preservation of excercise capacity has become the most meaningful definition of Prinzmetal's variant angina as pointed out by Opie [81]. Frequently, angina at rest is confused with unstable angina which merges into pre-infarction angina and threatened myocardial infarction. Both angina at rest and unstable angina are marked by spontaneous anginal pain at rest not evoked by any known external factor. Yet it is particularly important to distinguish angina at rest with short-lived episodes of chest pain usually less than 15 minutes from the longer lasting and much more serious attacks of true pre-infarction unstable angina. Ergonovine has been used as a diagnostic agent to provoke coronary artery spasm. Coronary angiography has revealed that a small dose of ergonovine given to patients with variant angina usually produced focal spasm caused by segmental abnormalities of the coronary artery [65] There are regional distribution of the sensitivity to ergonovine in patients with variant angina, the various regions of the coronary epicardial vessels presenting a different degree in responsiveness to ergonovine [85, 86, 124].

Clinical trials have been designed to test the action of diltiazem, nifedipine and verapamil in Prinzmetal's variant angina. In a randomized, double-blind crossover design, it was observed that diltiazem at a dosage of 240 mg daily decreased the frequency of episodes of variant angina and the number of nitroglycerin tablets required for pain relief, and increased the percentage of pain-free days compared with placebo [98, 99]. Similarly, Pepine et al. [91] found from angina diaries during a controlled two-week crossover trial that daily episodes of angina at rest decreased from 1.73 episodes with placebo to 0.3 episodes with diltiazem 120 mg daily and to 0.16 episodes with diltiazem 240 mg daily ($p < 0.05$). Similar decreases in nitroglycerin consumption were observed. In a multicenter clinical trial Schroeder et al. [107] also noted a dose-dependent decrease in anginal frequency and nitroglycerin consumption, although the magnitude of response was less than that observed in earlier studies. Tilmant et al. [131] reported that diltiazem (360 mg daily) abolished all spontaneous episodes of variant angina, although six of the 11 patients still developed vasospasm in response to ergonovine challenge. Waters et al. [135] had similarly observed that an ergonovine challenge could still provoke spasm in 16 of 27 patients pretreated with diltiazem 120 mg every eight hours, but that in 11 of theses 16 patients the dosage of ergonovine required to provoke vasospasm was much higher than that necessary when the patient was not treated with diltiazem. Variant angina occurred during none of the 30 treatment periods associated with a negative ergonovine test. These controlled studies illustrate the clinical efficacy of calcium antagonists in the treatment of variant angina. There are numerous confirmations, few of them are reported below. With a historical pre-treatment period as a baseline, Schroeder et al. [109] observed that prolonged treatment with diltiazem (mean daily dosage 270 mg, mean follow-up 19.6 months) decreased anginal frequency by 94% and decreased the incidence of cardiovascular events (myocardial infarction, sudden death or hospitalization to rule out myocardial infarction) by 91% in patients with variant angina. Previtali et al. [94] performed a double-blind, placebo controlled crossover trial comparing nifedipine (10 to 20 mg every four hours) with placebo in 14 patients with frequent angina at rest and ST-segment anomaly. Most of these patients probably had Prinzmetal's variant angina, although some others could suffer from unstable angina. In 13 patients, reversible ST-segment elevation was observed during angina at rest and an ergonovine challenge provoked vasospasm in seven of eight patients in whom the test was performed. The authors have observed that nifedipine produced a highly significant decrease in the mean daily number of episodes of myocardial ischaemia compared with results of placebo (mean 1.1 episodes/48 hours *versus* 20.9 episodes/48 hours, respectively, $p < 0.02$). Schick et al. [106] withdrew nifedipine therapy from 38 patients with Prinzmetal's variant angina in a randomized, placebo-controlled, double-blind manner. They reported that those patients randomized to placebo treatment experienced a significant increase in their angina episodes compared with the number observed during active therapy (increase of 2.8 episodes/week, $p < 0.003$), as well as an increase in nitroglycerin usage (increase of 0.5 tablets/week, $p < 0.03$). The randomized phase was terminated prematurely because of intolerable increases in angina frequency in seven to 19 patients taking placebo and only one of 19 patients taking nifedipine ($p = 0.02$). Double-blind therapy was considered to be effective in 16 out of 19 patients receiving nifedipine compared with only three out of 19 receiving placebo ($p < 0.001$).

Parodi et al. [89] treated 12 patients with frequent episodes of resting ischaemia associated with reversible ST-segment deviation with verapamil, most of whom manifested evidence of variant angina. Six of the patients exhibited ST-segment elevation with pain at rest. Six patients also underwent coronary angiography during an episode of angina and demonstrated coronary vasospasm in the coronary artery subserving the area of ST-segment change. Oral verapamil (480 mg daily) significantly decreased episodes of ischaemia regardless of whether the ST-segment became elevated or depressed during ischaemia, or whether or not symptoms of angina accompanied the ST-segment deviation. The total number of ischaemic episodes in a 48 hours period was decreased from 126 during placebo therapy to 24 during verapamil therapy ($p < 0.003$). In another study, the long-term response to verapamil therapy has been evaluated in 16 patients using a titrated dosage schedule (mean oral dosage 415 mg daily, range 240 to 480) and an eight-month, double-blind crossover design [47]. During treatment with verapamil, the frequency of anginal episodes per week decreased when compared with that observed during placebo treatment (from 12.6 to 1.7 episodes, $p < 0.01$) as did weekly nitroglycerin consumption (from 14.4 to 2.1 tablets, $p < 0.05$). The number of daily episodes of ST-segment deviation also was significantly decreased during verapamil therapy (from 33.1 to 7.7 episodes, $p < 0.01$). No major side-effects were observed.

Unstable angina and acute myocardial infarction

Unstable angina is a syndrome intermediate in severity between stable angina and myocardial infarction. According to Braunwald [13] unstable angina is a clinical syndrome, analogous to hypertension; it is not a specific disease, such as pneumococcal pneumonia. Unstable angina is commonly classified by use of simple clinical descriptors, such as the presence or absence of ischaemic chest discomfort at rest, as well as ECG changes and biochemical markers of myocardial injury during and after ischaemic episodes. Although these clinical descriptors are helpful in estimating prognosis and are used widely in determining the intensity of treatment, they provide little information regarding the cause of the syndrome. Causes of unstable angina, which are not mutually exclusive, some patients having two or more causes are the following: non-occlusive thrombus on pre-existing plaque, dynamic obstruction (coronary spasm or vasoconstriction), progressive mechanical obstruction, inflammation and/or infection, secondary unstable angina.

Electrocardiographic signs are compatible with ischaemia but not directly with diagnostic of infarction. Both postmortem investigations of coronary artery and coronary angiographies have given information on the coronary changes that cause instability in coronary artery disease and are responsible for unstable angina. It is agreed that the basic lesion in coronary artery disease is a slow deposition of atheromatous material leading to hardening or thickening of the arterial wall [51]. In the hard atherosclerotic arterial wall, a fissure or ulceration may suddenly develop without any warning or recognized triggering factor. This lesion will result in an intramural haemorrhage as well as an adhesion and aggregation of platelets as these become exposed to collagen in the vessel wall. The resulting platelet plug causes a further reduction of the coronary flow. This evolution may result in a definite occlusion of the vessels with a Q-wave myocardial infarction. In view of the complexity and of the crescendo of the pathology, the classical therapy includes bed rest and heart rate sedation in the case sub-endocardial (non Q-wave infarction) in which case there is no complete cessation of blood flow. It is agreed that patients, which in spite of medical therapy, still suffer from severe symptoms after two to four days, require investigation for emergency PTCA or surgery. Thrombolytic therapy and aspirin are also considered in such a case. Several trials have attempted to define the role of calcium antagonists. Some are summarized below.

Diltiazem: In early non-controlled trials of angina at rest, diltiazem has been effective in preventing episodes of resting pain [75, 138], although efficacy appeared to be greater in patients whose pain was accompanied by ST-segment elevation due perhaps to Prinzmetal's variant angina [75]. Andre-Fouet et al. [3] evaluated the response to diltiazem or propranolol therapy in 70 patients with unstable angina, defined as of recent (<1 month) appearance or aggravation of angina at rest; 24 patients (34%) had only angina at rest; the remaining 46 patients experienced angina both with exertion and at rest. Patients were divided into those who developed ST-segment elevation during pain [29] and those who developed ST-segment depression or T inversion during pain [41]. Therapy was then randomly assigned to each group to either diltiazem or propranolol in maximally tolerated dosages. Both diltiazem (mean daily dosage 282 mg) and propranolol (mean daily dosage 158 mg) evoked a 60% to 85% decrease in the frequency of daily angina episodes in the entire group of patients. Among the subset of patients who manifested only angina at rest without exertional angina, diltiazem treatment caused a 83% decrease in episodes of angina ($p < 0{,}001$), whereas propranolol had no therapeutic effect at all. This latter subgroup probably represents patients with Prinzmetal's variant angina in whom it is known that calcium antagonists, but no β-blockers, can prevent episodes of coronary vasospasm.

Theroux et al. [130] have reported the results of a randomized trial comparing diltiazem and propranolol in the treatment of unstable angina, in which patients with Prinzmetal's variant angina, defined as ST-segment elevation accompanying angina at rest, were distinctly excluded. Both diltiazem and propranolol decreased the daily frequency of angina by about 65% ($p < 0{,}05$ for each drug compared with baseline, difference not significant between the two treatments). During long-term follow-up (mean 5.1 months), the clinical outcome was similar for the calcium antagonist and the β-blocker treatment regimens (death 4%, development of infarction 10%, coronary artery bypass grafting 40% and angina 32%). This suggested that coronary artery spasm alone might not be the main factor determining the outcome in unstable angina when patients with Prinzmetal's variant angina are excluded. If vasospasm had been the principal pathophysiologic mechanism of unstable angina, then one would anticipate that effective treatment of vasospasm with diltiazem would favorably alter the outcome compared with the outcome in the patients treated with propranolol, which does not treat the vasospasm.

Nifedipine: Early uncontrolled studies [8, 44, 72, 113, 121] reported that the addition of nifedipine therapy in patients with unstable angina refractory to β-blockers and nitrates was associated with a dramatic decrease in the frequency of angina at rest. The role of nifedipine in the management of unstable angina has become clearer from the results of carefully designed clinical trials. For instance, Muller et al. [73] studied 126 patients with unstable angina who had initial therapy with either nifedipine or conventional therapy (β-blockers and nitrates), each in maximally-tolerated doses. There was no significant difference between the two groups in time to relief of pain, decrease in daily anginal frequency or daily nitroglycerin consumption, development of myocardial infarction or six-month mortality. However, among the 67 patients who were taking propranolol when they presented to the hospital, symptoms were more readily controlled when nifedipine was added to the regimen than when more propranolol was added. Conversely, among the other 59 patients who were taking nifedipine, treatment with propranolol and a nitrate led to rapid pain relief, very likely because nifedipine, as monotherapy, was associated with a reflex tachycardia increasing oxygen myocardial demand, this indicates that from earliest studies, the major side-effect of nifedipine on myocardial oxygen demand was already identified. The role of nifedipine in the treatment of patients with unstable angina refractory to maximal β-blockers and nitrate therapy is obvious from several studies. For instance, Gerstenblith et al. [30] have added nifedipine or placebo to the maximally-tolerated combination of β-blocker and nitrates in a randomized double-blind manner. They observed that the 68 patients who received nifedipine experienced a significant decrease in the symptoms of myocardial ischaemia compared with the 70 patients who received placebo. The magnitude of benefit was most marked among patients who manifested ST-segment elevation accompanying their angina, perhaps patients whose ischaemia was due to vasospasm. Despite the significant benefit in control of symptoms associated with nifedipine therapy, they observed no benefit in the occurence of sudden death or of myocardial infarction in either treatment group over a four-month follow-up (18% in nifedipine group, 20% in placebo group). Thus, nifedipine therapy improved symptoms of ischaemia in patients with unstable angina, especially those concomitantly treated with a β-blocker [34, 73], and also improved left ventricular performance because of its afterload reducing properties. However, it did not appear to influence the incidence of subsequent infarction or death [8, 84, 134]. Early symptomatic response to nifedipine did not appear to predict a decreased incidence of cardiac events.

Verapamil: In several studies, verapamil has been found to be effective as monotherapy in significantly decreasing episodes of ischaemia at rest associated with ST-segment elevation, depression or T wave inversion [7, 16, 66, 89, 90], although in theses studies the distinction was not obvious between patients with Prinzmetal's variant angina due to vasospasm and patients with unstable angina, which may be due to abnormalities in the atherosclerotic plaque or thrombus formation. As far as concerned the long-term efficacy of verapamil therapy for unstable angina, several studies have shown (see for instance Scheidt et al. [105]) that symptomatic improvement was generally well maintained for period of over a year, the incidence of infarction was about 12% and of death about 8%. These results are remarkably similar to the outcome of patients with unstable angina treated with nifedipine [30, 73], and those treated with the older conventional therapy of β-blockers and nitrates alone. It must be recognised that despite their potent action as antianginal agents, calcium antagonists of the first generation, including verapamil, nifedipine and diltiazem, were not demonstrated clearly to be efficient in acute myocardial infarction. However, in two trials [31, 45] from Gibson et al. (1986) and the Danish Study Group (DAVIT II, 1990), one with diltiazem, and the other with verapamil, patients with non Q-wave myocardial infarction and patients with myocardial infarction showed a reduced mortality [31, 32, 45]. Nevertheless, calcium antagonists are not recommended in myocardial infarction.

Iatrogenic ischaemia

Iatrogenic ischaemia may be considered as a cardiac ischaemic state evoked by medical or surgical maneuvers, for instance coronary artery bypass graft surgery (CABG). CABG, the most common cardiac surgical procedure, reduces morbidity and mortality from coronary artery disease [138a]. However, cardiac surgery remains associated with significant complications, including death, myocardial infarction (MI), neurocognitive dysfunction, and acute renal failure. The perioperative phase in patients undergoing coronary artery bypass graft surgery represents a very critical period. Despite improvement of anesthesia and of surgical techniques, incidence of perioperative myocardial ischaemia, such as myocardial infarction or transient myocardial ischaemia is relatively high. Strategies that reduce these events should therefore improve overall outcomes. Several authors have reported that the addition of nifedipine to cardioplegic solution reduced the incidence of myocardial damage. In a randomized study, Seitelberger et al. [111, 112] have divided patients in a group receiving continuous nifedipine infusion (10 µg/kg/hr) from the onset of extra corporal circulation until 24 hours after aortic cross-clamp time. During the same period of time, patients assigned to the control group had continuous nitroglycerin infusion (1 µg/kg/min). The authors have increased the infusion rate in both groups in case of postoperative hypertension. Plasma levels of nifedipine assessed 12 hours after the onset and before the end of the infusion were comprised between 15 and 33 ng/ml, corresponding to concentration ranging between 10^{-7} and 10^{-8} M. Major ischaemic events were significantly reduced by nifedipine, which however had no influence on arrhythmias. There was a significant difference in the serum levels of the cardiospecific enzyme CK-MB between nifedipine and control groups. The increase in the CK-MB levels during the first 4–6 hours after aortic cross-clamp time in both groups indicate a comparable extent of myocardial necrosis due to the surgical procedure itself. However, marked differences in CK-MB levels were observed during period of 36 hours after aortic cross-clamp time. The authors had previously published observations based on nifedipine treatment started at 2 hours after the onset of the reperfusion period showing a less efficient action of nifedipine.

In recent meta-analysis, Wijeysundera et al. [136] have reconsidered the use of CCBs in cardiac surgery. Out of the potential 1,813 studies, they eventually selected 41 studies for their meta-analysis. Of these, 28 studies related to intraoperative complications or those occurring during the first postoperative day. Other studies were for longer periods. Approximately one-half were given DHP therapy, mostly intravenous nifedipine or nicardipine; the rest were given either diltiazem or verapamil. They sought to determine the efficacy of calcium antagonists in reducing death, myocardial infarction (MI), ischaemia, and supraventricular tachyarrhythmia (SVT) after cardiac surgery. Their analysis showed that calcium antagonists significantly reduced MI (odds ratio [OR] 0.58, 95% confidence interval [CI] 0.37 to 0.91; $p = 0.02$) and ischaemia (OR 0.53, 95% CI 0.39 to 0.72; $p < 0.001$). Non-dihydropyridines significantly reduced SVT (OR 0.62, 95% CI 0.41 to 0.93; $p = 0.02$). Calcium antagonists were associated with trends toward decreased mortality during aorto-coronary bypass (OR 0.66, 95% CI 0.26 to 1.70, $p = 0.4$).

This meta-analysis has been carefully analyzed by Opie [79] who concluded that this surgical study fits into a general pattern: CCBs have anti-ischaemic properties for which they can safely be used, without there being sufficient long-term hard outcome data to be sure of effects on mortality. Nevertheless, Lionel Opie notes; 'the specific message of the present meta-analysis is quite clear: CCBs may be safer and have more benefit in cardiac surgery than often supposed'. As this will be examined later, ALLHAT [29] and major meta-analyses of outcome when CCBs were used for hypertension, all agree that there were no differences in major cardiac events or total mortality when CCBs were compared with conventional therapy by diuretics and/or beta-blockers.

This study is in agreement with data obtained from the trial named CAPARES. The Coronary Angioplasty Amlodipine Restenosis (CAPARES) Study was to investigate the effect of amlodipine on restenosis and clinical outcome in patients undergoing percutaneous transluminal coronary angioplasty (PTCA). In a prospective, double-blind design, 635 patients were randomized to 10 mg of amlodipine or placebo. Pre-treatment with the study drug started two weeks before PTCA and continued until four months after PTCA. The primary angiographic end-point was loss in minimal lumen diameter (MLD) from post-PTCA to follow-up, as assessed by quantitative coronary angiography (QCA). Clinical end-points were death, myocardial infarction, coronary artery bypass graft surgery and repeat PTCA (major adverse clinical events). There were no differences in clinical and angiographic baseline characteristics between the treatment groups. Ischaemia and angina were equally distributed before PTCA. Amlodipine therapy starting two weeks before PTCA did not reduce luminal loss, but the incidence of repeat PTCA and the composite major adverse clinical events were significantly reduced during the four-month follow-up period after PTCA with amlodipine as compared with placebo. Despite the fact that no difference in restenosis was found between the groups at follow-up, the incidence of angina was significantly lower in the amlodipine group compared with the placebo group both early and late after PTCA ($P = .04$ and .03). Exercise-induced ischaemia was reduced by 40% ($P = .009$) early and 34% ($P = .02$) late after PTCA in the amlodipine group, and ischaemia on ambulatory electrocardiography was reduced by 18% early and 28% late after PTCA compared with placebo (P = .06 and P = .009). Therefore, ischaemia and angina occurred after successful PTCA, but they were significantly reduced by amlodipine. [48, 49, 129].

These two studies are consistent with experimental data showing that CCBs are highly efficient when given before the ischaemic insult [33, 110].

Calcium antagonists in cardiac arrhythmias

In vitro studies have documented the action of calcium antagonist on impulse generation and conduction on the heart. Electrophysiological studies have differentiated the properties of L, N and T calcium currents and their relative sensitivity to various blocking molecules (see above Ca channel selectivity, page 114 [20]). Differences in action potentials according to the different anatomical regions of the heart are classical observations [33]. Atrial node and A-V node permeability changes during the action potential are marked for Ca and K. In atrium, Purkinje tissue and ventricles, permeability changes involve also marked changes in Na permeability. It may therefore be anticipated that S-A node and A-V node have the highest sensitivity to calcium channel blockade. This is particularly obvious with verapamil, which blocks K and Ca-channels within a same range of concentrations [35].

Arrhythmias may arise consecutively to abnormal impulse generation, abnormal conduction or both. The activity of the sinus node, the A-V node and the Purkinje tissue can be altered by autonomic activity. At the sinus node level, increased vagal activity can slow sinus node pacemakers by increasing potassium conductance. Gene-knockout experiments in mice have shown that $Ca_v1.3$ channels control sino-atrial node automaticity [63, 125]. Together with T-type Ca_v3 channels, they could contribute to cardiac pace maker function in human being, a hypothesis which still requires verification. The sympathetic system exerts opposite effects by accelerating the rate of phase 4 depolarization (pacemaker current). Impulse initiation by subsidiary pacemakers may arise in case of slowing or impairment of the dominant pacemaker. Augmented automaticity in the His Purkinje system is a common cause of arrhythmias.

Abnormal automaticity is a term used to refer to spontaneous diastolic depolarization that occurs at low (depolarized) level of membrane potentials in a cell that normally has a high level of membrane potential during diastole. Purkinje fibers, atrial and ventricular cells can show spontaneous diastolic depolarization and repetitive firing when the membrane potential is brought about to –60 mV. The ionic mechanisms involve alterations in calcium conductances. Altered extracellular conditions (acidosis, elevated extracellular K concentration, decreased p02 etc.) may induce heterogeneous action potential duration and lead to different levels of excitability in neighboring cells. Some depolarized cells are able to generate pacemaker and re-excite the cells recovering from refractory period and initiate an extrasystolic beat. Myocardial ischaemia, which shortens action potential duration, is a typical example of situations allowing such focal reexcitations that may be responsible for conduction disturbances. Furthermore, in ischaemic areas increased intracellular Na concentration and decreased intracellular K concentration cause partial depolarization in resting cells and slow Na channel reactivation favoring slow Ca currents. The slow depolarizing rate is responsible for decrement slowing of conduction velocity. Conduction blocks can occur in different regions of the heart (sinus node, A-V node, His Purkinje system, contractile myocardium) and play an essential role in the development of re-entrant pathways. The re-entry mechanism is usually involved in the occurrence of premature beats and ventricular tachycardia. To be initiated, both unidirectional block of conduction and slow conduction must occur. An anatomical and functional barrier may exist and form a circuit. Arrhythmias that result from such circus movements are self-sustained but are not self-initiated. They can be initiated by a single premature stimulus.

In 1971, Schamroth [102, 103] observed that verapamil (that was at that time considered as a β-blocker [115]) exhibited powerful antiarrhythmic action by reducing the ventricular rate in atrial fibrillation. This has stimulated interest for this drug and for the other agents also ranged later in Class IV antiarrhythmics [116]. If verapamil and diltiazem appear to be powerful antiarrhythmic agents *in vivo*, this is not the case for dihydropyridines, which usually evoke reflex tachycardia. Increase in sympathetic tone could overcome a slight negative chronotropic effect due to dihydropyridines. However, their lack of antiarrhythmic action might be due to their molecular interaction with cardiac calcium channels, which, as shown by *in vitro* studies, differs from the interaction achieved with verapamil and diltiazem. Blockade of currents by verapamil and diltiazem is increased when the frequency of stimulation is increased. This blocking action seems to be due to the fact that these charged drugs may reach their binding site, located at the intracellular site of Ca channels, when the channels are open. Dihydropyridine receptors are oriented extracellularly, their binding does not increase with repetitive fixing but only after long lasting depolarizing stimuli which evoke inactivation of Ca channels [35].

The action of verapamil and diltiazem has been well documented in supraventricular tachycardia (Tab. 1, modified from [74]). Intravenous verapamil is efficient in nearly 100% of trials for the acute conversion of re-entrant supraventricular tachycardia. Diltiazem is efficient in 80% of trials. Those percentages may be compared with 40 to 50% in the case of cardiac glycosides and of propranolol. However, chronic prophylaxis of paroxysmal supraventricular tachycardia with verapamil given *per os* (80 to 120 mg TID) has not been quite convincing [74].

In atrial fibrillation, intravenous injection of verapamil and diltiazem produces a reduction in the ventricular response and may tend to regularize the ventricular response [104]. It could diminish the amplitude of the fibrillatory waves and may uncommonly effect a conversion to sinus rhythm. The reduc-

Table 1. Clinical electrophysiologic effects of calcium antagonists modified from [74]

Effects[a]	Verapamil[b]	Nifedipine	Diltiazem	Bepridil
R-R Interval				
QRS	0	0	0	↑
Q-Tc	0	0	0	↑
PR	↑↑	0	↑	↑
A-H	↑↑↑	0	↑↑	↑
H-V	0	0	0	↑
Atrial ERP	0	0	0	↑
AV node ERP	↑↑↑	±	↑↑	↑↑
AV node FRP	↑↑↑	±	↑↑	↑↑
Ventricular FRP	0	0	0	↑↑
His-Purkinje ERP	0	0	0	↑
Bypass tact ERP	±	0	±	↑
Sinus node recovery time	0[c]	0	0[c]	0
Ventricular automaticity	0	0	0	↓

[a] ↓ = decrease; ↑ = increase; ± = variable effect; ERP = effective refractory period; FRP = functional refractory period.
[b] Effects of gallopamil and tiapamil are similar to those of verapamil.
[c] Prolonged in sick sinus syndrome.

tion in ventricular response is greatest in those patients with highest pre-treatments rate: the higher the pre-treatment rate, the greater the ensuing reduction in the ventricular response [104]). The reduction is additive to digitalis effect, an observation confirmed by several authors. The combination of verapamil (40 mg, three times daily) with digoxin (0.25 mg daily) is superior to digoxin alone [93]. It has been proposed that not only the calcium channel blocking action but also the sympatholytic properties are responsible for such beneficial effect of the combination.

Verapamil and diltiazem should not be given to patients in whom atrial fibrillation or flutter complicate the Wolff-Parkinson-White syndrome with anterograde conduction over the bypass tracts: indeed, in the presence of anomalous bundle, verapamil and diltiazem may accelerate the ventricular response.

Calcium antagonists in hypertension

The prevalence of hypertension in the human population is between 20% and 25%. Calcium antagonists are among the several drugs used to treat the disease. As pointed out by Zanchetti [140], the greater advantage of having a large spectrum of antihypertensive drugs available is that this choice makes it possible to find the most available agent for the individual patient. In clinical practice, the choice of a drug should be seen as tentative, to be confirmed, corrected or abandoned on the basis of the patient's response. Most aspects of a patient response are susceptible to clinical evaluation that is based not only on the blood pressure reduction, but on subjective and metabolic adverse effects and on the prevention of secondary cardiovascular changes. Evaluation of antihypertensive therapy has been made possible in large multicenter clinical trials such as ALLHAT [29].

Calcium antagonists have been proposed as antihypertensive drugs on the basis of their potent vasorelaxant properties. *In vivo*, they appear to act mainly on the arterial bed. They reduce the vascular resistance and evoke a fall in systolic and diastolic blood pressure. As was shown above (see page 136), they do preferentially dilate specific vascular beds. They evoke a much greater reduction in blood pressure in patients with essential hypertension than in normotensive subjects [52, 54, 55]. In hypertensive subjects, there is a significant correlation between pre-treatment blood pressure and the percentage fall in blood pressure after nifedipine, indicating that the effectiveness of the drug increases with higher pre-treatment levels of blood pressure. A similar observation has been reported with other calcium antagonists including verapamil, nitrendipine, diltiazem, tiapamil and isradipine but not with propranolol or captopril [15]. Animal studies have shown that the vessels of hypertensives have a higher affinity for CCBs than vessels of normotensives (see above, page 151). A higher vessel affinity for CCBs might be responsible for the higher effectiveness in hypertensive than in normotensive subjects.

The fall in blood pressure has been correlated with age, as shown in several but not all responses [39]. Such diversity in opinions may be related to variations in responsiveness among individuals, which also makes difficult the observation of the relation between dosage regimen and response, when studied in a population. Clinical trials of diltiazem showed that in some cases, the percentage of responders might just reach 50% [14]. This could be due to a too low dosage. Indeed, when single patients are examined, the relation between dose (or blood level) and reduction in blood pressure is obvious (Fig. 5) [39]. According to some authors [15], the fall in blood pressure after calcium antagonists is inversely correlated with plasma renin activity and their efficacy in patients with low renin activity is likely one of the determinants for their action in patients whose hypertension is insensitive to beta-blockers.

In contrast to a pronounced arteriolar effect, no haemodynamically significant venous relaxation has been found after calcium antagonists. This is consistent with an absence of orthostatic hypotension in patients treated with those drugs. Arteriolar vasodilators such as hydralazine evoke a sustained stimulation of renin secretion [34]. The interaction of calcium antagonists with the renin-angiotensin system is complex, as observed in animal experiments discussed above (page 185). According to some authors [4, 95], CCBs evoked only a transitory increase in renin secretion, which returned to normal values when the administration was continued. Millar et al. [68] have shown that nifedipine inhibited in humans angiotensin-II induced aldosterone secretion. Another interesting difference between calcium antagonist and arteriolar vasodilators

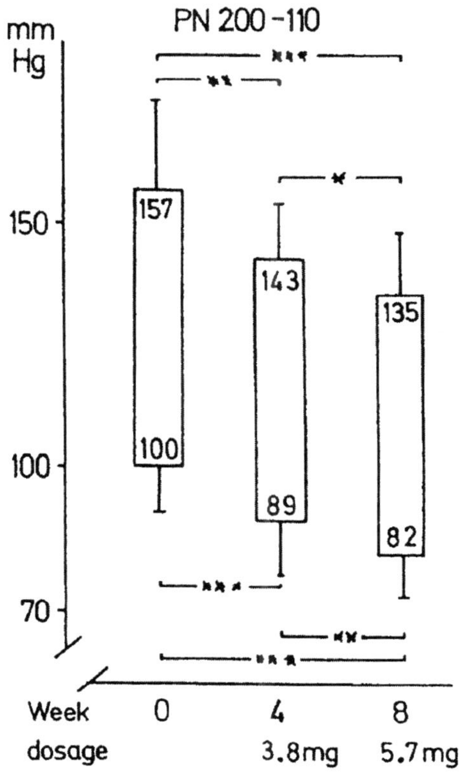

Figure 5. Average supine blood pressure in 20 patients while receiving placebo, then receiving two sequential dosage levels of PN 200-110 (isradipine); modified from [40].

used to treat hypertension is their contrasting effect on renal electrolyte and water excretion. It has been demonstrated several times that the decrease of blood pressure by hydralazine, minoxidil or diazoxide is associated with water and sodium retention, which offset their antihypertensive action. By contrast, calcium antagonists have a natriuretic effect. This action is greater in patients with high blood pressure than in normotensive ones. This action has been shown to occur without substantial alteration in renal plasma flow or in glomerular filtration rate [56, 142]. This natriuretic action may justify the use of calcium antagonists in monotherapy of hypertension. It is masked after prolonged treatment but may be revealed by a fall in natriuresis observed after calcium antagonist withdrawal. Experimental studies have shown that calcium antagonists inhibit renal tubular reabsorption of water and sodium in the distal tubule and collecting duct and that potassium metabolism is unaffected.

Using continuous 24-hour blood pressure monitoring, it has been observed that circadian variation of systolic and diastolic blood pressure persisted during treatment with calcium antagonists.

Long-term administration of calcium antagonists to spontaneously hypertensive rats protects the heart against pathological remodeling and is also able to induce substantial regression of established left ventricular hypertrophy and to improve cardiac function. Regression or prevention of hypertrophy was initially attributed to normalization of blood pressure and left ventricular systolic load. As discussed above (see the Chapter entitled: 'Blood pressure-independent effects of calcium antagonists), even if the role of blood pressure reduction in protection against end organ damage appears indisputable, experimental data strongly suggest that additional mechanisms, unrelated to this haemodynamic action, could contribute to the tissue protective effects of calcium antagonists. A similar hypothesis has been advocated in the case of ACE inhibitors. The beneficial effects of cardiac antagonists might involve several mechanisms including reduction of elevated blood pressure, blunting of "hypertrophic genes" activation in myocardial and vascular cells as a consequence of long-term inhibition of Ca entry, protection against renal damage and the subsequent activation of the RAS, and, possibly, reduction of oxidative stress in cardiovascular tissues. These two latter mechanisms of action take a variable part in the cardiovascular protection evoked by individual CCBs. Prevention of RAS activation by low doses of long-acting CCBs results in beneficial anti-remodeling effects, which are also associated with the use of ACE inhibitors or of Ang II receptor blockers. However, the cardioprotective effect of long-acting CCBs at high doses might be blunted by their capacity to promote renin secretion by the kidney, independently of their nephroprotective action.

Cardiac hypertrophy is a long-term response of the heart submitted to an increased hemodynamic burden. The increase in mass is due to the hypertrophy of existing myocytes rather than to hyperplasia. Physiological cardiac hypertrophy occurs during pregnancy and in trained athletes, and it meets the requirement for increased stroke volume and cardiac output arising in these particular circumstances. Thus, an increase in left ventricular (LV) mass by itself does not result in muscle dysfunction. In response to pressure overload in conditions such as hypertension, the parallel addition of sarcomeres causes an increase in myocyte width, which in turn increases wall thickness. When both thickness and mass increase, the resulting remodeling is concentric hypertrophy (increase in ratio of wall thickness/chamber dimension). Under prolonged pathological stress, LV hypertrophy is followed by maladaptive changes, including interstitial fibrosis, contractile dysfunction, altered gene expression pattern and changes in energy metabolism, which could lead to abnormal electrophysiological properties and heart failure. Thus, although cardiac hypertrophy in itself may be considered as a compensatory event, it is also part of a pathological process that triggers the onset of heart failure.

In an early meta-analysis of antihypertensive treatment trials, Dahlof et al. [18c] reported that ACE inhibitors reduced LV more than CCBs or other treatments when induced BP reduction and baseline LV mass were taken into account. At that time, this opinion was in agreement with another study [18b] suggesting that 1,4-DHP CCBs had little effect on LV hypertrophy. However, more recent analyses found no difference between LV effects of ACE inhibitors and newer, long-acting CCBs [24a, 50b]. Quite recently, the prospective randomized enalapril study evaluating regression of ventricular enlargement (PRESERVE) trial showed that regimens based on once-daily administration of enalapril or long-acting nifedipine significantly reduced left ventricular mass index during 1 year of treatment, and that there was no significant difference between the two treatment regimens. The PRESERVE trial [21a] provides the largest prospective, randomized, double-blind study to date comparing cardiac effects of ACE inhibition and calcium channel blockade in patients with hypertensive LV hypertrophy. This trial was designed to test primarily the following hypothesis: antihypertensive treatment with enalapril induces greater regression of LV hypertrophy than treatment with nifedipine by a prognostically meaningful amount on a population basis despite equivalent blood pressure reduction. Blinded treatment began with 10 mg enalapril or 30 mg nifedipine GITS (gastrointestinal treatment system) and matching placebo. During clinic visits over a 12-week titration phase, enalapril or nifedipine could be increased blindly to 20 mg or 60 mg, respectively, once daily. If maximum dose did not control BP, hydrochlorothiazide (25 mg) and then atenolol (25 mg) were recommended. More enalapril-treated than nifedipine-treated patients required supplemental treatment with hydrochlorothiazide (59% versus 34%, P,0.001) but not with atenolol (27% versus 22%, NS). The most important result of the study is that regimens based on once-daily administration of enalapril or long-acting nifedipine significantly reduced LV mass index and relative wall thickness during 1 year of treatment. LV mass index was reduced to the normal range in 56% of enalapril-treated patients and 48% of nifedipine-treated patients, with no significant difference in LV mass index between the two treatment regimens.

The results of PRESERVE suggest that disappointing results in early studies with 1,4-DHP CCBs may have been caused by side-effects that could have been predicted from physiological reflexes to acute fall of blood pression, including induction of volume overload and sympathetic activation. These deleterious effects are not associated with lower drug dosage regimens and with subsequently introduced longer-acting preparations. In line with conclusion from experimental studies, clinical studies indicate that excessive lowering of blood pressure might be detrimental in ischemic hypertensives by increasing the risk of myocardial infarction [18a]. In this therapeutic field, appropriate titration of dosage regimen need to be improved in order to gain the full beneficial action of CCBs. As pointed out by Frohlich [26a], well-controlled, and prospectively conducted multicenter clinical studies are still required in the field of hypertension.

Calcium antagonists and atherosclerosis

Experimental data

Several studies have shown that raised plasma lipid levels constitute an important risk factor for arteries and clinical evidence suggests that sustained lipid-lowering therapy can inhibit the progression of the disease. Clinical studies have been designed in order to examine if a similar clinical result could be achieved with calcium antagonists that do not influence plasma lipids levels. Rationale for those clinical trials came from experimental studies in animals. As this is reported by Tulenko et al. [133], atherosclerotic disease has been present in the human population apparently from the beginning of time. However, it has only been in the 20th century that improvements in the control of infectious diseases have allowed the average life span to increase to the point where atherosclerosis has been able to affect the general population. By the middle of the 20th Century, atherosclerosis had reached epidemic levels, and it is currently pandemic and increasing worldwide. Current thinking holds that an unchecked chronic inflammatory process involving the cells of the arterial wall and their interaction with LDL and various inflammatory cells causes atherosclerosis. Considerable evidence suggests that the principal insults underlying atherogenesis are serum dyslipidemias and oxidative stress mediated primarily by oxidized LDL. At least two processes are involved in the initiation of the atherogenic cascade: an enhanced focal endothelial transcytosis of low-density lipoprotein that accumulates in the proteoglycan-rich subendothelial space is associated with the preferential recruitment of blood monocytes to the intima—a process that is augmented by even, short periods of hyperlipidemia. In lesion progression, cellular necrosis with lipid release from foam cells and lysosomal enzymes are important events because such release further modifies or injures the surrounding intimal cells and interstitial components and induces a second cascade of inflammatory responses within the arterial intima. The smooth muscle cell (SMC) membrane becomes enriched in unesterified cholesterol soon after the development of serum hypercholesterolemia. With excess membrane cholesterol, the membrane becomes thicker and develops distinct cholesterol domains. These alterations in the membrane increase the permeability of SMC to calcium and induce a variety of alterations in SMC function that contribute to cellular atherogenic processes during plaque genesis. Dzau and his colleagues have elegantly described the various steps involved in the atherosclerotic process [23]. They have shown how VSMC has a central role in the process. The alteration of smooth muscle function, associated with an increase in cell calcium is the background of search for a role of calcium antagonists. Among CCBs, dihydropyridines have been the most studied as antiatherogenic drugs devoid of action on the plasma levels of cholesterol. Their mechanisms of action may result from their anti-oxidant properties and their pharmacological actions including the reduction in vascular tone/vasospasm in coronary arteries and elsewhere, the inhibition of smooth muscle cell proliferation within the intima, the inhibition of smooth muscle cell migration from the media to the intima, the reduction in ischaemia-induced endothelial permeability and their interaction with the L-arginine-NO pathway. The initial molecular and cellular events in atherogenesis are triggered by endothelial dysfunction, resulting in decreased nitric oxide production, increased cyclooxygenase activity and inflammation [57]. The early inflammatory response to atherosclerosis is designed to be beneficial, yet often progresses with adverse consequences. Pro-inflammatory factors, such as oxidized low-density lipoprotein (LDL) and infectious agents, stimulate the release of cytokines from the diseased vessel and other peripheral sites. This process leads to the accumulation of mononuclear cells, migration and proliferation of smooth muscle cells, and formation of fibrous tissue that eventually results in the formation of the mature atherosclerotic plaque. As a number of these cellular and inflammatory processes are mediated by disruption in calcium homeostasis, this has prompted experimental studies on the potential role of CCBs as antiatherogenic agents [41]. This hypothesis has been extensively tested in a variety of cellular and animal models of atherosclerosis [64, 88].

Initially, studies were performed on animals fed high cholesterol diet, later with transgenic animals, which do not express proteins such as ApoE or LDL receptors, showing lesions which closely resemble the inflammatory-fibrous plaques seen in humans. The protective effect of drugs was tested with various methodologies, incuding morphological and physiological ones. A variety of animal models have been used to determine whether calcium channel blockers exert an inhibitory effect on atherosclerotic lesion formation. These models include the cholesterol-fed rabbit, in which the lesions resemble the fatty-streak stage of atherosclerotic lesion development in humans [22, 117, 118]. Diet-induced atherosclerosis in monkeys is also used and, in this case, the lesions resemble those found in humans, both in pathology and distribution. Other models involve mechanical injury superimposed on cholesterol feeding. Cellular and subcellular preparations are being used to investigate the mechanisms involved in the antiatherosclerotic activity of the calcium channel blockers [12, 38, 60, 137]. The ability of calcium channel blockers to slow atherosclerotic lesion formation is accompanied by a reduction in vessel wall cholesterol and calcium and this slowed calcium uptake is associated with restoration of endothelium-dependent relaxation.

For instance the activity of the calcium antagonist lacidipine has been investigated in hamsters fed an atherogenic diet containing 2% cholesterol and 5% butter. Animals were examined at 14, 20 and 24 weeks of treatment. At 14 weeks, in hamsters fed the atherogenic diet and without lacidipine treatment, there were significant increases in serum levels of total cholesterol, triglycerides and lipoproteins; these values were approximately similar at week 24. Lacidipine treatment at 0.3, 1.0 and 3.0 mg/kg/d did not affect levels of serum cholesterol, triglycerides and lipoproteins. At 24 weeks, in hyperlipidemic hamsters fed the atherogenic diet, the area of the fatty streak in the aortic arch covered a mean area of $375 \pm 145\ \mu^2 \times 100$, which accounted for 2.7% of the total surface area of the aortic arch. In hamsters fed the atherogenic diet and treated with lacidipine at 0.3, 1.0 and 3.0 mg/kg, at 24 weeks, the surface area of the aortic arch lesion was significantly reduced by 41 to 71%. In the thoracic aorta at 24 weeks, in lacidipine-treated animals, both the incidence and degree of severity of the lesions was reduced, the area of the fatty streak being lowered by 78 to 97% in comparison with non-lacidipine-treated control animals. Ultrastructural examination demonstrated that the early changes in the aorta in hamsters fed the atherogenic diet involved the intima and smooth muscle cells; lacidipine treatment reduced the severity of the intimal lesions significantly [17, 18]. Cristofori et al. [18] investigated the antiatherosclerotic potential of lacidipine in the apoE-deficient mouse, an experimental model of atherosclerosis showing progressively complex and widespread lesions, as already mentioned above, they closely resemble the inflammatory-fibrous plaques seen in humans. Lacidipine was administered daily by gavage for 10 weeks at dose levels of 0 (control), 0.3, 1.0 and 3.0 mg/kg. The authors reported that lacidipine administration reduced the extension of atherosclerotic lesions in the aorta of the apoE-deficient mouse without affecting plasma lipid levels. They also showed that apoE-deficient mice have four-fold higher values of the proatherogenic peptide, endothelin, compared with the wild-type C57BL/6 mouse and that lacidipine administration reduced, in a dose-dependent manner, the concentrations of plasma endothelin.

Calcium antagonist drugs have also been reported to reverse the impairment in endothelium-dependent, nitric oxide (NO)-mediated vasorelaxation in hypercholesterolemic rabbits [6, 37]. Such an increase in NO availability may also attenuate the aforementioned early events in atherogenesis [69, 70].

Clinical studies

Clinical trials such as INTACT performed in humans with predominantly mild coronary disease confirmed the inhibitory effect of nifedipine on the progression of atherosclerosis found in animal experiment. In 1990, Lichtlen et al. [58, 59] have designed a multicenter, placebo (PL)-controlled, randomized, double-blind study, to test the effect of 80 mg nifedipine (NIF) per day *versus* placebo on the progression of mild coronary artery disease (CAD) (further development of existing stenoses, especially formation of new stenoses and occlusions) over a duration of three years. Progression of CAD was assessed by coronary angiograms performed at entrance and at completion of the study, using a computer-assisted analysis system (CAAS) to quantitate various stenosis parameters (percent degree of stenosis and minimal stenosis diameter). Of the 425 patients enrolled, 348 (82%) underwent a second angiogram; 66 of them, however, terminated treatment prematurely after an average of 359 (placebo) and 467 days (nifedipine). A total of 282 patients (148 on placebo, 134 on nifedipine) completed the trial with full-length treatment. There were no differences between the two groups in the progression of the existing stenoses. Patients on nifedipine, however, demonstrated significantly fewer new lesions than those on placebo. In the 282 patients undergoing the full-length treatment, there were 73 patients on placebo (49%) with 118 new lesions (0.8/patient) and 54 patients on nifedipine (40%) with 78 new lesions (0.58/patient), a difference of –27% ($p = 0.031$ by Cochran's linear trend test).

The difference was greatest in the left anterior descending branch, with 28 patients on placebo developing 33 new lesions (0.22/patient), *versus* 16 patients on nifedipine with 18 new lesions (0.13/patient) (-40%; p = 0.045), as well as in the left circumflex branch, where 34 patients on placebo exhibited 39 new lesions (0.26/patient) *versus* 23 patients on nifedipine with 22 new lesions (0.16/patient) (-38%, p = 0.033). No differences were observed in the right coronary artery, the vessel with the highest number of existing and new lesions. Hence, INTACT confirmed the previous experimental studies and demonstrated a significant reduction in newly formed coronary lesions in patients on nifedipine when compared with those on placebo, especially in the presence of early coronary artery disease. In contrast, arteriograms showed no significant differences in the progression or regression of existing lesions over three years, once fibrosis and calcification have begun. Risk factors were similar in placebo and nifedipine group both at entry and after three years. During the period of this trial with two groups of patients which were well matched for age, sex and risk factors, no statistically significant differences were evident in the relative frequencies of non-fatal myocardial infarction, unstable angina and the need for revascularisation between the treated and untreated patients. However, experience gained from studies with lipid lowering procedure indicates that significant clinical advantage is unlikely to become apparent until treatment has been continued for five to seven years. Furthermore, the role of reduction of blood pressure on atherosclerosis was not evaluated by INTACT when nifedipine was studied against a placebo. This is not the case with MIDAS, a study comparing isradipine and hydrochlorothiazide [11]. The rate of progression of mean maximum intimal-medial thickness (IMT) in carotid arteries has been followed using quantitative B-mode ultrasound imaging, during antihypertensive therapy. This study was a randomized, double-blind, positive-controlled trial performed in nine medical center clinics on a total of 883 patients with baseline mean ± SD systolic and diastolic blood pressure (SBP and DBP, respectively) of 149.7 ± 16.6 and 96.5 ± 5.1 mm Hg, age of 58.5 ± 8.5 years, and maximum IMT of 1.17 ± 0.20 mm. They received twice daily doses of isradipine (2.5–5.0 mg) or hydrochlorothiazide (12.5–25 mg). The primary end point was the rate of progression of mean maximum IMT in 12 carotid focal points over three years. The results show that there was no difference in the rate of progression of mean maximum IMT between isradipine and hydrochlorothiazide over three years (P = .68). There was a higher incidence of major vascular events (e.g., myocardial infarction, stroke, congestive heart failure, angina, and sudden death) in isradipine (n = 25; 5.65%) *versus* hydrochlorothiazide (n = 14; 3.17%) (P = .07), and a significant increase in non-major vascular events and procedures (e.g., transient ischaemic attack, dysrhythmia, aortic valve replacement, and femoral popliteal bypass graft) in isradipine (n = 40; 9.05%) *versus* hydrochlorothiazide (n = 23; 5.22%) (P = .02). At 6 months, mean DBP decreased by 13.0 mm Hg in both groups, and mean SBP decreased by 19.5 mm Hg in hydrochlorothiazide and 16.0 mm Hg in isradipine (P = .002); the difference in SBP between the two groups persisted throughout the study but did not explain the increased incidence of vascular events in patients treated with isradipine. The rate of progression of mean maximum IMT in carotid arteries, the surrogate end point in this study, did not differ between the two treatment groups.

As pointed out above, long duration seems to be required in order to characterize an action of CCBs over other antihypertensive agents. A support to this hypothesis is provided by the Verapamil-Hypertension Atherosclerosis Study (VHAS) [97, 144]. In 498 hypertensive patients in eight Italian centers, randomized to either verapamil (240 mg once a day) or chlorthalidone (25 mg once a day), a B-mode ultrasound scan was performed according to a standardized procedure at baseline and after 3, 12, 24, 36 and 48 months of treatment. The maximum intima-media thicknesses of the far walls of common, bifurcation and internal carotid arteries were measured bilaterally, and the following indices calculated: the mean thickness at the six measured sites, the mean thickness at the common and bifurcation sites and the single maximum thickness. The primary endpoint for treatment efficacy was the slope of the change over four years (rate of change, mm/year), corrected by using the initial mean over the six sites (baseline + three months) as a covariate (mm/year per mm). The patients were also classified into three strata according to their baseline single maximum thickness: those with normal carotid arteries (single maximum (1 mm)), those with thickened carotid arteries (single maximum >1 and < or = 1.5 mm), and those with carotid plaques (single maximum >1.5 mm). Among the 456 patients with satisfactory baseline ultrasound readings, 33% were classified with normal carotid arteries, 27% with thickened carotid arteries and 40% with plaques. In the intention-to-treat population (377 patients with ultrasound measurements taken on at least three different occasions over a period of at least two years), the rate of change in the mean thickness at the six sites measured was rather small (0.015 mm/year), but significantly ($P < 0.05$) smaller in patients with plaques (0.003 mm/year) than in patients with thickened or with normal carotids (0.023 and 0.025 mm/year, respectively). When related to initial values, the rate of change in the mean thickness at the six sites had a negative slope (–0.059 mm/year per mm, $P < 0.01$). Although rates of change in the carotid intima-media thickness in unstratified patients were not different in those treated with verapamil or with chlorthalidone, when changes in the mean thickness of six sites were related to the initial value, the slope of this relationship was significantly different in the two treatment groups (verapamil –0.082 *versus* chlorthalidone –0.037 mm/year per mm, $P < 0.02$). The blood pressure-lowering effect of the two randomized treatments was similar. Taking fatal and non-fatal, major and minor cardiovascular events together, there were 19 events in the verapamil group and 35 in the chlorthalidone group, with a significantly ($P < 0.01$) greater incidence in patients with plaques, and among patients with plaques in those who were randomized to chlorthalidone ($P < 0.05$). In accord with evidence from animal models of atherosclerosis, the calcium antagonist verapamil was more effective than the diuretic chlorthalidone in promoting regression of thicker carotid lesions. Changes in the carotid intima-media thickness were small in both groups. According to the authors, the observation that these small differences in carotid wall changes were paralleled by differences in the incidence of cardiovascular events (better intima-media thickness regression with verapamil paralleled by a lower cardiovascular event rate) suggests that even small effects on carotid plaques may have clinical and prognostic relevance.

The results of angiographic studies have suggested that calcium channel-blocking agents may prevent new coronary lesion formation, the progression of minimal lesions, or both. The Prospective Randomized Evaluation of the Vascular Effects of Norvasc Trial (PREVENT) [92] was a multicenter, randomized, placebo-controlled, double-masked clinical trial designed to test whether amlodipine would slow the progression of early coronary atherosclerosis in 825 patients with angiographically documented coronary artery disease. The primary outcome was the average 36-month angiographic change in mean minimal diameters of segments with a baseline diameter stenosis of 30%. A secondary hypothesis was whether amlodipine would reduce the rate of atherosclerosis in the carotid arteries as assessed with B-mode ultrasonography, which measured intimal-medial thicknesses (IMT). The rates of clinical events were also monitored. The placebo and amlodipine groups had nearly identical average 36-month reductions in the minimal diameter: 0.084 *versus* 0.095 mm, respectively ($P = 0.38$). In contrast, amlodipine had a significant effect in slowing the 36-month progression of carotid artery atherosclerosis: the placebo group experienced a 0.033 mm increase in IMT, whereas there was a 0.0126 mm decrease in the amlodipine group ($P = 0.007$). There was no treatment difference in the rates of all-cause mortality or major cardiovascular events, although amlodipine use was associated with fewer cases of unstable angina and coronary revascularization. Although amlodipine had no demonstrable effect on angiographic progression of coronary atherosclerosis or the risk of major cardiovascular events but was associated with fewer hospitalizations for unstable angina and revascularization.

Randomized trials of antihypertensive therapy showed smaller progression or greater regression of carotid lesions in patients treated with a calcium antagonist rather than a diuretic, but the changes were small and the trials had limited power to detect these differences. Whether different CCBs vary in their capacity to slow the progression of carotid atherosclerosis is clinically relevant. Studies with various molecules are justified on the basis of experimental data showing differences in their pharmacological profile. The European Lacidipine Study on Atherosclerosis (ELSA) [141] was planned with sufficient power to test whether long-term (four years) antihypertensive therapy using the calcium antagonist lacidipine was equally effective as therapy with the β-blocker atenolol on carotid IMT changes. ELSA was a randomized, double-blind trial in 2,334 patients with hypertension that compared the effects of a four-year treatment based on either lacidipine or atenolol on the mean of the maximum intima-media thicknesses (IMT) in far walls of common carotids and bifurcations, an index of carotid atherosclerosis (CBM_{max}). This index has been shown by epidemiological studies to be predictive of cardiovascular events. A significant ($P < 0.0001$) effect of lacidipine was found compared with atenolol, with a treatment difference in four-year CBM_{max} progression of 20.0227 mm (intention-to-treat population) and 20.0281 mm (completers). The intention-to-treat (ITT) population consisted of all patients randomized to double-blind medication who had the baseline ultrasound scan and at least one follow-up scan, including scans performed after withdrawal (mean follow-up 3.75 years). The completer population was made up of patients who actually completed the four-years of the study under randomized medication. The yearly IMT progression rate was 0.0145 mm/y in atenolol-treated and 0.0087 mm/y in lacidipine-treated patients (completers, 40% reduction; $P = 0.0073$). Patients with plaque progression were significantly less common, and patients with plaque regression were significantly more common in the lacidipine group. Clinic blood pressure reductions were identical with both treatments, but 24-hour ambulatory systolic/diastolic blood pressure changes were greater with atenolol (210/29 mm Hg) than with lacidipine (27/25 mm Hg). No significant difference between treatments was found in any cardiovascular events, although the relative risk for stroke, major cardiovascular events, and mortality showed a trend favoring lacidipine. According to the authors, the greater efficacy of lacidipine on carotid IMT progression and number of plaques per patient, despite a smaller ambulatory blood pressure reduction, indicates an antiatherosclerotic action of lacidipine independent of its antihypertensive action. This conclusion is consistent with CCBs properties reported above.

ALLHAT and meta-analyses

Psaty and Furberg who concluded from a meta-analysis that in patients with coronary disease, the use of short-acting nifedipine in moderate to high doses caused an increase in total mortality have questioned the safety of CCBs in therapy in 1995. The authors added that other calcium antagonists may have similar adverse effects, in particular those of the dihydropyridine type and that long-term safety data were lacking for most calcium antagonists for the treatment of hypertension [28]. Several authors have re-evaluated the conclusions of this meta-analysis. For instance, Opie et al. [83] pointed out that safety and efficacy are ultimately linked to each other and that both must be evaluated especially in the therapy of angina and hypertension, the main clinical indications for CCBs. Opie and his colleagues pointed out that structural, functional, and pharmacokinetic heterogeneity of CCBs means that the efficacy and dangers of one subclass, such as the short-acting dihydropyridines (DHPs), in one situation, such as unstable angina, do not necessarily apply in other clinical situations. Therefore, these authors reviewed one hundred studies according to Furberg's methods of data collection: case series, case control, cohort, randomized controlled trials (RCTs), and meta-analyses. Opie et al. [83] observed that regarding safety, both observational studies and RCTs suggest that adverse effects of CCBs may be linked to short-acting agents, specifically short-acting nifedipine and that incomplete but increasing overall evidence favors the safety of longer-acting DHPs. Their analysis confirmed that heart failure remains a class contraindication to the use of CCBs, with some exceptions shown by DAVIT II trial [45]. One of their main conclusions was that the future aim with CCBs must be to obtain a large database gathered from RCTs, which will give the same certainty about efficacy and safety that already holds for use of the diuretics in hypertension. Some of ALLHAT conclusions are meeting this expectation.

The "antihypertensive and lipid lowering to prevent heart attack trial" (ALLHAT), the largest ever randomized trial of antihypertensive treatment was designed to determine whether the choice of first line treatment for hypertension influenced cardiovascular outcome [1]. The trial was sufficiently large to examine cause specific outcomes and was the first hypertension study to have sufficient power to examine the combined incidence of fatal coronary heart disease and non-fatal myocardial infarction as the primary end point. It was a randomized double blind controlled clinical trial conducted in 623 centers in North America. The trial randomized 42,418 patients with mild to moderate hypertension aged 55 years or older (mean age 67 years) with one additional cardiovascular risk factor to one of four antihypertensive treatments: the diuretic chlorthalidone (12.5–25 mg daily), the ACE inhibitor lisinopril (10–40 mg daily), the calcium channel blocker amlodipine (2.5–10 mg daily), or the α-blocker doxazosin (1–8 mg daily). The doxazosin arm was stopped prematurely in 2000 after a reported excess of cardiovascular events (principally congestive heart failure) compared with the reference drug, chlorthalidone. This left 33,357 patients who completed the trial for a mean follow up of 4.9 years. The design of the trial ensured the inclusion of large numbers of patients' groups, previously under-represented in trials of blood pressure—notably women (47%), black Americans (35%), Hispanics (19%), and people with diabetes mellitus (36%). The primary outcome occurred in 2956 participants, and no differences were found between the rates with the reference drug chlorthalidone (11.5%), and amlodipine (11.3%) and lisinopril (11.4%). Moreover, this conclusion is valid irrespective of the patient's sex, ethnicity, or the presence or absence of diabetes. There has been a large debate as to whether the duration of the trial was sufficient to identified differences in secondary outcomes not initially expected. According to Zanchetti and Mancia, there are questions that ALLHAT trial has not answered and that are still left open. These are mostly those inherent in the nature of large event based trials. Can the results of 4–5 years of treatment be extrapolated to the much longer life expectation of middle-aged hypertensive patients? Can some of the metabolic changes differently occurring with different drug regimens have some impact on a longer time course than the five-year duration of a trial? Did the peculiar and unusual combination therapy required by the ALLHAT design have some influence on the results, and did it cause some disadvantage [5, 139, 143].

It is remarkable that Allhat [1] has prompted about 115 other commentary papers before [27] and after [2, 50, 67, 71] its publication in December 2002. But it is highly worth noting that the new information provided by ALLHAT dismisses previous concerns about the safety and efficacy of calcium channel blockers. It reinforces the interpretation of Staessen et al. [119, 120] who compared to treatments with older drugs (diuretics and β-blockers), those with calcium-channel blockers and angiotensin converting-enzyme inhibitors in 62,605 patients. They concluded from their meta-analysis that blood pressure control is important, all approved antihypertensive drugs having similar long-term efficacy and safety, but that calcium channel blockers might be especially effective in stroke prevention [80, 82, 120]. Nevertheless, the question is still open whether CCBs may have therapeutic effects unrelated to blood pressure reduction.

References

1 Major outcomes in high-risk hypertensive patients randomized to angiotensin-converting enzyme inhibitor or calcium channel blocker vs diuretic: The Antihypertensive and Lipid-Lowering Treatment to Prevent Heart Attack Trial (ALLHAT). *Jama* 288: 2981–2997, 2002

2 Alderman MH. Allhat and beyond. *Am J Hypertens* 16: 512–514, 2003

3 Andre-Fouet X, Usdin JP, Gayet C, Wilner C, Thizy JF, Viallet M, Apoil E, Vernant P and Pont M. Comparison of short-term efficacy of diltiazem and propranolol in unstable angina at rest—a randomized trial in 70 patients. *Eur Heart J* 4: 691–698, 1983

4 Bambauer R, Jutzler GA, Weber U, Walter R and Keller HE. Nitrendipine in patients with end-stage renal disease and hypertension. *J Cardiovasc Pharmacol* 12 Suppl 4: S133–135, 1988

5 Bath P, Chalmers J, Powers W, Beilin L, Davis S, Lenfant C, Mancia G, Neal B, Whitworth J and Zanchetti A. International Society of Hypertension (ISH): statement on the management of blood pressure in acute stroke. *J Hypertens* 21: 665–672, 2003

6 Becker RH, Linz W, Wiemer G and Nordlander M. Low-dose felodipine treatment attenuates endothelial dysfunction in rabbits fed an atherogenic diet. *J Cardiovasc Pharmacol* 18 Suppl 10: S36–41, 1991

7 Biagini A, Mazzei MG, Carpeggiani C, Testa R, Antonelli R, Michelassi C, L'Abbate A and Maseri A. Vasospastic ischemic mechanism of frequent asymptomatic transient ST-T changes during continuous electrocardiographic monitoring in selected unstable angina patients. *Am Heart J* 103: 13–20, 1982

8 Blaustein AS, Heller GV and Kolman BS. Adjunctive nifedipine therapy in high-risk, medically refractory, unstable angina pectoris. *Am J Cardiol* 52: 950–954, 1983

9 Boon D, Piek JJ and van Montfrans GA. Silent ischaemia and hypertension. *J Hypertens* 18: 1355–1364, 2000

10 Boon D, van Goudoever J, Piek JJ and van Montfrans GA. ST segment depression criteria and the prevalence of silent cardiac ischemia in hypertensives. *Hypertension* 41: 476–481, 2003

11 Borhani NO, Mercuri M, Borhani PA, Buckalew VM, Canossa-Terris M, Carr AA, Kappagoda T, Rocco MV, Schnaper HW, Sowers JR and Bond MG. Final outcome results of the Multicenter Isradipine Diuretic Atherosclerosis Study (MIDAS). A randomized controlled trial. *Jama* 276: 785–791, 1996

12 Bossaller C, Habib GB, Yamamoto H, Williams C, Wells S and Henry PD. Impaired muscarinic endothelium-dependent relaxation and cyclic guanosine 5'-monophosphate formation in atherosclerotic human coronary artery and rabbit aorta. *J Clin Invest* 79: 170–174, 1987

13 Braunwald E. Unstable angina: an etiologic approach to management. *Circulation* 98: 2219–2222, 1998

14 Buckley MM, Grant SM, Goa KL, McTavish D and Sorkin EM. Diltiazem. A reappraisal of its pharmacological properties and therapeutic use. *Drugs* 39: 757–806, 1990

15 Bühler F, Bolli W, Müller F and Erne P. Calcium antagonists for identification of mechanisms and

treatment of patients with essential hypertension. In: *Cardiovascular effects of dihydropyridine-type calcium antagonists and agonists.*, edited by Fleckenstein A, Van Breemen C, Gross R and Hoffmeister F. Berlin Heidelberg New York: Springer, 1985, p. 445–457

16 Capucci A, Bassein L, Bracchetti D, Carini G, Maresta A and Magnani B. Propranolol v. verapamil in the treatment of unstable angina. A double-blind cross-over study. *Eur Heart J* 4: 148–154, 1983

17 Cristofori P, Lanzoni A, Gaviraghi G, Turton J and Sbarbati A. Anti-atherosclerotic activity of the calcium antagonist lacidipine in cholesterol-fed hamsters. *Biomed Pharmacother* 54: 93–99, 2000

18 Cristofori P, Lanzoni A, Quartaroli M, Pastorino AM, Zancanaro C, Cominacini L, Gaviraghi G and Turton J. The calcium-channel blocker lacidipine reduces the development of atherosclerotic lesions in the apoE-deficient mouse. *J Hypertens* 18: 1429–1436, 2000

18a Cruickshank JM. Antihypertensive treatment and the J-curve. *Cardiovasc Drugs Ther* 14: 373-379, 2000

18b Cruickshank JM, Lewis J, Moore V and Dodd C. Reversibility of left ventricular hypertrophy by differing types of antihypertensive therapy. *J Hum Hypertens* 6: 85-90, 1992

18c Dahlof B, Pennert K, and Hansson L. Reversal of left ventricular hypertrophy in hypertensive patients. A metaanalysis of 109 treatment studies. *Am J Hypertens* 5: 95-110, 1992

19 Dargie HJ, Lynch PG, Krikler DM, Harris L and Krikler S. Nifedipine and propranolol: a beneficial drug interaction. *Am J Med* 71: 676–682, 1981

20 De Paoli P, Cerbai E, Koidl B, Kirchengast M, Sartiani L and Mugelli A. Selectivity of different calcium antagonists on T- and L-type calcium currents in guinea-pig ventricular myocytes. *Pharmacol Res* 46: 491–497, 2002

21 de Ponti C and Vincenzi M. Acute and chronic effect of verapamil in exercise-induced angina p 148–158. In: *Calcium antagonism in cardiovascular therapy: experience with verapamil.* Zanchetti, A. and Krikler, DM (Ed). Amsterdam, Oxford, Princetown: Excerpta Medica, 1981

21a Devereux RB, Palmieri V, Sharpe N, De Quattro V, Bella JN, de Simone G, Walker JF, Hahn RT and Dahlof B. Effects of once-daily angiotensin-converting enzyme inhibition and calcium channel blockade-based antihypertensive treatment regimens on left ventricular hypertrophy and diastolic filling in hypertension: the prospective randomized enalapril study evaluating regression of ventricular enlargement (preserve) trial. *Circulation* 104: 1248-1254, 2001

22 Donetti E, Fumagalli R, Paoletti R and Soma MR. Direct antiatherogenic activity of isradipine and lacidipine on neointimal lesions induced by perivascular manipulation in rabbits. *Pharmacol Res* 35: 417–422, 1997

23 Dzau VJ, Braun-Dullaeus RC and Sedding DG. Vascular proliferation and atherosclerosis: new perspectives and therapeutic strategies. *Nat Med* 8: 1249–1256, 2002

24 Eichelbaum M and Somogyi A. *Verapamil distribution in health and the diseased state. p 64–71. In: Calcium channel blocking agents in the treatment of cardiovascular disorders. Stone, PH and Antman EM (Eds).* Mount Kisco, New York: Futura Publishing Company, Inc., 1983

24a Fagard RH. Reversibility of left ventricular hypertrophy by antihypertensive drugs. *Neth J Med* 47: 173-179, 1995

25 Findlay IN, MacLeod K, Gillen G, Elliott AT, Aitchison T and Dargie HJ. A double blind placebo controlled comparison of verapamil, atenolol, and their combination in patients with chronic stable angina pectoris. *Br Heart J* 57: 336–343, 1987

25a Fleckenstein A, Tritthart H, Fleckenstein B, Herbst A and Grun G. A new group of competitive divalent Ca-antagonists (iproveratril, D 600, prenylamine) with potent inhibitory effects on electromechanical coupling in mammalian myocardium. *Pflugers Arch* 307: R25, 1969

26 Frishman WH, Klein NA, Strom JA, Willens H, LeJemtel TH, Jentzer J, Siegel L, Klein P, Kirschen N, Silverman R et al. Superiority of verapamil to propranolol in stable angina pectoris: a double-blind, randomized crossover trail. *Circulation* 65: I51–59, 1982

26a Frohlich ED. Local hemodynamic changes in hypertension: insights for therapeutic preservation of target organs. *Hypertension* 38: 1388-1394, 2001

27 Furberg CD. A new era in hypertension research: discussing the findings of ALLHAT. *Curr Control Trials Cardiovasc Med* 2: 249–250, 2001

28 Furberg CD, Psaty BM and Meyer JV. Nifedipine. Dose-related increase in mortality in patients with coronary heart disease. *Circulation* 92: 1326–1331, 1995

29 Furberg CD, Psaty BM, Pahor M and Alderman MH. Clinical implications of recent findings from the antihypertensive and lipid-lowering treatment to prevent heart attack trial (ALLHAT) and other studies of hypertension. *Ann Intern Med* 135: 1074–1078, 2001

30 Gerstenblith G, Ouyang P, Achuff SC, Bulkley BH, Becker LC, Mellits ED, Baughman KL, Weiss JL, Flaherty JT, Kallman CH et al. Nifedipine in unstable angina: a double-blind, randomized trial. *N Engl J Med* 306: 885–889, 1982

31 Gibson RS, Boden WE, Theroux P, Strauss HD, Pratt CM, Gheorghiade M, Capone RJ, Crawford MH, Schlant RC, Kleiger RE et al. Diltiazem and reinfarction in patients with non-Q-wave myocardial infarction. Results of a double-blind, randomized, multicenter trial. *N Engl J Med* 315: 423–429, 1986

32 Gibson RS, Hansen JF, Messerli F, Schechtman KB and Boden WE. Long-term effects of diltiazem and verapamil on mortality and cardiac events in non-Q-wave acute myocardial infarction without pulmonary congestion: *post hoc* subset analysis of the multicenter diltiazem postinfarction trial and the second danish verapamil infarction trial studies. *Am J Cardiol* 86: 275–279, 2000

33 Godfraind T, Miller R and Wibo M. Calcium antagonism and calcium entry blockade. *Pharmacol Rev* 38: 321–416, 1986

34 Gottlieb TB, Katz FH and Chidsey CA, 3rd. Combined therapy with vasodilator drugs and beta-adrenergic blockade in hypertension. A comparative study of minoxidil and hydralazine. *Circulation* 45: 571–582, 1972

35 Grace AA and Camm AJ. Voltage-gated calcium-channels and antiarrhythmic drug action. *Cardiovasc Res* 45: 43–51, 2000

36 Haas H and Hartfelder G. Alpha-isopropylalpha{(N-metyl-N-homoveratriyl).-gamma-aminopropyl}-3,4-dimethoxyphenylacetonitils, einer Substanz mit coronargefässerweiternden Eigenschaften. *Arzneim-Forsch* 12: 549–558, 1962

37 Habib J, Bossaller C, Wells S, Williams C, Morrisett J and Henry P. Preservation of endothelium-dependent vascular relaxation in cholesterol-fed rabbit by treatment with the calcium blocker PN 200110. *Circ Res* 58: 305–309, 1986

38 Habib JB, Bossaller C, Wells S, Williams C, Morrisett JD and Henry PD. Preservation of endothelium-dependent vascular relaxation in cholesterol-fed rabbit by treatment with the calcium blocker PN 200110. *Circ Res* 58: 305–309, 1986

39 Hansson L and Dahlof B. Antihypertensive effect of a new dihydropyridine calcium antagonist, PN 200-110 (isradipine), combined with pindolol. *Am J Cardiol* 59: 137B-140B, 1987

40 Hansson L and Dalhof B. Antihypertensive effect of a new dihydropyridine calcium antagonist, PN 2OO-110 (Isradipine) combined with pindolol. *Am J Cardiol* 59: 137b-140b, 1987

41 Henry P. Atherosclerosis, calcium and calcium antagonists. *Circulation* 72: 456–459, 1985

42 Higginbotham MB, Morris KG, Coleman RE and Cobb FR. Chronic stable angina monotherapy. Nifedipine *versus* propranolol. *Am J Med* 86: 1–5, 1989

42a Higginbotham MB, Morris KG, Coleman RE and Cobb FR. Comparison of nifedipine alone with propranolol alone for stable angina pectoris including hemodynamics at rest and during exercise. *Am J Cardiol* 57: 1022-1028, 1986

43 Hopf R, Dowinsky S and Kaltenbach M. Use of the calcium blocking agents in the treatment of classic exertional angina. In: *Calcium blocking agents in the treatment of cardiovascular disorders.* p 241–268. Stone, P.H. and Antman, E.M. (Eds). Mount Kisco, New York: Futura Publishing Company, 1983

44 Hugenholtz PG, Michels HR, Serruys PW and Brower RW. Nifedipine in the treatment of unstable angina, coronary spasm and myocardial ischemia. *Am J Cardiol* 47: 163–173, 1981

45 II D. Effect of verapamil on mortality and major events after acute myocardial infarction (the Danish Verapamil Infarction Trial II—DAVIT II). *Am J Cardiol* 66: 779–785, 1990

46 Johnson SM, Mauritson DR, Corbett JR, Woodward W, Willerson JT and Hillis LD. Double-blind, randomized, placebo-controlled comparison of propranolol and verapamil in the treatment of patients with stable angina pectoris. *Am J Med* 71: 443–451, 1981

47 Johnson SM, Mauritson DR, Willerson JT and Hillis LD. A controlled trial of verapamil for Prinzmetal's variant angina. *N Engl J Med* 304: 862–866, 1981

48 Jorgensen B, Simonsen S, Endresen K, Forfang K, Vatne K, Hansen J, Webb J, Buller C, Goulet G, Erikssen J and Thaulow E. Restenosis and clinical outcome in patients treated with amlodipine after angioplasty: results from the Coronary AngioPlasty Amlodipine REStenosis Study (CAPARES). *J Am Coll Cardiol* 35: 592–599, 2000

49 Jorgensen B and Thaulow E. Effects of amlodipine on ischemia after percutaneous transluminal coronary angioplasty: secondary results of the Coronary Angioplasty Amlodipine Restenosis (CAPARES) Study. *Am Heart J* 145: 1030–1035, 2003

50 Kaplan NM. The meaning of ALLHAT. *J Hypertens* 21: 233–234, 2003

50a Kaltenbach M and Zimmermann D. The effect of iproveratril on angina pectoris and the adrenergic beta-receptors of man. *Dtsch Med Wochenschr* 93: 25–28, 1968
50b Klingbeil AU, Schneider M, Martus P, Messerli FH and Schmieder RE. A meta-analysis of the effects of treatment on left ventricular mass in essential hypertension. *Am J Med* 115: 41–46, 2003
51 Kragel AH, Reddy SG, Wittes JT and Roberts WC. Morphometric analysis of the composition of coronary arterial plaques in isolated unstable angina pectoris with pain at rest. *Am J Cardiol* 66: 562–567, 1990
52 Lederballe Pedersen O, Christensen CK, Mikkelsen E and Ramsch KD. Relationship between the antihypertensive effect and steady-state plasma concentration of nifedipine given alone or in combination with a beta-adrenoceptor blocking agent. *Eur J Clin Pharmacol* 18: 287–293, 1980
53 Leon MB, Rosing DR, Bonow RO, Lipson LC and Epstein SE. Clinical efficacy of verapamil alone and combined with propranolol in treating patients with chronic stable angina pectoris. *Am J Cardiol* 48: 131–139, 1981
54 Leonetti G, Cuspidi C, Sampieri L, Terzoli L and Zanchetti A. Comparison of cardiovascular, renal, and humoral effects of acute administration of two calcium channel blockers in normotensive and hypertensive subjects. *J Cardiovasc Pharmacol* 4 Suppl 3: S319–324, 1982
55 Leonetti G, Magnani B, Pessina AC, Rappelli A, Trimarco B and Zanchetti A. Tolerability of long-term treatment with lercanidipine *versus* amlodipine and lacidipine in elderly hypertensives. *Am J Hypertens* 15: 932–940, 2002
56 Leonetti G, Rupoli L, Gradnik R and Zanchetti A. Effects of a low-sodium diet on antihypertensive and natriuretic responses to acute administration of nifedipine. *J Hypertens Suppl* 5: S57–60, 1987
57 Libby P. Molecular bases of the acute coronary syndrome. *Circulation* 91: 2844–2850, 1995
58 Lichtlen PR, Hugenholtz PG, Rafflenbeul W, Hecker H, Jost S and Deckers JW. Retardation of angiographic progression of coronary artery disease by nifedipine. Results of the International Nifedipine Trial on Antiatherosclerotic Therapy (INTACT). INTACT Group Investigators. *Lancet* 335: 1109–1113, 1990
59 Lichtlen PR, Hugenholtz PG, Rafflenbeul W, Hecker H, Jost S, Nikutta P and Deckers JW. Retardation of coronary artery disease in humans by the calcium-channel blocker nifedipine: results of the INTACT study (International Nifedipine Trial on Antiatherosclerotic Therapy). *Cardiovasc Drugs Ther* 4 Suppl 5: 1047–1068, 1990
60 Lichtor T, Davis HR, Vesselinovitch D, Wissler RW and Mullan S. Suppression of atherogenesis by nifedipine in the cholesterol-fed rhesus monkey. *Appl Pathol* 7: 8–18, 1989
61 Livesley B, Catley PF, Campbell RC and Oram S. Double-blind evaluation of verapamil, propranolol, and isosorbide dinitrate against a placebo in the treatment of angina pectoris. *Br Med J* 1: 375–378, 1973
62 Lynch P, Dargie H, Krikler S and Krikler D. Objective assessment of antianginal treatment: a double-blind comparison of propranolol, nifedipine, and their combination. *Br Med J* 281: 184–187, 1980
63 Mangoni ME, Couette B, Bourinet E, Platzer J, Reimer D, Striessnig J and Nargeot J. Functional role of L-type $Ca_V1.3$ Ca^{2+} channels in cardiac pacemaker activity. *Proc Natl Acad Sci USA* 100: 5543–5548, 2003
64 Mason RP. Mechanisms of plaque stabilization for the dihydropyridine calcium channel blocker amlodipine: review of the evidence. *Atherosclerosis* 165: 191–199, 2002
65 Matsuda Y, Moritani K, Ogawa H, Kohno M, Kohtoku S, Miura T, Hiro T, Yano M, Matsuda M and Kusukawa R. Response of the coronary artery to a small dose of ergonovine in variant angina. *Am Heart J* 112: 947–952, 1986
66 Mauritson DR, Johnson SM, Winniford MD, Cary JR, Willerson JT and Hillis LD. Verapamil for unstable angina at rest: a short-term randomized, double-blind study. *Am Heart J* 106: 652–658, 1983
67 McInnes GT. ALLHAT: a saga of missed opportunities. *J Hum Hypertens* 17: 373–377, 2003
68 Millar JA, Struthers AD, Beastall GH and Reid JL. Effect of nifedipine on blood pressure and adrenocortical responses to trophic stimuli in humans. *J Cardiovasc Pharmacol* 4 Suppl 3: S330–334, 1982
69 Moncada S and Higgs A. The L-arginine-nitric oxide pathway. *N Engl J Med* 329: 2002–2012, 1993
70 Moncada S, Martin JF and Higgs A. Symposium on regression of atherosclerosis. *Eur J Clin Invest* 23: 385–398, 1993
71 Moser M. Results of ALLHAT: is this the final answer regarding initial antihypertensive drug

therapy? *Arch Intern Med* 163: 1269–1273, 2003

72 Moses JW, Wertheimer JH, Bodenheimer MM, Banka VS, Feldman M and Helfant RH. Efficacy of nifedipine in rest angina refractory to propranolol and nitrates in patients with obstructive coronary artery disease. *Ann Intern Med* 94: 425–429, 1981

73 Muller JE, Turi ZG, Pearle DL, Schneider JF, Serfas DH, Morrison J, Stone PH, Rude RE, Rosner B, Sobel BE et al. Nifedipine and conventional therapy for unstable angina pectoris: a randomized, double-blind comparison. *Circulation* 69: 728–739, 1984

74 Nademanee K and Singh BN. Control of cardiac arrhythmias by calcium antagonism. *Ann NY Acad Sci* 522: 536–552, 1988

75 Nakamura M and Koiwaya Y. Beneficial effect of diltiazem, a new antianginal drug, on angina pectoris at rest. *Jpn Heart J* 20: 613–621, 1979

76 Nayler WG, McInnes I and Swann JB. Some effects of iproveratril (Isoptin) on the cardiovascular system. *J Pharmacol Exp Ther* 161: 247–251, 1968

77 Nesto RW and Phillips RT. Silent myocardial ischemia: clinical characteristics, underlying mechanisms, and implications for treatment. *Am J Med* 81: 12–19, 1986

78 Nesto RW, Phillips RT, Kett KG, McAuliffe LS, Roberts M and Hegarty P. Effect of nifedipine on total ischemic activity and circadian distribution of myocardial ischemic episodes in angina pectoris. *Am J Cardiol* 67: 128–132, 1991

79 Opie L. Anti-ischemic properties of calcium-channel blockers: lessons from cardiac surgery. *J Am Coll Cardiol* 41: 1506–1509, 2003

80 Opie LH. Calcium channel blockers in hypertension: reappraisal after new trials and major meta-analyses. *Am J Hypertens* 14: 1074–1081, 2001

81 Opie LH. *Clinical use of calcium channel antagonist drugs.* Boston, Dordrecht, London: Kluwer Academic Publishers, 1989

82 Opie LH and Schall R. Evidence-based evaluation of calcium channel blockers for hypertension: equality of mortality and cardiovascular risk relative to conventional therapy. *J Am Coll Cardiol* 39: 315–322, 2002

83 Opie LH, Yusuf S and Kubler W. Current status of safety and efficacy of calcium channel blockers in cardiovascular diseases: a critical analysis based on 100 studies. *Prog Cardiovasc Dis* 43: 171–196, 2000

84 Ouyang P, Brinker JA, Mellits ED, Weisfeldt ML and Gerstenblith G. Variables predictive of successful medical therapy in patients with unstable angina: selection by multivariate analysis from clinical, electrocardiographic, and angiographic evaluations. *Circulation* 70: 367–376, 1984

85 Ozaki Y, Keane D and Serruys PW. Fluctuation of spastic location in patients with vasospastic angina: a quantitative angiographic study. *J Am Coll Cardiol* 26: 1606–1614, 1995

86 Ozaki Y, Keane D and Serruys PW. Relation of basal coronary tone and vasospastic activity in patients with variant angina. *Heart* 75: 267–273, 1996

87 Pahor M, Psaty BM, Alderman MH, Applegate WB, Williamson JD, Cavazzini C and Furberg CD. Health outcomes associated with calcium antagonists compared with other first-line antihypertensive therapies: a meta-analysis of randomised controlled trials. *Lancet* 356: 1949–1954, 2000

88 Paoletti R, Corsini A, Soma MR and Bernini F. Calcium, calcium antagonists and experimental atherosclerosis. *Blood Press Suppl* 4: 12–15, 1996

89 Parodi O, Maseri A and Simonetti I. Management of unstable angina at rest by verapamil. A double-blind cross-over study in coronary care unit. *Br Heart J* 41: 167–174, 1979

90 Parodi O, Simonetti I, Michelassi C, Carpeggiani C, Biagini A, L'Abbate A and Maseri A. Comparison of verapamil and propranolol therapy for angina pectoris at rest: a randomized, multiple-crossover, controlled trial in the coronary care unit. *Am J Cardiol* 57: 899–906, 1986

91 Pepine CJ, Feldman RL, Whittle J, Curry RC and Conti CR. Effect of diltiazem in patients with variant angina: a randomized double-blind trial. *Am Heart J* 101: 719–725, 1981

92 Pitt B, Byington RP, Furberg CD, Hunninghake DB, Mancini GB, Miller ME and Riley W. Effect of amlodipine on the progression of atherosclerosis and the occurrence of clinical events. PREVENT Investigators. *Circulation* 102: 1503–1510, 2000

93 Pomfret SM, Beasley CR, Challenor V and Holgate ST. Relative efficacy of oral verapamil and digoxin alone and in combination for the treatment of patients with chronic atrial fibrillation. *Clin Sci (Lond)* 74: 351–357, 1988

94 Previtali M, Salerno JA, Tavazzi L, Ray M, Medici A, Chimienti M, Specchia G and Bobba P. Treatment of angina at rest with nifedipine: a short-term controlled study. *Am J Cardiol* 45: 825–830, 1980

95 Reid JL, Millar JA and Struthers AD. Nifedipine—studies on its mechanism of action and interaction with other circulatory control mechanisms in man. *Postgrad Med J* 59 Suppl 2: 98–103, 1983
96 Reuschel-Janetschek E, Erath A and Armin T. *Effects of oral nisoldipine on transient ischemia uring Holter monitoring. p 174–182. In: Recent aspects in calcium antagonism: Nisoldipine. Lichtlen, PR and Hugenholtz PG (Eds).* New York, Stuttgart: Schattauer, 1988
97 Rosei EA, Dal Palu C, Leonetti G, Magnani B, Pessina A and Zanchetti A. Clinical results of the Verapamil in Hypertension and Atherosclerosis Study. VHAS Investigators. *J Hypertens* 15: 1337–1344, 1997
98 Rosenthal SJ, Ginsburg R, Lamb IH, Baim DS and Schroeder JS. Efficacy of diltiazem for control of symptoms of coronary arterial spasm. *Am J Cardiol* 46: 1027–1032, 1980
99 Rosenthal SJ, Lamb IH, Schroeder JS and Ginsburg R. Long-term efficacy of diltiazem for control of symptoms of coronary artery spasm. *Circ Res* 52: I153–157, 1983
100 Sadick NN, Tan AT, Fletcher PJ, Morris J and Kelly DT. A double-blind randomized trial of propranolol and verapamil in the treatment of effort angina. *Circulation* 66: 574–579, 1982
101 Sandler G, Clayton GA and Thornicroft SG. Clinical evaluation of verapamil in angina pectoris. *Br Med J* 3: 224–227, 1968
102 Schamroth L. Calcium ion antagonists in supraventricular and ventricular arrhythmias. *Cardiology* 69 Suppl: 140–143, 1982
103 Schamroth L. Immediate effects of intravenous verapamil on atrial fibrillation. *Cardiovasc Res* 5: 419–424, 1971
104 Schamroth L and Antman E. *Calcium channel blocking agents in tghe treatment of cardiac arrhythmias, p 347–375. In: Calcium channel blocking agents in the treatment of cardiovascular disorders. Stone, PH and Antman, EM (Eds).* Mount Cisco, New York: Futura Publishing Company, Inc., 1983
105 Scheidt S, Frishman WH, Packer M, Mehta J, Parodi O and Subramanian VB. Long-term effectiveness of verapamil in stable and unstable angina pectoris. One-year follow-up of patients treated in placebo-controlled double-blind randomized clinical trials. *Am J Cardiol* 50: 1185–1190, 1982
106 Schick EC, Jr, Liang CS, Heupler FA, Jr, Kahl FR, Kent KM, Kerin NZ, Noble RJ, Rubenfire M, Tabatznik B and Terry RW. Randomized withdrawal from nifedipine: placebo-controlled study in patients with coronary artery spasm. *Am Heart J* 104: 690–697, 1982
107 Schroeder JS, Feldman RL, Giles TD, Friedman MJ, DeMaria AN, Kinney EL, Mallon SM, Pit B, Meyer R, Basta LL et al Multiclinic controlled trial of diltiazem for Prinzmetal's angina. *Am J Med* 72: 227–232, 1982
108 Schroeder JS, Hung J, Lamb IH, Connolly SJ, Jutzy KR and Goris ML. Diltiazem and propranolol, alone and in combination, on exercise performance and left ventricular function in patients with stable effort angina: a double-blind, randomized, and placebo-controlled study. *Acta Pharmacol Toxicol (Copenh)* 57 Suppl 2: 55–60, 1985
109 Schroeder JS, Lamb IH, Bristow MR, Ginsburg R, Hung J and McAuley BJ. Prevention of cardiovascular events in variant angina by long-term diltiazem therapy. *J Am Coll Cardiol* 1: 1507–1511, 1983
110 Segawa D, Sjoquist PO, Wang QD, Gonon A and Ryden L. Time-dependent cardioprotection with calcium antagonism and experimental studies with clevidipine in ischemic-reperfused pig hearts: part II. *J Cardiovasc Pharmacol* 40: 339–345, 2002
111 Seitelberger R, Zwolfer W, Binder TM, Huber S, Peschl F, Spatt J, Schwarzacher S, Holzinger C, Coraim F, Weber H et al. Infusion of nifedipine after coronary artery bypass grafting decreases the incidence of early postoperative myocardial ischemia. *Ann Thorac Surg* 49: 61–67; discussion 67–68, 1990
112 Seitelberger R, Zwolfer W, Huber S, Schwarzacher S, Binder TM, Peschl F, Spatt J, Holzinger C, Podesser B, Buxbaum P et al. Nifedipine reduces the incidence of myocardial infarction and transient ischemia in patients undergoing coronary bypass grafting. *Circulation* 83: 460–468, 1991
113 Serruys PW, Steward R, Booman F, Michels R, Reiber JH and Hugenholtz PG. Can unstable angina pectoris be due to increased coronary vasomotor tone? *Eur Heart J* 1: 71–85, 1980
114 Sherman LG and Liang CS. Nifedipine in chronic stable angina: a double-blind placebo-controlled crossover trial. *Am J Cardiol* 51: 706–711, 1983
115 Singh B. A fourth class of anti-dysrhythmic action? Effect of verapamil and ouabain toxicity, on atrial and ventricular intracellular potentials, and on other features of cardiac function.

Cardiovasc Res 45: 39–42, 2000
116 Singh BN. A fourth class of anti-dysrhythmic action? Effect of verapamil on ouabain toxicity, on atrial and ventricular intracellular potentials, and on other features of cardiac function. *Cardiovasc Res* 6: 109–119, 1972
117 Soma MR, Donetti E, Parolini C, Barberi L, Paoletti R, Fumagalli R and Catapano AL. Effect of lacidipine on the carotid intimal hyperplasia induced by cuff injury. *J Cardiovasc Pharmacol* 23 Suppl 5: S71–74, 1994
118 Soma MR, Donetti E, Seregni R, Barberi L, Fumagalli R, Paoletti R and Catapano AL. Effect of lacidipine on fatty and proliferative lesions induced in hypercholesterolaemic rabbits. *Br J Pharmacol* 118: 215–219, 1996
119 Staessen JA, Wang JG and Thijs L. Calcium-channel blockade and cardiovascular prognosis: recent evidence from clinical outcome trials. *Am J Hypertens* 15: 85S-93S, 2002
120 Staessen JA, Wang JG and Thijs L. Cardiovascular protection and blood pressure reduction: a meta-analysis. *Lancet* 358: 1305–1315, 2001
121 Stone PH and Muller JE. Nifedipine therapy for recurrent ischemic pain following myocardial infarction. *Clin Cardiol* 5: 223–230, 1982
122 Stone PH, Muller JE, Turi ZG, Geltman E, Jaffe AS and Braunwald E. Efficacy of nifedipine therapy in patients with refractory angina pectoris: significance of the presence of coronary vasospasm. *Arq Bras Cardiol* 41: 469–476, 1983
123 Striessnig J. Targeting voltage-gated Ca^{2+} channels. *Lancet* 357: 1294, 2001
124 Szlachcic J, Waters DD, Miller D and Theroux P. Ventricular arrhythmias during ergonovine-induced episodes of variant angina. *Am Heart J* 107: 20–24, 1984
125 Takimoto K, Li D, Nerbonne JM and Levitan ES. Distribution, splicing and glucocorticoid-induced expression of cardiac alpha 1C and alpha 1D voltage-gated Ca^{2+} channel mRNAs. *J Mol Cell Cardiol* 29: 3035–3042, 1997
126 Tan AT, Sadick N, Kelly DT, Harris PJ, Freedman SB and Bautovich G. Verapamil in stable effort angina: effects on left ventricular function evaluated with exercise radionuclide ventriculography. *Am J Cardiol* 49: 425–430, 1982
127 Taylor CR, Hodge EM and White DA. Circadian rhythm of angina: similarity to circadian rhythms of myocardial infarction, ischemic ST segment depression, and sudden cardiac death. The Amlodipine Angina Study Group. *Am Heart J* 118: 1098–1099, 1989
128 Terry RW. Nifedipine therapy in angina pectoris: evaluation of safety and side-effects. *Am Heart J* 104: 681–689, 1982
129 Thaulow E and Jorgensen B. Results and clinical implications of the CAPARES trial. *Can J Cardiol* 16 Suppl D: 8D–11D, 2000
130 Theroux P, Taeymans Y, Morissette D, Bosch X, Pelletier GB and Waters DD. A randomized study comparing propranolol and diltiazem in the treatment of unstable angina. *J Am Coll Cardiol* 5: 717–722, 1985
131 Tilmant PY, Lablanche JM, Thieuleux FA, Dupuis BA and Bertrand ME. Detrimental effect of propranolol in patients with coronary arterial spasm countered by combination with diltiazem. *Am J Cardiol* 52: 230–233, 1983
132 Tshirdewahn B and Klepzig H. Clinical Studies on the effect of Isoptin and Isoptin S in patients with coronary insufficiency (in German). *Deutsche Med Wochensch* 88: 1702–1710, 1963
133 Tulenko TN, Sumner AE, Chen M, Huang Y, Laury-Kleintop L and Ferdinand FD. The smooth muscle cell membrane during atherogenesis: a potential target for amlodipine in atheroprotection. *Am Heart J* 141: S1–11, 2001
134 van der Wall EE, Kerkkamp HJ, Simoons ML, van Rijk PP, Reiber JH, Bom N, Lubsen JC and Lie KI. Effects of nifedipine on left ventricular performance in unstable angina pectoris during a follow-up of 48 hours. *Am J Cardiol* 57: 1029–1033, 1986
135 Waters DD, Theroux P, Szlachcic J and Dauwe F. Provocative testing with ergonovine to assess the efficacy of treatment with nifedipine, diltiazem and verapamil in variant angina. *Am J Cardiol* 48: 123–130, 1981
136 Wijeysundera DN, Beattie WS, Rao V and Karski J. Calcium antagonists reduce cardiovascular complications after cardiac surgery: a meta-analysis. *J Am Coll Cardiol* 41: 1496–1505, 2003
137 Willis AL, Nagel B, Churchill V, Whyte MA, Smith DL, Mahmud I and Puppione DL. Antiatherosclerotic effects of nicardipine and nifedipine in cholesterol-fed rabbits. *Arteriosclerosis* 5: 250–255, 1985
138 Yasue H, Nagao M, Omote S, Takizawa A, Miwa K and Tanaka S. Coronary arterial spasm and

Prinzmetal's variant form of angina induced by hyperventilation and Tris-buffer infusion. *Circulation* 58: 56–62, 1978

138aYusuf S, Zucker D, Peduzzi P, Fisher LD, Takaro T, Kennedy JW, Davis K, Killip T, Passamani E, Norris R et al. Effect of coronary artery bypass graft surgery on survival: overview of 10-year results from randomised trials by the Coronary Artery Bypass Graft Surgery Trialists Collaboration. *Lancet* 344: 563-570, 1994

139 Zanchetti A. Emerging data on calcium-channel blockers: the COHORT study. *Clin Cardiol* 26: II17–20, 2003

140 Zanchetti A. Role of calcium antagonists in systemic hypertension. *Am J Cardiol* 59: 130B–136B, 1987

141 Zanchetti A, Bond MG, Hennig M, Neiss A, Mancia G, Dal Palu C, Hansson L, Magnani B, Rahn KH, Reid JL et al. Calcium antagonist lacidipine slows down progression of asymptomatic carotid atherosclerosis: principal results of the European Lacidipine Study on Atherosclerosis (ELSA), a randomized, double-blind, long-term trial. *Circulation* 106: 2422–2427, 2002

142 Zanchetti A and Leonetti G. Natriuretic effects of calcium antagonists. Clinical implications. *Drugs* 40 Suppl 2: 15–21, 1990

143 Zanchetti A and Mancia G. The ALLHAT trial: a verdict or a challenge? *J Hypertens* 21: 223, 2003

144 Zanchetti A, Rosei EA, Dal Palu C, Leonetti G, Magnani B and Pessina A. The Verapamil in Hypertension and Atherosclerosis Study (VHAS): results of long-term randomized treatment with either verapamil or chlorthalidone on carotid intima-media thickness. *J Hypertens* 16: 1667–1676, 1998

Beyond the cardiovascular system

As discussed in former chapters blockade of L-type calcium channels by dihydropyridines, phenylalkylamines and benzothiazepines forms the basis for treatment of cardiovascular diseases. A number of other agents that either unselectively or selectively target neuronal and other calcium channels have been described. Some of them have been introduced in therapy to treat gastrointestinal or neuronal disorders and more recently, blockers of Ca_V2 channels have become the subject of intense interest regarding their potentiality for the treatment of chronic and neuropathic pain, this appears promising for a variety of pain conditions. The purpose of this section is to review already established non-cardiovascular therapies and to point to further possibilities.

Calcium antagonists and gastrointestinal pharmacology

Motor activity of the gastrointestinal tract

Synchronized circumferential contractions and propagating phasic contractile activity are important components of gastrointestinal motility involved in propulsion of food and food residues. These contractions are initiated and regulated by electrical activity (slow-wave-type action potentials or slow waves) of the smooth muscle cell membranes. Periodically electrical pacemaker potentials are generated by specialized pacemaker cells [a network of interstitial cells of Cajal (ICC) and smooth muscle cells] and propagated into the rest of the smooth muscle layer. Slow-wave-type action potentials generated in the smooth muscle layers consist of an upstroke phase and a plateau phase with or without superimposed spikes. Calcium channels play a role in both the initiation of the slow-wave and in the generation of the plateau phase, the latter being associated with generation and regulation of contraction. Pharmacological manipulation of calcium channel activity influences the slow wave frequency and propagation, determining the characteristics of propulsion and synchronization, as well as the duration and amplitude of the slow wave plateau phase, determining the force of the individual phasic contractions. Colonic circular smooth muscle of the dog is electrically dominated by pacemaker activity generated by a network of ICC located at its submucosal border. This activity (a six-cycles-per-minute depolarizing pulse) is transmitted to the circular muscle cells where it activates L-type calcium channels that lead to the creation of a slow-wave-type action potential. It is the plateau phase of the action potential, generated through L-type calcium channels, that is associated with generation of contraction. The amplitude and duration of the plateau phase depends on the level of excitation. Modification of this plateau potential by excitatory or inhibitory drugs is directly related to modification of force of contraction. At high levels of excitation, activity of L-type calcium channels creates spikes superimposed on the plateau phase of the slow waves further increasing force of contraction. L-type calcium channel blockers affect the slow-wave-type action potential in gastrointestinal smooth muscle in a very characteristic manner. They inhibit the plateau potential without affecting the frequency of the activity. In many intestinal tissues, force of contraction is enhanced through development of spiking activity superimposed on the slow waves. Calcium channel blockers inhibit spike activity at concentrations lower than those needed to inhibit the slow-wave plateau [4, 33]. In conscious dogs, intravenous infusions not only of nifedipine but also of verapamil and diltiazem, exert profound inhibitory effects on intestinal motility [16]. Nifedipine and nilvadipine reduced activity in the proximal colon of the dog. Oral or sublingual administration of nifedipine also decreased lower esophageal sphincter (LES) pressure and partially inhibited the LES response to tetragastrin or bethanechol in dogs [31].

Because L-type calcium channel blockers were already used in gastrointestinal motor disorders such as esophageal spasm and excessive postprandial colonic contractions [47] but that their actions on the cardiovascu1ar system and the vasculature have prevented widespread acceptance, Huizinga and his colleagues [44] have compared the action of pinaverium to the action of classical CCBs (diltiazem, nicardipine and D600) on canine circular smooth muscle. Indeed, pinaverium bromide was found to interact with the dihydropyridine site, at the external surface of the plasma membrane, in a competitive manner [21, 45] and could substitute to classical CCBs. Data obtained from different experimental conditions provide a rationale for the clinical use of pinaveriun bromide to decrease the force of contraction in the colon. Oral intake of pinaverium bromide does not lead to significant blood levels and consequently is without effects on the cardiovascular system. Pinaverium bromide is hypothesized to be absorbed into the muscle wall of the colon, directly from the gut [12].

Clinical studies

Upper GI tract

In normal human volunteers, LES pressure was reduced by nifedipine (10–40 mg), but only by about 40% at the highest dose administered [6], and nifedipine generally had a much less pronounced effect on contraction amplitude in the body of the esophagus. Nifedipine (20 mg, sublingually) reduced LES pressure by about 30–35% in achalasia patients. Thus, in both healthy and achalasia humans, oral nifedipine reduces LES pressure. Nifedipine also showed some promise (reduced esophageal pressure) in patients with "nutcracker esophagus," very high LES pressures, or diffuse esophageal spasm, but symptoms were not improved and adverse cardiovascular side-effects occurred in some cases [60]. It was concluded that nifedipine could be useful in treating elderly achalasia patients possessing risk factors that would render pneumatic dilatation or surgery inappropriate. A placebo-controlled, double-blind crossover study was performed to compare the effects of oral nifedipine (up to 20 mg) and verapamil (160 mg) on LES pressure, esophageal contraction amplitude, and clinical symptomatology in patients with achalasia. Both nifedipine and verapamil significantly decreased mean LES pressure, but only nifedipine caused a significant decrease in the amplitude of esophageal contractions. No statistically significant improvement in overall clinical symptomatology was observed with these drugs, but some individual improvements in dysphagia and chest pain were noted in these achalasia patients [80]. In another trial, the effect of sublingual nifedipine (mean dose, 55 mg/day; I.e., 10–20 mg, 30 minutes before meals) and pneumatic dilatation were compared in patients suffering from mild or moderate esophageal achalasia. Significant decreases in LES pressure were produced by both treatments, and excellent or good clinical results were observed in 75% of the dilated patients and in 77% of the patients treated with nifedipine. One of the 14 patients treated with nifedipine could not tolerate the drug. It was concluded that long-term treatment with sublingual nifedipine and pneumatic dilatation are equally effective in treating mild-to-moderate esophageal achalasia [13]. In contrast to these positive results, Robertson et al. [63] had not found that nifedipine (10 mg, 15 minutes before meals) produced detectable decrease in LES pressure in achalasia patients. However, the methods used by these latter workers differed from Coccia et al. [13]; e.g., the dose of nifedipine (10 mg) that was administered was lower and it was given at shorter intervals before meals.

Lower GI tract

Nifedipine (30 mg, p.o.) did not affect fasting or postprandial duodenal or jejunal motility, and did not alter gastric emptying in normal subjects [66], but similar doses inhibited colonic spike activity induced by eating and decreased the abnormal colonic motor response to distension in patients afflicted with irritable bowel syndrome (IBS). In the practice of gastroenterology, organic disease, peptic ulcer, cholelithiasis, pancreatitis, diverticulitis (definite structural anatomical problems) account for about 50% of the practice referral base. The other 50% involves such upper gastrointestinal symptoms such as dyspepsia, indigestion, esophageal problems, so-called functional disease, and in turn a large part of that overlaps the spectrum of irritable bowel syndrome (IBS). Irritable bowel syndrome (IBS) involves a heterogenous group of entities. Patients can have varying bowel habits, either diarrhea or constipation, sometimes alternating, are exquisitely sensitive to bowel distention, have a very low threshold for pain, and some have an enhanced gastrocolic reflex [31]. There may be stress factors, there may be psychological implications in some of these patients, and indeed there may be different sensitivities in the right side of the large bowel compared to the transverse colon, and compared to the left side of the bowel [6]. Sublingually-administered nifedipine and intravenously-administered nicardipine reduced colonic motor responses to a standard meal in IBS patients. Paired controlled studies were conducted in normal volunteers and patients with IBS to examine the effect of standard nicardipine (20 mg, p.o.) and sustained-release nicardipine (30 mg, t.i.d.) on the responses of the anorectum to rectal distension and a meal [77]. In normal volunteers, standard nicardipine did not affect rectal responses to distension but did significantly reduce the postprandial motility index. In IBS patients, standard nicardipine caused a significant reduction in distention-induced rectal motor activity and increased the rectal sensory thresholds for desire to defecate and discomfort. Both formulations of nicardipine significantly reduced the postprandial motility index and symptoms, supporting the contention that Ca^{2+} -antagonists may be useful in managing IBS [77]. The most pronounced change with the largest increase in motility occurs in the sigmoid colon, which also seems to be the site of most symptoms in IBS patients [32]. Each of the segments has a sensitivity to eating, perhaps least so in the ascending colon which is the part of the colon where fecal contents of the stool are rather liquidy and perhaps less distending. Is there a rationale for calcium channel blockers in IBS? Nifedipine has been shown to decrease the rectosigmoid motility index, which occurs in response to distention; in other words, it will decrease or minimize the contraction and pain related to distention of the bowel [58]. Nifedipine will also decrease the postprandial rectosigmoid gastrocolic reflex. Huizinga's experiments reported above support clinical studies that have indicated effectiveness of pinaverium in irritable bowel syndrome [3, 57].

Calcium antagonists and neuropharmacology

When considering neuropharmacological indications, a review of 1986 [22], mentioned the beneficial effect of flunarizine and nimodipine in the treatment of common and classical migraine. The pharmacological target for this action (cerebral arteries or neurones) remained controversial. Clinical trials examined the protective action of specific calcium entry blockers in ischaemic brain damage. Current data in patients with aneurysmal subarachnoid hemorrhage indicated that nimodipine, a calcium entry blocker with a predilective action on the cerebral circulation, could improve the clinical situation of patients at risk. Clinical reports have demonstrated a beneficial action of cinnarizine and flunarizine in the treatment of vertigo and in sleep disorders, in aged patients. Preliminary data suggested a possible action in some forms of epilepsia. An interaction of neuroleptics with calcium channels has been clearly demonstrated [67]. Therefore, calcium channels might be targets for therapeutic actions beyond the cardiovascular system.

Migraine (with a note on vertigo)

As far as migraine treatment is concerned, there is a large body of information confirming the efficacy of flunarizine and nimodipine for the prevention of the migraine attacks, which are reduced in frequency in patients treated with these drugs [18, 42]. In comparative studies, it has been reported that flunarizine was more effective than nimodipine in prophylactic treatment. For instance in a trial, flunarizine was given for a six-month treatment at the dose of 10 mg once daily and nimodipine for the same period at a dose of 40 mg. The authors observed that the frequency of migraine attacks was reduced to 20% with flunarizine and to 50% with nifedipine. Furthermore, the therapeutic effect persisted after discontinuation of the treatment: during eight months with flunarizine and five months with nimodipine; these differences were statistically significant [49]. It has also been reported that flunarizine reduced cortical spreading depression [19].

Such agents, therefore, appear to be active in disseminated nervous disorders. Recent studies in patients suffering from migraines [8, 26] have provided evidence that the visual aura is the result of cortical spreading depression (CSD), a wave of neuronal depolarization that spreads slowly across the cerebral cortex. Investigations in animal models and humans indicate that the headache is a consequence of activation of trigeminovascular afferents innervating the meninges, causing neurogenic inflammation and activation of trigeminal nucleus caudalis and brainstem nuclei involved in the perception of pain [46]. It has been reported [7] that CSD in the rat cortex activates trigeminovascular afferents and evokes a series of alterations in the meninges and brainstem consistent with the development of headache. These data, together with earlier pharmacological work, point to CSD as a critical event in the pathogenesis of migraine with aura. Some authors have proposed that nitrergic nerves are involved in this process [52, 78].

Tottene et al. [79] have studied a familial hemiplegic migraine (FHM), a dominantly inherited subtype of migraine with aura associated with ictal hemiparesis associated with a mutations in the gene encoding the pore-forming a_1-subunit of $Ca_V2.1$ (voltage- gated P-Q-type) channels. They expressed FHM mutants in $Ca_V2.1$-deficient neurons. They uncovered two common changes in $Ca_V2.1$ function caused by FHM mutations: an increased single-channel Ca^{2+} influx and a decreased maximal $Ca_V2.1$ current density in neurons. According to the authors, these functional alterations should favor the spontaneous occurrence of CSD in the brain of patients. Therefore a role for $Ca_V2.1$ channels could be dominant in the pathogenesis of migraine aura, indicating a potential molecular target for unspecific calcium channel blockers such as flunarizine. Alternatively, Ca_V1 channels (L-type) may also be involved, since they are upregulated in mouse brain subjected to episodes of CSD [11]. There are other targets, which could account for an action of CCBs, one of them could be NF-kappaB, which has recently been proposed to play a role in migraine [59]. It appears that the precise mechanism of action of CCBs in migraine remains conjectural, but identified targets support the clinical observations of their therapeutic benefit.

Note on vertigo

Vertigo associated with migraine may also be reduced by CCBs [27]. Similarly, cinnarizine and nimodipine were efficacious in otological vertigo [56]. This is also true for the action of flunarizine in vestibular neuritis [15]. It might be that such therapeutics effects are related to a vascular action.

Pain

CCBs and opioids

There have been several experimental reports showing that CCBs may potentiate the analgesic effects of opioid. For instance, in animal studies by using the acetic acid writhing test in mice, it appeared that subcutaneous injections of diltiazem, verapamil, nicardipine, flunarizine and cinnarizine produced a dose-dependent antinociception. This activity of diltiazem was stereospecific; d-cis-diltiazem was more potent than 1-cis-diltiazem. All the calcium channel blockers studied increased morphine analgesia and displaced to the left the morphine dose-response curve. The effect of diltiazem being stereospecific, this indicates that calcium channel blockers may induce analgesia and do increase morphine analgesia.[17]. Caro et al. have examined the effects of two enantiomers of diltiazem (l-cis and d-cis) on naloxone-precipitated morphine abstinence after acute morphine dependence *in vivo* in mice. d-cis-diltiazem (10–40 mg/kg) produced a dose-dependent inhibition of the jumping and body weight loss induced by naloxone in acutely morphine dependent mice. By contrast, l-cis-diltiazem 40 mg/kg did not significantly inhibit jumping and produced a much lower inhibition of body weight loss than the same dose of d-cis-diltiazem [9]. Contreras et al. have observed that the administration of nifedipine, flunarizine and verapamil reduced the intensity of the tolerance induced by a single dose of morphine administered in a slow release preparation [14]. Kishioka et al. examined the interaction between calcium channel blockade with drug-induced analgesia and respiratory depression in rhesus monkey. The antinociceptive effects of the drugs were evaluated using a warm-water (50 °C) tail-withdrawal assay in rhesus monkeys, and the respiratory depressant effects were evaluated using a pressure-displacement plethysmograph. Pre-treatment with diltiazem (10–40 mg/kg, i.m.) 30 min before administration of morphine (0.3 to 10 mg/kg) or heroin (0.03 to 1.0 mg/kg) produced a dose-dependent potentiation of the opioid-induced analgesia. The analgesic potency of morphine and heroin was increased by approximately 0.5 log unit in the presence of 40 mg/kg diltiazem. However, diltiazem failed to alter the analgesic potencies of μ-opioid and κ-opioid receptor agonists or the non-opioid, clonidine. Respiratory frequency, minute volume, and tidal volume were suppressed by morphine, heroin, and fentanyl, but these effects were not modified by pre-treatment with diltiazem (40 mg/kg) indicating the specific action of CCBs on morphine- and heroin-induced analgesia. At variance, Gullapalli and Ramarao observed a potentiation by nimodipine and lercanidipine of the analgesia of κ-opioid receptor agonist in rats [24]. This indicates that they may be species and/or methodology variations. Further studies have confirmed interaction between CCBs and opioids at the biochemical level. Gullapalli et al. observed that nimodipine reversed the down-regulation of CCBs binding sites evoked by naloxone in rats treated by naloxone (1 mg/kg) during 10 days [24, 25, 38].

Similar observations have been done in patients. For instance, Santillan et al. have examined the ability of nimodipine to reduce the daily dose of oral morphine in cancer patients who had developed dose escalation, in patients under randomized, double-blind, placebo-controlled conditions [68]. They selected patients that required at least two successive increments of morphine to maintain pain relief. They observed that the dose of morphine was reduced from 313 ± 52 to 174 ± 33 mg/day ($P < 0.001$) in the nimodipine group, and from 254 ± 26 to 218 ± 19 mg/day (not significant) in the placebo group. However, in another clinical trial, Nitahara et al. found that continuous *i.v.* infusion of diltiazem did not reduce epidural fentanyl consumption when administered at dosages having minimal haemodynamic depressant effects [48, 68]. However pharmacokinetics conditions and the site of action of tested drugs are different in the two trials here summarized, therefore the actions of nimodipine and diltiazem cannot be compared in those two settings. Furthermore, as was shown in an experiment comparing verapamil and flunarizine, the opioid receptor sub-types involved in their action are not identical [83].

Neuropathic pain

Pain is usually an indication of tissue injury and is usually temporary in duration. With healing, the pain associated with the injury will resolve. Its major role is to warn the individual from further injury. However, in some individuals, this painful experience can result in chronic pain that persists for months or even years after the initial insult as a result of disruption of the nervous system. This abnormality of the peripheral, central, and sympathetic nervous system can result in a painful state termed neuropathic. Hence, neuropathic pain represents a chronic pain syndrome group with a diverse etiology and perhaps an anatomical cause. L-, N- and P/Q-types Ca^{2+} channel types (see page 27 for IUPHAR nomenclature) are expressed in the spinal cord and studies summarized based on the spinal delivery of specific antagonists to high-threshold calcium channels reveal that blockade of L-type, P/Q-type and particularly, N-type channels can prevent, attenuate, or both, subjective pain as well as primary and/or secondary hyperalgesia and allodynia in a variety of experimental and clinical conditions. In various animal models, the selective block of N-type currents via intrathecal administration of ϖ-conotoxin GVIA or ϖ-conotoxin MVIIA significantly depresses the formalin Phase 2 response, thermal hyperalgesia, mechanical allodynia and post-surgical pain [81].

Ziconotide, a synthetic form of the 25 amino acid cationic *Conus magus* peptide toxin, MVIIA, is a selective antagonist of the N-type $Ca_v2.2$ channel. Ziconotide has been shown to be antinociceptive in animal models of persistent, postoperative and neuropathic pain. It is up to several orders of magnitude more potent than morphine on intrathecal administration and does not appear to exhibit tolerance or addiction characteristics. Its probable site of action is the high concentration of N-type $Ca_v2.2$-channels found in the superficial laminae of the spinal cord dorsal horn, although there is also some evidence for efficacy on injured peripheral nerves upon subcutaneous administration. Intrathecal bolus injection of ziconotide is significantly more potent and long-lasting for the inhibition of heat hyperalgesia and mechanical allodynia in a rat model of post-operative pain. In addition, ziconotide appears to be more specific in its action compared to morphine. Pre-treatment with intrathecal ziconotide was also shown to prevent the establishment of allodynia and hyperalgesia [55, 61, 71, 82].

Gabapentin, 1-(aminomethyl) cyclohexaneacetic acid, is a novel anticonvulsant drug found to be active in a variety of animal seizure models. It is considered as an important and effective drug in the management of neuropathic pain syndromes. The efficacy of gabapentin in preventing hyperalgesia has been demonstrated in a number of different animal models of neuropathic pain It appears to have a unique effect on voltage-dependent calcium ion channels at the post-synaptic dorsal horns and may, therefore, interrupt the series of events that possibly leads to the experience of a neuropathic pain sensation. Gabapentin is especially effective at relieving allodynia and hyperalgesia in animal models. It has been shown to be efficacious in numerous small clinical studies and case reports in a wide variety of pain syndromes. Gabapentin has been clearly demonstrated to be effective for the treatment of neuropathic pain in diabetic neuropathy and postherpetic neuralgia. This evidence, combined with its favourable side-effect profile in various patient groups (including the elderly) and lack of drug interactions, makes it an attractive agent [64]. The gabapentin binding site has been purified from pig brain and gabapentin was identified as the first ligand to interact with the $\alpha_2\delta$ subunit of high-threshold Ca^{2+} channels. Both the $\alpha_2\delta$ subunit protein and [^{3}H]+gabapentin binding sites are up-regulated in the dorsal horn following sciatic nerve chronic constriction injury. The association of $\alpha_2\delta$ with the pore-forming α_1 subunit of the Ca^{2+} channel modulates channel function. This indicates that gabapentin could affect Ca channel function indirectly, thereby modulating neuronal excitability [72]. The exact mode of action of gabapentin still needs to be better evaluated. No doubt that this investigation shall improve our knowledge about interaction of drugs alleviating pain with calcium channels.

Dementia

Confirming earlier claims a recent Harvard Health Letter (of May 2003) announced that calcium channel blockers may prevent dementia. The authors mentioned the fact that for years, doctors have known about a possible connection between high blood pressure and dementia, a correlation found nowadays statistically significant. They referred to Systeur trial [73] designed to test whether active treatment could reduce cardiovascular complications of isolated systolic hypertension. According to Atkinson, targeting cerebral circulation is an option for therapy in dementia [2]. Fatal and non-fatal stroke combined was the primary endpoint of Systeur trial. After stratification for centre, sex, and previous cardiovascular complications, 4,695 patients were randomly assigned to nitrendipine 10–40 mg daily, with the possible addition of enalapril 5–20 mg daily and hydrochlorothiazide 12.5–25.0 mg daily, or matching placebos. The authors of this trial observed that active treatment reduced the total rate of stroke from 13.7 to 7.9 endpoints per 1,000 patient-years (42% reduction; $p = 0.003$). Non-fatal stroke decreased by 44% ($p = 0.007$). In the active treatment group, all fatal and non-fatal cardiac endpoints, including sudden death, declined by 26% ($p = 0.03$). Non-fatal cardiac endpoints decreased by 33% ($p = 0.03$) and all fatal and non-fatal cardiovascular endpoints by 31% ($p < 0.001$). Cardiovascular mortality was slightly lower on active treatment (-27%, $p = 0.07$), but all-cause mortality was not influenced (–14%; $p = 0.22$). They concluded that among elderly patients with isolated systolic hypertension, antihypertensive drug treatment starting with nitrendipine reduces the rate of cardiovascular complications and that treatment of 1,000 patients for five years with this type of regimen may prevent 29 strokes or 53 major cardiovascular endpoints. In a further analysis they examined the problem of dementia and found that participants initially assigned to take the calcium-channel blocker were 55% less likely to develop dementia, in particular Alzheimer's disease than those given a placebo [74].

Lopez-Arrieta et al. aimed to assess the clinical efficacy of nimodipine for the manifestations of dementia, in unclassified disease and in the major subtypes—Alzheimer's disease, cerebrovascular disease, and mixed Alzheimer's and cerebrovascular disease. Their search was based on the Cochrane Dementia and Cognitive Improvement Group's Specialized Register, which contains reports of trials from all major medical databases and many trial databases. Data were extracted independently by the reviewers and the odds ratio (95% CI) or the average difference (95% CI) were estimated. Both intention-to-treat and on-treatment results were extracted. Fourteen trials were included which tested two treatment regimes, 90 and 180 mg/day of nimodipine for 12 and 24 weeks. Two trials included only patients with Alzheimer's disease (AD), nine trials included only patients with cerebrovascular dementia (CVD), and three trials included patients with AD, CVD and mixed disease. Available outcome data from nine trials (2,492 patients) cover the domains of cognitive function, activities of daily living, global clinical state, safety and tolerability.

By pooling available data from all trials, whatever the diagnosis of the patients included, the reviewers found benefit associated with nimodipine (90 mg/day at 12 weeks) compared with placebo. When the AD trials and the VD trials were pooled separately similar significant results were found for the 90 mg/day dose of nimodipine at 12 weeks. The authors concluded that nimodipine can be of some benefit in the treatment of patients with features of dementia due to unclassified disease or to Alzheimer's disease, cerebrovascular disease, or mixed Alzheimer's and cerebrovascular disease [43].

In a multinational, double-blind, placebo-controlled study, Pantoni et al. evaluated the safety and efficacy of nimodipine administered for as long as 26 weeks in improving cognition or slowing cognitive deterioration in patients defined as having multi-infarct dementia (DSM-III-R criteria). Two hundred and fifty-nine patients were included (128 nimodipine, 131 placebo), and 251 were available for the intention-to-treat analysis. This study failed to show a significant effect of nimodipine on cognitive, social or global assessments in patients defined as affected by multi-infarct dementia according to the DSM-III-R criteria. However, a lower incidence of cerebrovascular and cardiac events was observed in the nimodipine-treated patients in comparison with the placebo group. A *post hoc* analysis (presented in an accompanying paper) suggests that nimodipine may have a favorable effect in the subgroup of patients defined as affected by subcortical (small vessel) vascular dementia [53, 54].

This brief review shows that calcium channel blockers may have benefits for the brain that other blood pressure medications do not have. In a large meta-analysis, Staessen et al. [15] concluded that all antihypertensive drugs have similar long-term efficacy and safety. Calcium channel blockers might be especially effective in stroke prevention. They did not find that converting-enzyme inhibitors or a-blockers affect cardiovascular prognosis beyond their antihypertensive effects [75]. Calcium channel blockers cross the blood-brain barrier and reduce the turnover of some neurotransmitters deficient in dementia. Since they have been shown to have neuroprotective effects in animal experiments. By slowing the movement of calcium into cells, they may be a boost to aging brain cells, which have a hard time maintaining regular calcium levels [40].

Subarachnoid haemorrhage

Brain ischaemia, which may be related to vasospasm, is a frequent cause of poor outcome in patients with subarachnoid haemorrhage. Although the pathogenesis of delayed cerebral vasospasm after subarachnoid haemorrhage remains quite unclear [34, 41], experimental studies have indicated that calcium antagonists can prevent or reverse vasospasm [28]. In ischaemic tissues, high-energy phosphate depletion is thought to cause rundown of ionic gradients and membrane depolarization, leading to excessive Ca^{2+} influx. When this excess of free Ca^{2+} can no longer be rapidly sequestered into intracellular stores or removed from the cell, it provokes a wide array of metabolic changes, which can result in cell death. Moreover, with reperfusion, extracellular Ca^{2+} increases, and cells not initially damaged by the ischaemia may be affected by the injurious effects of rapid Ca^{2+} overload [36, 69, 70]. Membrane stabilization, improvement of the rheology and inhibition of neurotransmitter release constitute putative mechanisms for cellular protection. However, blocking the deleterious Ca^{2+} accumulation by damaged tissues is probably the most effective way to improve the cell survival. CCBs have been reported to be an important class of drug in the prophylactic and therapeutic managements of cardiac and cerebral ischaemia. Moreover, beside their preventive action on excessive Ca^{2+} influx into the cells, these drugs promote the relaxation of cerebral vascular smooth muscle and thereby restore the cerebral blood flow. The neuroprotective effect of CCBs has been documented after both global and focal ischaemia in animal experiments [1, 5, 50, 51]. Studies with cells in culture have shown the ability of nervous cells to adapt to and recover from insult. Excitable cells, when submitted to prolonged or intermittent membrane depolarization occurring in brain ischaemia [35], could react by adapting the functional activity of their own voltage-dependent Ca^{2+} channels. Feron and Godfraind [20] have examined the regulation of L-type calcium channels in chronically depolarized neuronal and vascular smooth muscle cells. Their study revealed that the two cell types are differently regulated by a chronic treatment with high K^+ concentrations. Neuron-type cells exhibited a reversible down-regulation of L-type Ca^{2+} channels whereas vascular smooth muscle cells were characterized by a long-term inactivation of Ca^{2+} channels without modification of their expression. They also observed that nifedipine protected isolated cells from the deleterious effects of prolonged depolarization.

Calcium antagonists have been studied in several clinical trials, but data are conflicting. Rinkel et al. [62] have searched the Cochrane Stroke Group Trials Register in order to determine whether calcium antagonists improve outcome in patients with aneurysmal subarachnoid haemorrhage (SAH). They selected all completed, unconfounded, truly randomised controlled trials comparing any calcium antagonist with control, within ten days of SAH onset. Eleven trials that met the inclusion criteria were included in the overview, totaling 2,804 randomised patients with subarachnoid haemorrhage (1,376 in the treatment and 1,428 in the control group). The drugs analysed were: nimodipine (eight trials, 1,574 patients), nicardipine (two trials, 954 patients), and AT877 (one trial, 276 patients). In 92% of the patients aneurysms were confirmed by angiography or autopsy. They concluded that calcium antagonists reduce the proportion of patients with poor outcome and ischaemic neurological deficits after aneurysmal SAH. The results for 'poor outcome' are statistically robust, but depend largely on one large trial with oral nimodipine; the evidence for nicardipine is inconclusive. The evidence for nimodipine is not beyond every doubt, but given the potential benefits and modest risks associated with this treatment, against the background of a devastating natural history, oral nimodipine (60 mg every four hours) is indicated in patients with aneurysmal SAH. For oral nimodipine uncertainty remains regarding patients in poor clinical condition on admission or in patients with established cerebral ischaemia, since there is an optimal time window. Furthermore, the concentration of the CCB in the vicinity of the spastic artery is of great importance as shown by the study of Kasuya et al. [34]. These authors have conducted a study to examine the efficacy and safety of nicardipine prolonged-release implants (NPRI) for humans, which have already been proven in dogs. Twenty consecutive subarachnoid haemorrhage patients with thick subarachnoid clot were treated with NPRI (a pellet of diameter 2 mm, length 10 mm, containing 4 mg of nicardipine) during surgery after clipping of their aneurysm. The number and location of pellets depended on the amount and site of subarachnoid clot on pre-operative CT and on craniotomy. Two to 10 pellets were implanted in the cistern of the internal carotid, middle cerebral, and/or anterior cerebral artery, where thick clots existed and therefore vasospasm related to delayed ischaemic neurological deficits was highly likely. Delayed ischaemic neurological deficits and cerebral infarctions were seen in one patient. Angiography performed on days seven to 12 revealed no vasospasm in any arteries near which NPRI were placed. No complications were experienced. They concluded that vasospasm being completely prevented for the arteries in thick clot cisterns, when NPRI were placed adjacent to the arteries during surgery. According to the authors, this drug-delivery system offers a promising approach for preventing vasospasm. Further studies are required in order to better clarify the pharmacology of the vasospasm resulting from subarachnoid haemorrhages.

Perspectives

As shown along this book, ion channels play critical roles in the regulation of excitable cell physiology. In recent years, ion channel regulation of non-excitable cell function has also been recognized to be important. In Chapter 2, Figure 1 (page 12) illustrates that several pathways may contribute to the regulation of calcium entry into animal cells. Interest in ion channels as drug targets continues to grow with the hope to identify novel and more specific therapeutic agents. Although the future is by definition imperceptible, there are indications for identification of powerful medicines within a novel generation of calcium channel blockers. Calcium channels represent a rich class of validated targets for discovery of new therapeutic agents for treatment of central nervous system and cardiovascular disorders. In the recent years, much attention has been paid to subtypes and/or splice-variants of ion channels, although limited progress has been made towards discovery of new molecules that modulate these targets. Combinatorial chemistry is playing an increasingly important role as one of the modern medicinal chemistry tools for rapid discovery of new leads. The generation of combinatorial libraries of peptides and oligonucleotides is now well established, however, preparation of libraries of small organic molecules is an evolving area of research. An important feature of combinatorial chemistry is the synthesis of compounds on solid support to be employed for library construction. Gordeev et al. [23] have reported the preparation of a 300-member DHP library and its iterative screening for the identification of 1,4-dihydropyridines with potent calcium channel binding activity. By using competition of ^{3}H-nitrendipine binding, they have successfully identified in the DHP library, by rank ordering of the crude pools and components thereof, in addition to nifedipine, new potent calcium channel blockers.

A cornerstone in current drug discovery is high throughput screening assays (HTS), which allow examination of the activity of specific ion channels. Specific radioligand competition assays and patch clamp studies are techniques with sensitivity required for recognition of appropriate interaction with channels. Patch clamp presents sufficiently high time resolution for precise and direct characterization of ion channel properties. However, patch clamp is a slow, labor-intensive, and thus expensive, technique. The full pharmacological potential of ion channel active drugs is far from realized when using inadequate screening methods. Fortunately, automated ion channel screening technology is under development. Chip-based technology enables automated and parallel patch clamp assays. For instance, The Nanion Patch Clamp chips contain multiple apertures for cell positioning and seal formation. The microstructured glass chips enable whole cell as well as single channel recordings. The cell and compound application as well as the experimental protocol are fully automated. This technology overcomes the biggest hurdle in drug-screening assays evaluating ion channels, which has been to generate enough throughputs with high information content and reliability. The IonWorks HT system overcomes the major drawbacks to traditional patch clamp techniques. It performs high throughput whole cell patch clamping of multiple cells simultaneously using a 48-channel detection system to reach throughputs of up to 3,000 patches per day. Thus, new techniques combining the reliability and high information content of patch clamping with the virtues of high throughput screening are emerging and predicted to make a number of ion channel targets accessible for drug screening. According to Willumsen et al. the introduction of new powerful HTS electrophysiological techniques is predicted to cause a revolution in ion channel drug discovery [84].

We are entering the era of systems biology, where to understand a disease we feel obliged to understand its causes from the molecular level to the organism level. The whole biological molecules involved and the complex nature of their interactions are yet unidentified. Therefore, technology-driven science has not provided yet substitute for serendipity. During the drug discovery process, once the lead compound is identified, there is a need for a lead optimization phase during which the identified lead is subjected to methodical synthetic modification by medicinal chemists in order to optimize activity. At this stage it is crucial to develop drug assays providing therapeutically-relevant data in order to change the molecular structure of the drug to obtain the most appropriate activity. As pointed out by Kenakin, the use of recombinant systems as lead-optimization assays, although being a tremendous boon to drug discovery in terms of obviating species differences, still does not eliminate the leap of faith required in going from the laboratory to the clinic [37]. This faith is also required when searching for novel CCBs. Indeed, the pressure of 'déjà vu' could discard promoters of research from this field, despite evidences for potentialities with novel compounds having clinically valid indications in epilepsy, migraine, pain and other pathologies. Developing a comprehensive analytical pharmacology within this field could improve the drug discovery process by disclosing the most appropriate targets for the lead-optimization assays. For instance, the novel piperazines dotarizine and lomerizine [30, 65] share some properties with flunarizine, but a comparative pharmacological profile, considering also their interaction with VOCs, has not been performed. Therefore, it cannot be assumed that dotarizine is an optimized flunarizine and could have better clinical indications particularly in epilepsy, where despite positive experimental results [29, 39, 67, 72, 76], clinical applications are not as successful [10].

The jump from pharmacological experiments to clinical trials remains hazardous and once a chemical agent has become a drug, a long time might be required before being universally recognized as a safe medicine. Twenty years after the earliest clinical trials and after many controversies, ALLHAT has proven the safety of calcium channel blockers! A long time ago, Withering wrote about digitalis: 'Time will fix the real value upon this discovery, and determine whether I imposed upon myself and others, or contributed to the benefit of science and mankind' [85].

References

1 Alps BJ. Drugs acting on calcium channels: potential treatment for ischaemic stroke. *Br J Clin Pharmacol* 34: 199–206, 1992
2 Atkinson J. Cerebrovascular structure and dementia: new drug targets. *Trends Pharmacol Sci* 22: 630–635, 2001
3 Awad R, Dibildox M and Ortiz F. Irritable bowel syndrome treatment using pinaverium bromide as a calcium channel blocker. A randomized double-blind placebo-controlled trial. *Acta Gastroenterol Latinoam* 25: 137–144, 1995
4 Barajas-Lopez C and Huizinga JD. Different mechanisms of contraction generation in circular muscle of canine colon. *Am J Physiol* 256: G570–580, 1989
5 Bentahila S, Atkinson J and Capdeville C. Protective effects of antihypertensive treatment with isradipine on the consequences of cerebral ischaemia in the spontaneously hypertensive rat. *J Hypertens* 9: 121–129, 1991
6 Blackwell JN, Holt S and Heading RC. Effect of nifedipine on oesophageal motility and gastric emptying. *Digestion* 21: 50–56, 1981
7 Bolay H, Reuter U, Dunn AK, Huang Z, Boas DA and Moskowitz MA. Intrinsic brain activity triggers trigeminal meningeal afferents in a migraine model. *Nat Med* 8: 136–142, 2002
8 Bowyer SM, Aurora KS, Moran JE, Tepley N and Welch KM. Magnetoencephalographic fields from patients with spontaneous and induced migraine aura. *Ann Neurol* 50: 582–587, 2001
9 Caro G, Barrios M and Baeyens JM. Dose-dependent and stereoselective antagonism by diltiazem of naloxone-precipitated morphine abstinence after acute morphine-dependence *in vivo* and *in vitro*. *Life Sci* 43: 1523–1527, 1988

10 Chaisewikul R, Baillie N and Marson AG. Calcium antagonists as an add-on therapy for drug-resistant epilepsy. *Cochrane Database Syst Rev*: CD002750, 2001
11 Choudhuri R, Cui L, Yong C, Bowyer S, Klein RM, Welch KM and Berman NE. Cortical spreading depression and gene regulation: relevance to migraine. *Ann Neurol* 51: 499–506, 2002
12 Christen MO. Action of pinaverium bromide, a calcium-antagonist, on gastrointestinal motility disorders. *Gen Pharmacol* 21: 821–825, 1990
13 Coccia G, Bortolotti M, Michetti P and Dodero M. Prospective clinical and manometric study comparing pneumatic dilatation and sublingual nifedipine in the treatment of oesophageal achalasia. *Gut* 32: 604–606, 1991
14 Contreras E, Tamayo L and Amigo M. Calcium channel antagonists increase morphine-induced analgesia and antagonize morphine tolerance. *Eur J Pharmacol* 148: 463–466, 1988
15 Corvera J, Corvera-Behar G, Lapilover V and Ysunza A. Objective evaluation of the effect of flunarizine on vestibular neuritis. *Otol Neurotol* 23: 933–937, 2002
16 De Ponti F, D'Angelo L, Frigo GM and Crema A. Inhibitory effects of calcium channel blockers on intestinal motility in the dog. *Eur J Pharmacol* 168: 133–144, 1989
17 Del Pozo E, Caro G and Baeyens JM. Analgesic effects of several calcium channel blockers in mice. *Eur J Pharmacol* 137: 155–160, 1987
18 Diener HC, Matias-Guiu J, Hartung E, Pfaffenrath V, Ludin HP, Nappi G and De Beukelaar F. Efficacy and tolerability in migraine prophylaxis of flunarizine in reduced doses: a comparison with propranolol 160 mg daily. *Cephalalgia* 22: 209–221, 2002
19 Dora B, Balkan S and Tercan E. Normalization of high interictal cerebrovascular reactivity in migraine without aura by treatment with flunarizine. *Headache* 43: 464–469, 2003
20 Feron O and Godfraind T. Regulation of the L-type calcium channel alpha-1 subunit by chronic depolarization in the neuron-like PC12 and aortic smooth muscle A7r5 cell lines. *Pflugers Arch* 430: 323–332, 1995
21 Feron O, Wibo M, Christen MO and Godfraind T. Interaction of pinaverium (a quaternary ammonium compound) with 1,4-dihydropyridine binding sites in rat ileum smooth muscle. *Br J Pharmacol* 105: 480–484, 1992
22 Godfraind T, Miller R and Wibo M. Calcium antagonism and calcium entry blockade. *Pharmacol Rev* 38: 321–416, 1986
23 Gordeev MF, Patel DV, England BP, Jonnalagadda S, Combs JD and Gordon EM. Combinatorial synthesis and screening of a chemical library of 1,4-dihydropyridine calcium channel blockers. *Bioorg Med Chem* 6: 883–889, 1998
24 Gullapalli S and Ramarao P. L-type Ca^{2+} channel modulation by dihydropyridines potentiates kappa-opioid receptor agonist induced acute analgesia and inhibits development of tolerance in rats. *Neuropharmacology* 42: 467–475, 2002
25 Gullapalli S and Ramarao P. Regulation of dihydropyridine-sensitive Ca^{2+} channels during naloxone-induced opioid supersensitivity in rats. *Eur J Pharmacol* 451: 271–277, 2002
26 Hadjikhani N, Sanchez Del Rio M, Wu O, Schwartz D, Bakker D, Fischl B, Kwong KK, Cutrer FM, Rosen BR, Tootell RB et al. Mechanisms of migraine aura revealed by functional MRI in human visual cortex. *Proc Natl Acad Sci USA* 98: 4687–4692, 2001
27 Hain TC and Uddin M. Pharmacological treatment of vertigo. *CNS Drugs* 17: 85–100, 2003
28 Hall ED and Wolf DL. A pharmacological analysis of the pathophysiological mechanisms of posttraumatic spinal cord ischemia. *J Neurosurg* 64: 951–961, 1986
29 Hanson GR, Jensen M, Johnson M and White HS. Distinct features of seizures induced by cocaine and amphetamine analogs. *Eur J Pharmacol* 377: 167–173, 1999
30 Hara H, Shimazawa M, Sasaoka M, Yamada C, Iwakura Y, Sakai T, Maeda Y, Yamaguchi T, Sukamoto T and Hashimoto M. Selective effects of lomerizine, a novel diphenylmethylpiperazine Ca^{2+} channel blocker, on cerebral blood flow in rats and dogs. *Clin Exp Pharmacol Physiol* 26: 870–876, 1999
31 Hongo M. [Effect of nifedipine on canine LESP (author's transl)]. *Nippon Heikatsukin Gakkai Zasshi* 17: 47–51, 1981
32 Hongo M, Traube M, McAllister RG, Jr and McCallum RW. Effects of nifedipine on esophageal motor function in humans: correlation with plasma nifedipine concentration. *Gastroenterology* 86: 8–12, 1984
33 Huizinga JD and Barajas-Lopez C. Ionic and cellular basis for slow-wave-type and spike-like action potentials. *Prog Clin Biol Res* 327: 605–615, 1990
34 Kasuya H, Onda H, Takeshita M, Okada Y and Hori T. Efficacy and safety of nicardipine pro-

longed-release implants for preventing vasospasm in humans. *Stroke* 33: 1011–1015, 2002
35 Katsura K, Rodriguez de Turco EB, Folbergrova J, Bazan NG and Siesjo BK. Coupling among energy failure, loss of ion homeostasis, and phospholipase A2 and C activation during ischemia. *J Neurochem* 61: 1677–1684, 1993
36 Katsura K, Rodriguez de Turco EB, Kristian T, Folbergrova J, Bazan NG and Siesjo BK. Alterations in lipid and calcium metabolism associated with seizure activity in the postischemic brain. *J Neurochem* 75: 2521–2527, 2000
37 Kenakin T. Predicting therapeutic value in the lead optimization phase of drug discovery. *Nat Rev Drug Discov* 2: 429–438, 2003
38 Kishioka S, Ko MC and Woods JH. Diltiazem enhances the analgesic but not the respiratory depressant effects of morphine in rhesus monkeys. *Eur J Pharmacol* 397: 85–92, 2000
39 Kiura Y, Hanaya R, Serikawa T, Kurisu K, Sakai N and Sasa M. Involvement of Ca^{2+} channels in abnormal excitability of hippocampal CA3 pyramidal cells in noda epileptic rats. *J Pharmacol Sci* 91: 137–144, 2003
40 Kobayashi T and Mori Y. Ca^{2+} channel antagonists and neuroprotection from cerebral ischemia. *Eur J Pharmacol* 363: 1–15, 1998
41 Lefranc F, Golzarian J, Chevalier C, DeWitte O, Pochet R, Heizman C, Decaestecker C, Brotchi J, Salmon I and Kiss R. Expression of members of the calcium-binding S-100 protein family in a rat model of cerebral basilar artery vasospasm. *J Neurosurg* 97: 408–415, 2002
42 Leone M, Grazzi L, La Mantia L and Bussone G. Flunarizine in migraine: a minireview. *Headache* 31: 388–391, 1991
43 Lopez-Arrieta JM and Birks J. Nimodipine for primary degenerative, mixed and vascular dementia. *Cochrane Database Syst Rev*: CD000147, 2002
44 Malysz J, Farraway LA, Christen MO and Huizinga JD. Pinaverium acts as L-type calcium channel blocker on smooth muscle of colon. *Can J Physiol Pharmacol* 75: 969–975, 1997
45 Morel N, Buryi V, Feron O, Gomez JP, Christen MO and Godfraind T. The action of calcium channel blockers on recombinant L-type calcium channel alpha1-subunits. *Br J Pharmacol* 125: 1005–1012, 1998
46 Moskowitz MA and Macfarlane R. Neurovascular and molecular mechanisms in migraine headaches. *Cerebrovasc Brain Metab Rev* 5: 159–177, 1993
47 Narducci F, Bassotti G, Gaburri M, Farroni F and Morelli A. Nifedipine reduces the colonic motor response to eating in patients with the irritable colon syndrome. *Am J Gastroenterol* 80: 317–319, 1985
48 Nitahara K, Matsunaga M, Katori K, Yotsui H, Higuchi H and Higa K. Effect of continuous low-dose intravenous diltiazem on epidural fentanyl analgesia after lower abdominal surgery. *Br J Anaesth* 90: 507–509, 2003
49 Nuti A, Lucetti C, Pavese N, Dell'Agnello G, Rossi G and Bonuccelli U. Long-term follow-up after flunarizine or nimodipine discontinuation in migraine patients. *Cephalalgia* 16: 337–340, 1996
50 Oka M, Itoh Y and Ukai Y. Preferential inhibition by a novel Na^+/Ca^{2+} channel blocker NS-7 of severe to mild hypoxic injury in rat cerebrocortical slices: A possible involvement of a highly voltage-dependent blockade of Ca^{2+} channel. *J Pharmacol Exp Ther* 293: 522–529, 2000
51 Oka M, Itoh Y, Ukai Y and Kimura K. Blockade by NS-7, a neuroprotective compound, of both L-type and P/Q-type Ca^{2+} channels involving depolarization-stimulated nitric oxide synthase activity in primary neuronal culture. *J Neurochem* 72: 1315–1322, 1999
52 Olesen J and Jansen-Olesen I. Nitric oxide mechanisms in migraine. *Pathol Biol (Paris)* 48: 648–657, 2000
53 Pantoni L, Bianchi C, Beneke M, Inzitari D, Wallin A and Erkinjuntti T. The Scandinavian Multi-Infarct Dementia Trial: a double-blind, placebo-controlled trial on nimodipine in multi-infarct dementia. *J Neurol Sci* 175: 116–123, 2000
54 Pantoni L, Rossi R, Inzitari D, Bianchi C, Beneke M, Erkinjuntti T and Wallin A. Efficacy and safety of nimodipine in subcortical vascular dementia: a subgroup analysis of the Scandinavian Multi-Infarct Dementia Trial. *J Neurol Sci* 175: 124–134, 2000
55 Penn RD and Paice JA. Adverse effects associated with the intrathecal administration of ziconotide. *Pain* 85: 291–296, 2000
56 Pianese CP, Hidalgo LO, Gonzalez RH, Madrid CE, Ponce JE, Ramirez AM, Moran LM, Arenas JE, Rubio AT, Uribe JO et al. New approaches to the management of peripheral vertigo: efficacy and safety of two calcium antagonists in a 12-week, multinational, double-blind study. *Otol Neurotol* 23: 357–363, 2002

57 Poynard T, Naveau S, Mory B and Chaput JC. Meta-analysis of smooth muscle relaxants in the treatment of irritable bowel syndrome. *Aliment Pharmacol Ther* 8: 499–510, 1994
58 Prior A, Harris SR and Whorwell PJ. Reduction of colonic motility by intravenous nicardipine in irritable bowel syndrome. *Gut* 28: 1609–1612, 1987
59 Reuter U, Chiarugi A, Bolay H and Moskowitz MA. Nuclear factor-kappaB as a molecular target for migraine therapy. *Ann Neurol* 51: 507–516, 2002
60 Richter JE, Dalton CB, Bradley LA and Castell DO. Oral nifedipine in the treatment of noncardiac chest pain in patients with the nutcracker esophagus. *Gastroenterology* 93: 21–28, 1987
61 Ridgeway B, Wallace M and Gerayli A. Ziconotide for the treatment of severe spasticity after spinal cord injury. *Pain* 85: 287–289, 2000
62 Rinkel GJ, Feigin VL, Algra A, Vermeulen M and van Gijn J. Calcium antagonists for aneurysmal subarachnoid haemorrhage. *Cochrane Database Syst Rev*: CD000277, 2002
63 Robertson CS, Hardy JG and Atkinson M. Quantitative assessment of the response to therapy in achalasia of the cardia. *Gut* 30: 768–773, 1989
64 Rose MA and Kam PC. Gabapentin: pharmacology and its use in pain management. *Anaesthesia* 57: 451–462, 2002
65 Ruiz-Nuno A, Villarroya M, Cano-Abad M, Rosado A, Balfagon G, Lopez MG and Garcia AG. Mechanisms of blockade by the novel migraine prophylactic agent, dotarizine, of various brain and peripheral vessel contractility. *Eur J Pharmacol* 411: 289–299, 2001
66 Santander R, Mena I, Gramisu M and Valenzuela JE. Effect of nifedipine on gastric emptying and gastrointestinal motility in man. *Dig Dis Sci* 33: 535–539, 1988
67 Santi CM, Cayabyab FS, Sutton KG, McRory JE, Mezeyova J, Hamming KS, Parker D, Stea A and Snutch TP. Differential inhibition of T-type calcium channels by neuroleptics. *J Neurosci* 22: 396–403, 2002
68 Santillan R, Hurle MA, Armijo JA, de los Mozos R and Florez J. Nimodipine-enhanced opiate analgesia in cancer patients requiring morphine dose escalation: a double-blind, placebo-controlled study. *Pain* 76: 17–26, 1998
69 Siesjo BK. Historical overview. Calcium, ischemia, and death of brain cells. *Ann NY Acad Sci* 522: 638–661, 1988
70 Siesjo BK. Mechanisms of ischemic brain damage. *Crit Care Med* 16: 954–963, 1988
71 Smith MT, Cabot PJ, Ross FB, Robertson AD and Lewis RJ. The novel N-type calcium channel blocker, AM336, produces potent dose-dependent antinociception after intrathecal dosing in rats and inhibits substance P release in rat spinal cord slices. *Pain* 96: 119–127, 2002
72 Snutch TP, Sutton KG and Zamponi GW. Voltage-dependent calcium channels—beyond dihydropyridine antagonists. *Curr Opin Pharmacol* 1: 11–16, 2001
73 Staessen JA, Fagard R, Thijs L, Celis H, Arabidze GG, Birkenhager WH, Bulpitt CJ, de Leeuw PW, Dollery CT, Fletcher AE et al. Randomised double-blind comparison of placebo and active treatment for older patients with isolated systolic hypertension. The Systolic Hypertension in Europe (Syst-Eur) Trial Investigators. *Lancet* 350: 757–764, 1997
74 Staessen JA, Wang JG and Thijs L. Calcium-channel blockade and cardiovascular prognosis: recent evidence from clinical outcome trials. *Am J Hypertens* 15: 85S-93S, 2002
75 Staessen JA, Wang JG and Thijs L. Cardiovascular protection and blood pressure reduction: a meta-analysis. *Lancet* 358: 1305–1315, 2001
76 Subramanyam K, David J and Joseph T. Interaction of flunarizine with sodium valproate or ethosuximide in gamahydroxybutyrate induced absence seizures in rats. *Indian J Exp Biol* 39: 998–1001, 2001
77 Sun WM, Edwards CA, Prior A, Rao SS and Read NW. Effect of oral nicardipine on anorectal function in normal human volunteers and patients with irritable bowel syndrome. *Dig Dis Sci* 35: 885–890, 1990
78 Toda N and Okamura T. The pharmacology of nitric oxide in the peripheral nervous system of blood vessels. *Pharmacol Rev* 55: 271–324, 2003
79 Tottene A, Fellin T, Pagnutti S, Luvisetto S, Striessnig J, Fletcher C and Pietrobon D. Familial hemiplegic migraine mutations increase Ca^{2+} influx through single human $Ca_V2.1$ channels and decrease maximal $Ca_V2.1$ current density in neurons. *Proc Natl Acad Sci USA* 99: 13284–13289, 2002
80 Triadafilopoulos G, Aaronson M, Sackel S and Burakoff R. Medical treatment of esophageal achalasia. Double-blind crossover study with oral nifedipine, verapamil, and placebo. *Dig Dis Sci* 36: 260–267, 1991

81 Vanegas H and Schaible H. Effects of antagonists to high-threshold calcium channels upon spinal mechanisms of pain, hyperalgesia and allodynia. *Pain* 85: 9–18, 2000
82 Wang YX, Gao D, Pettus M, Phillips C and Bowersox SS. Interactions of intrathecally administered ziconotide, a selective blocker of neuronal N-type voltage-sensitive calcium channels, with morphine on nociception in rats. *Pain* 84: 271–281, 2000
83 Weizman R, Getslev V, Pankova IA, Schrieber S and Pick CG. Pharmacological interaction of the calcium channel blockers verapamil and flunarizine with the opioid system. *Brain Res* 818: 187–195, 1999
84 Willumsen NJ, Bech M, Olesen SP, Jensen BS, Korsgaard MP and Christophersen P. High throughput electrophysiology: new perspectives for ion channel drug discovery. *Receptors Channels* 9: 3–12, 2003
85 Withering W. *An Account of the Foxglove and some of its Medical Uses with practical remarks on dropsy and other diseases*. London: G.G.J. and J. Robison, 1785

Index

MIX
Papier aus verantwortungsvollen Quellen
Paper from responsible sources
FSC® C105338

If you have any concerns about our products,
you can contact us on
ProductSafety@springernature.com

In case Publisher is established outside the EU,
the EU authorized representative is:
Springer Nature Customer Service Center GmbH
Europaplatz 3, 69115 Heidelberg, Germany

Printed by Libri Plureos GmbH
in Hamburg, Germany